Recent Advances on the Pathogenesis and Management of Diabetes Mellitus

Recent Advances on the Pathogenesis and Management of Diabetes Mellitus

Proceedings of the 9th Korea-Japan Symposium on Diabetes Mellitus, Kyongju, Korea, 11–12 April 1997

Editors:

S.H. Shinn
Department of Internal Medicine
College of Medicine
Chung-Ang University
Seoul, Korea

M. Shichiri
Department of Metabolic Medicine
Kumamoto University School of Medicine
Kumamoto, Japan

K.-W. Kim
Department of Internal Medicine
Samsung Medical Center
Sung Kyun Kwan University College of Medicine
Seoul, Korea

1998

ELSEVIER

Amsterdam – Lausanne – New York – Oxford – Shannon – Singapore – Tokyo

International Congress Series No. 1149
ISBN 0 444 82856 7

This book is printed on acid-free paper.

Published by:
Elsevier Science (Singapore) Pte Ltd.
No. 1 Temasek Ave.
#17-01 Millenia Tower
Singapore 039192

Printed in the Netherlands

President's opening address

It is my great pleasure and honor to publish the proceedings of the 9th Korea-Japan Symposium on Diabetes Mellitus, held on April 11–12, 1997 in Kyongju, Korea. Since the very first symposium in 1981, the subsequent meetings (held every 2 years in Korea and Japan alternately) have promoted scientific achievement and friendship between the two countries.

Recently diabetes research has advanced remarkably, especially in the aspects of pathogenesis and management, and has contributed to the understanding of pathophysiology and the proper management of diabetes mellitus. This was one reason that we selected the title "Recent Advances on the Pathogenesis and Management" as the main theme of this symposium. This symposium would help in the understanding of the recent advances in diabetes mellitus.

The symposium venue of Kyongju city was the capital city of the Shilla Dynasty for more than 1,000 years. It has a diverse cultural heritage as well as the antique fragrance of ancient history, and provides long-lasting memories.

Lastly, I would like to express my sincere gratitude to the guest speakers, Prof Lebovitz from the USA and Prof Lefebvre from Belgium, as well as the many speakers and participants for presenting their valuable scientific papers. I would also like to thank the Organizing Committee for the organization of this fruitful symposium, and Servier Korea, Ltd. and Nihon Servier for their financial support towards the publication of this Proceedings.

Soon Hyun Shinn MD

President
The 9th Korea-Japan Symposium on Diabetes Mellitus

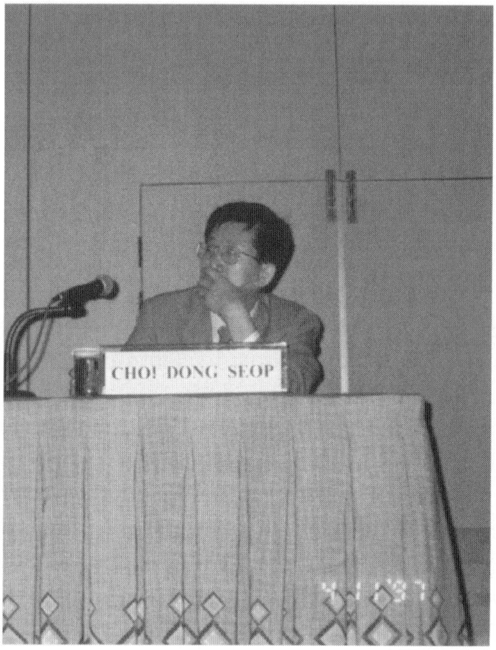

Dr. Dong Seop Choi.

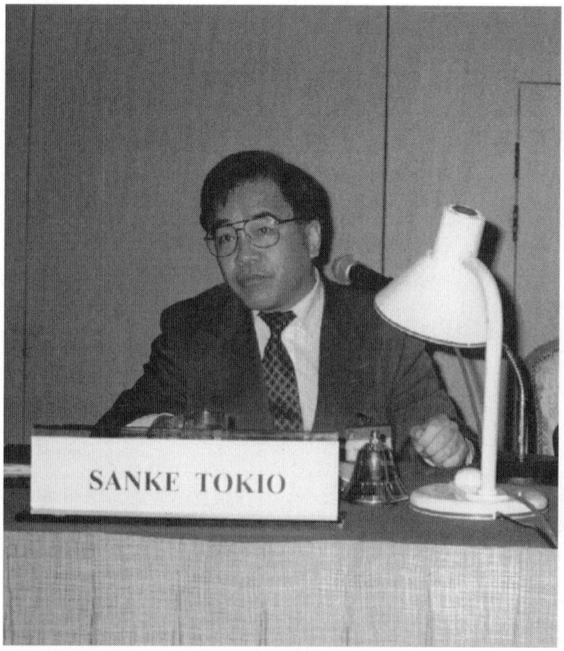

Dr. Sanke Tokio.

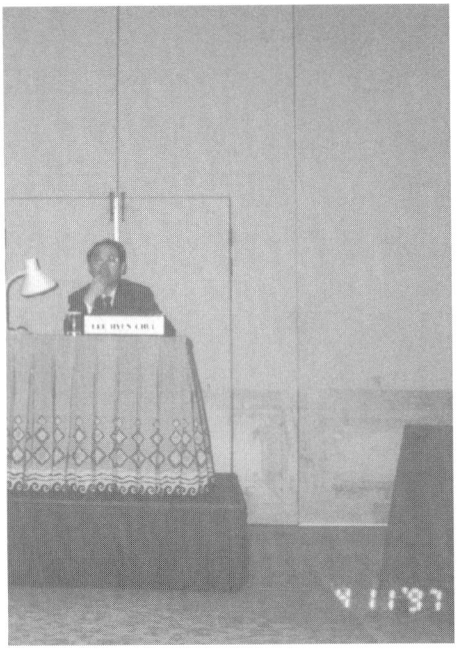

Dr. Hyn Chul Lee.

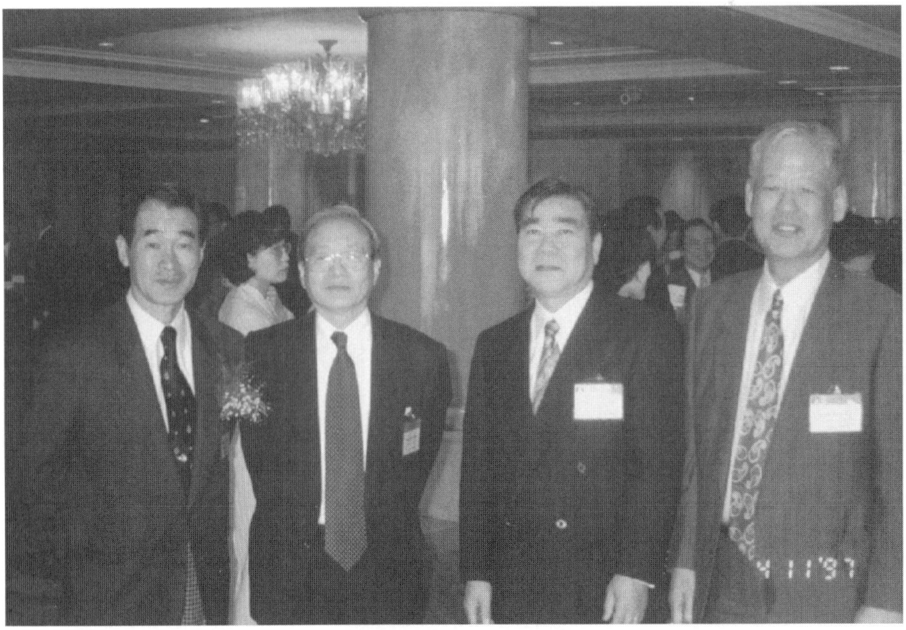

(From left) Drs. Tae Hee Lee, Young Kil Choi, Kaneko Toshio and Sang Jong Lee.

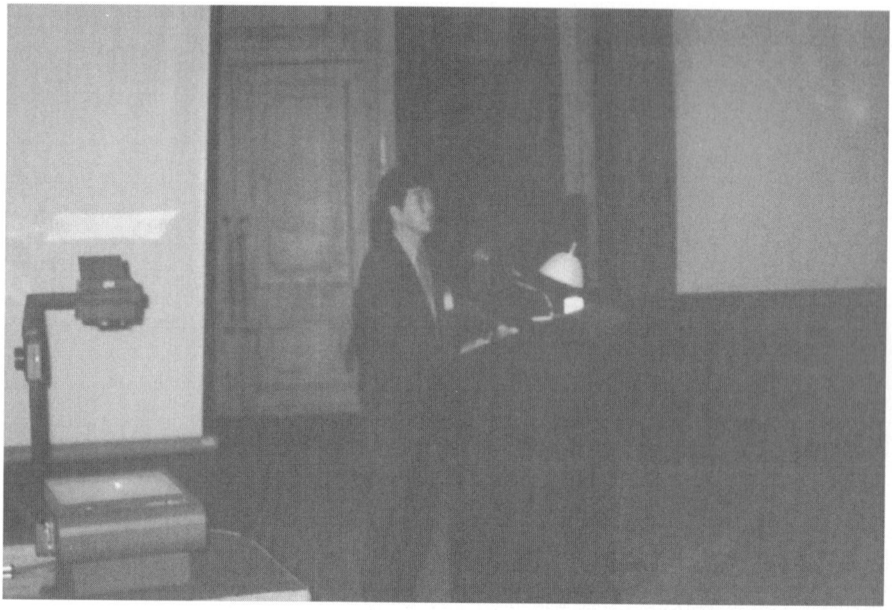

Dr. Yu Bae Ahn.

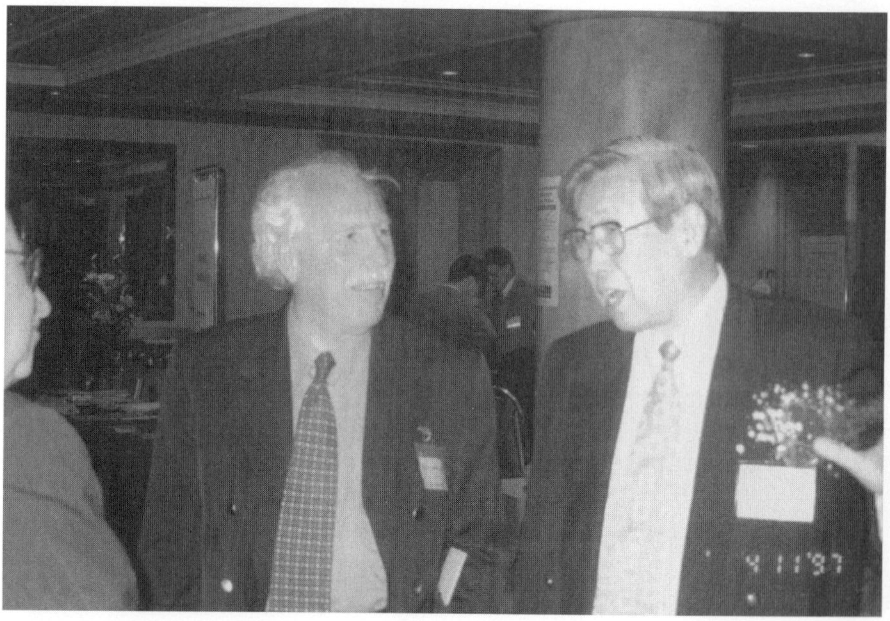

(From left) Drs. P.J. Lefebvre and Hun Ki Min.

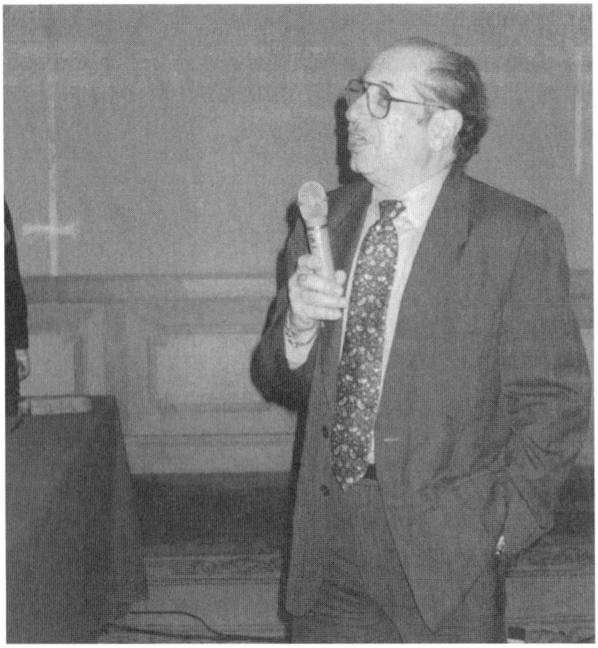

Dr. H.E. Lebovitz.

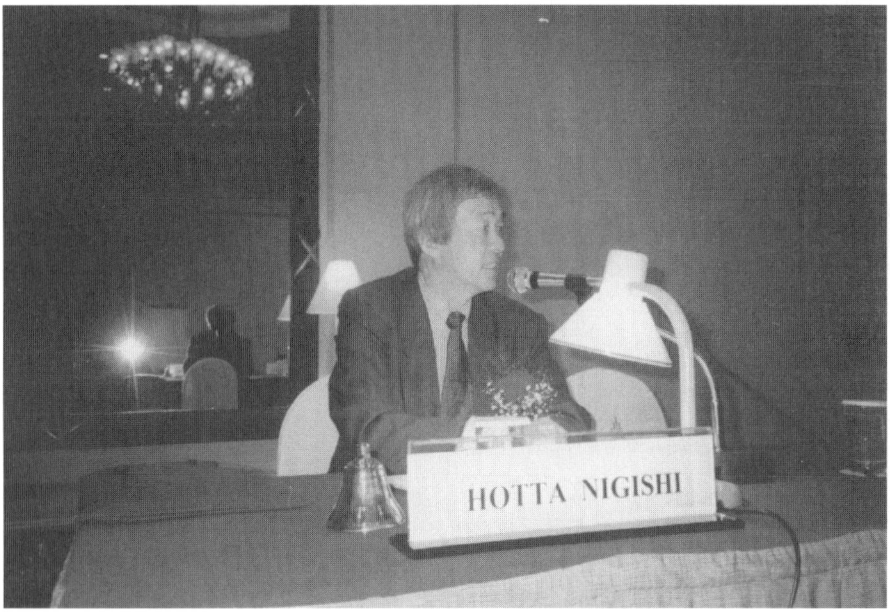

Dr. Hotta Nighishi.

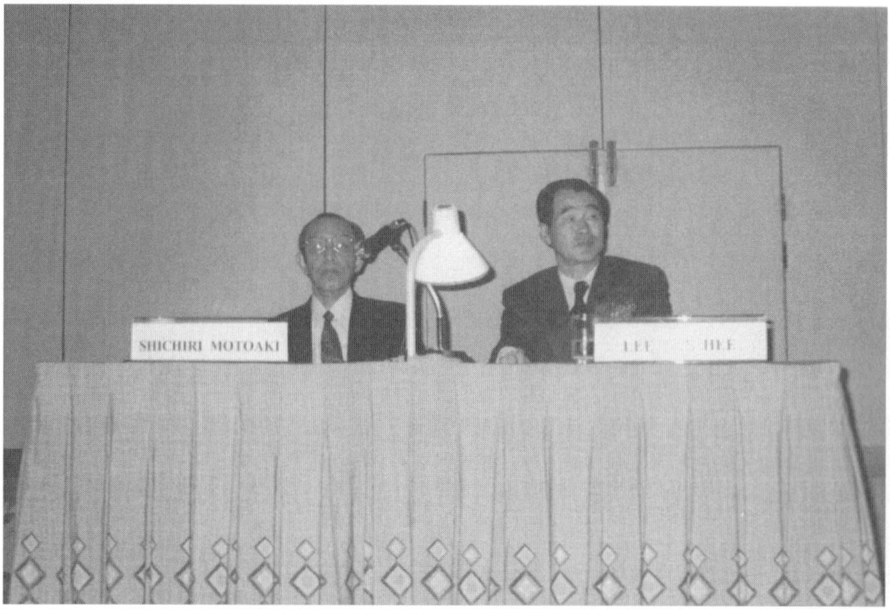

(From left) Drs. Shichiri Motoaki and Tae Hee Lee.

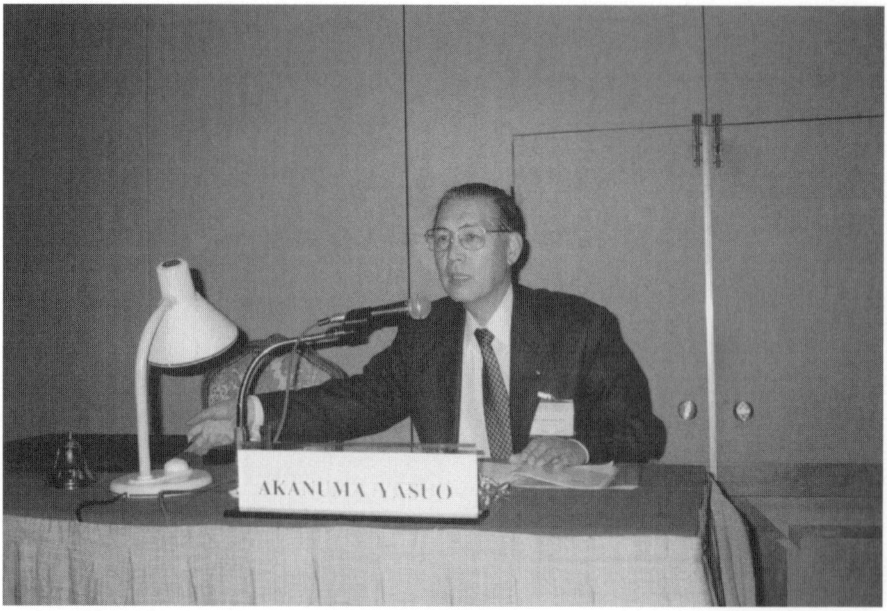

Dr. Akanuma Yasuo.

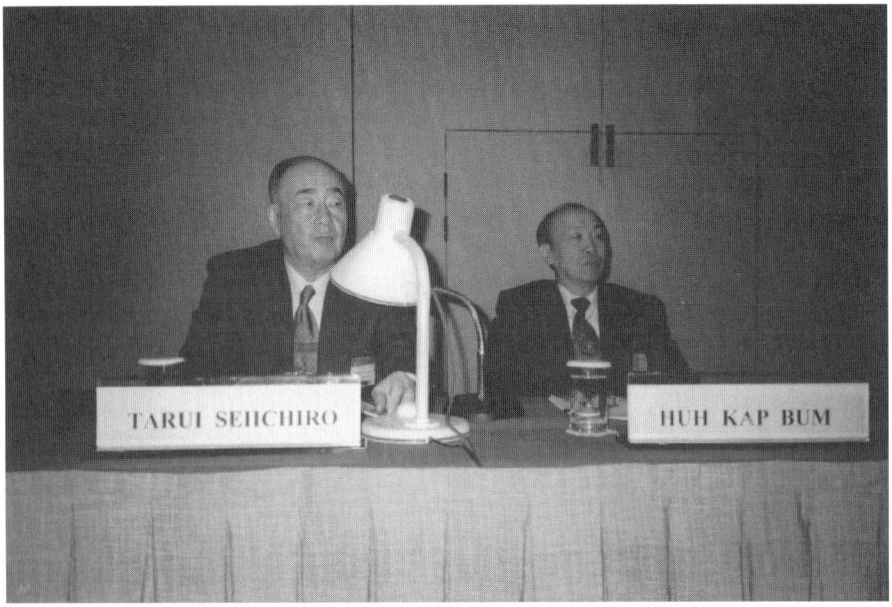

(From left) Drs. Tarui Seiichiro and Kap Bum Huh.

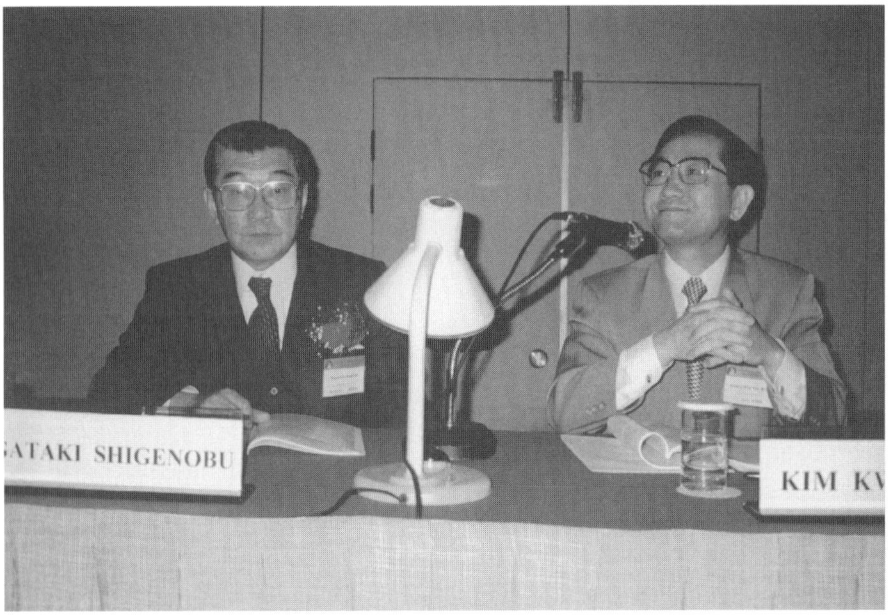

(From left) Drs. Nagataki Shigenobu and Kwang-Won Kim.

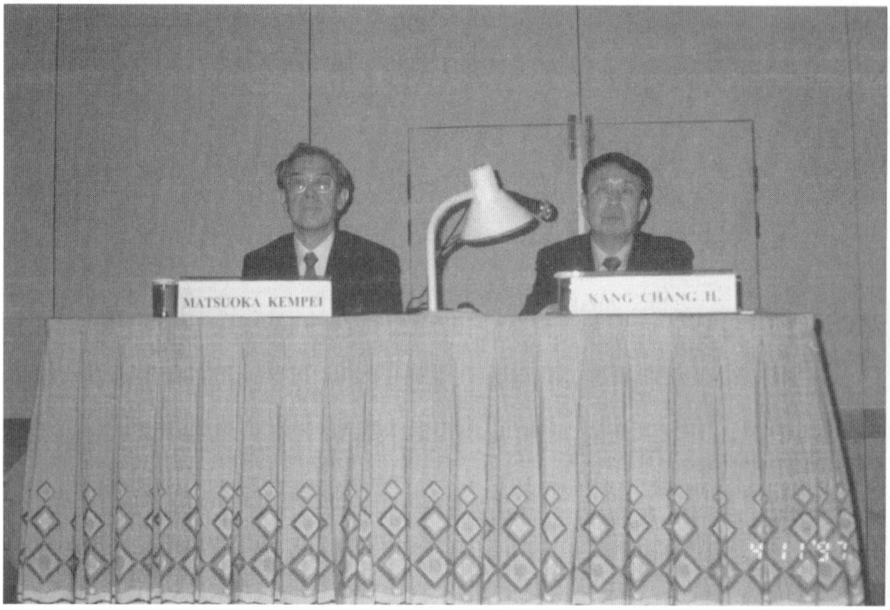

(From left) Drs. Matsuoka Kempei and Chang Il Kang.

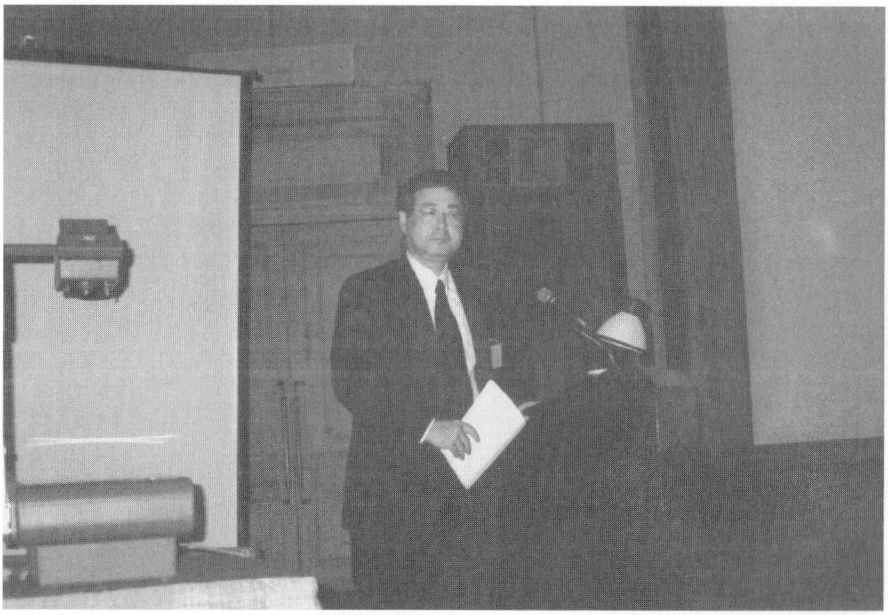

Dr. Hong Kyu Lee.

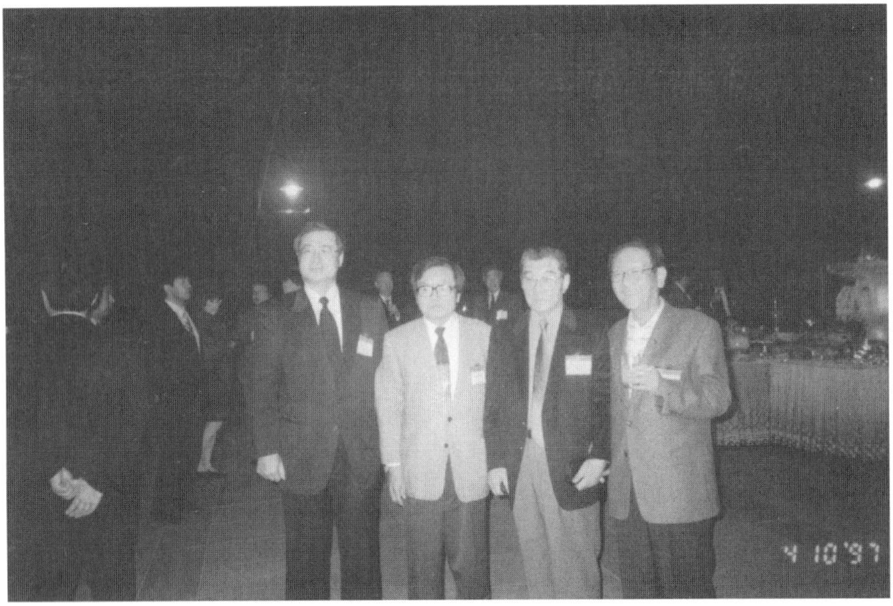

(From left) Drs. Hong Kyu Lee, Soon Hyn Shinn, Nagataki Shigenobu and Mok Hyun Kim.

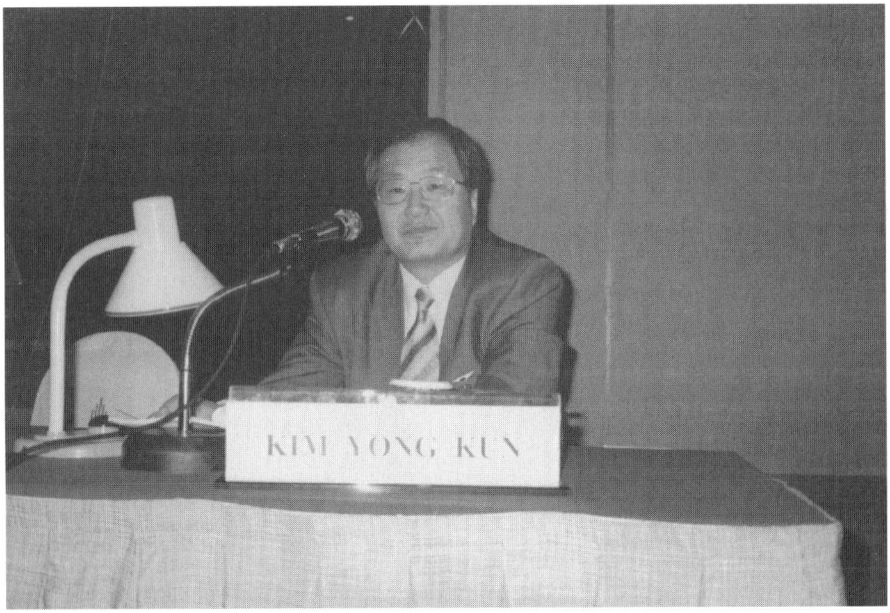

Dr. Young Kun Kim.

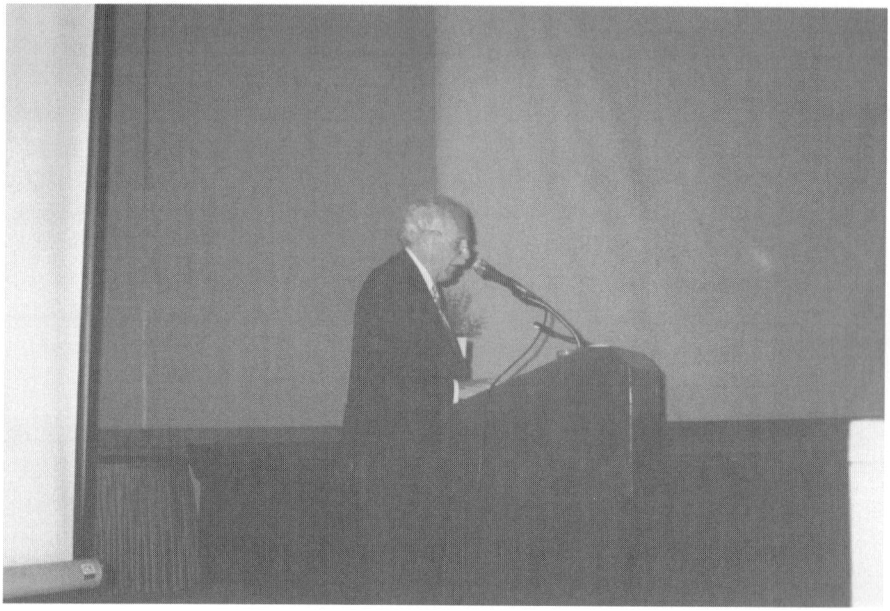

Dr. P.J. Lefebvre.

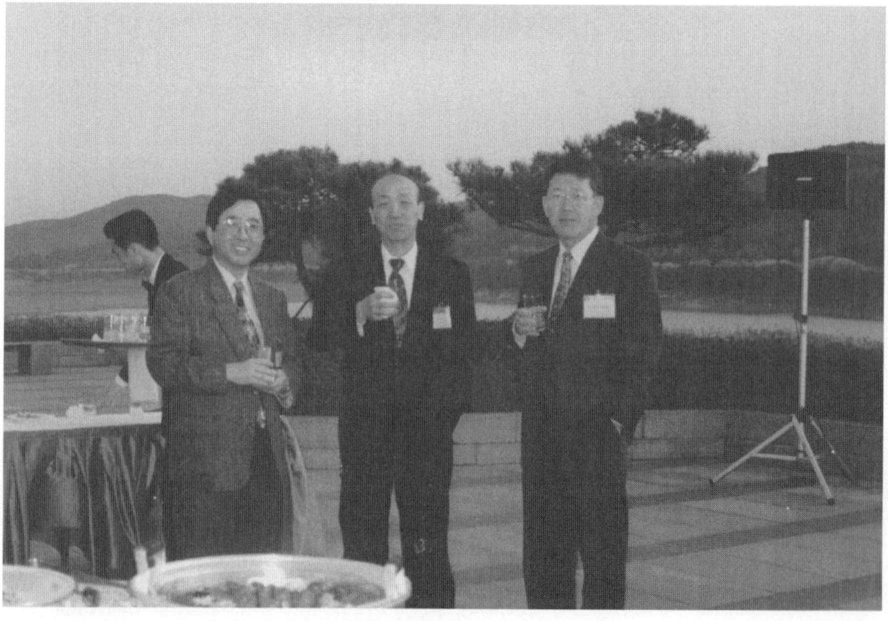

(From left) Drs. Ho Young Son, Kap Bum Huh and Kwang Woo Lee.

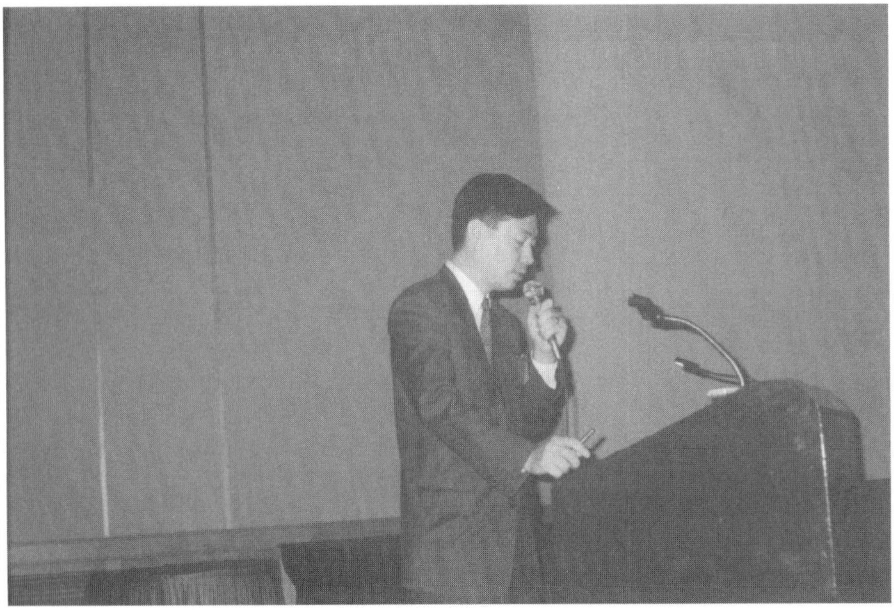

Dr. Chan Soo Shin.

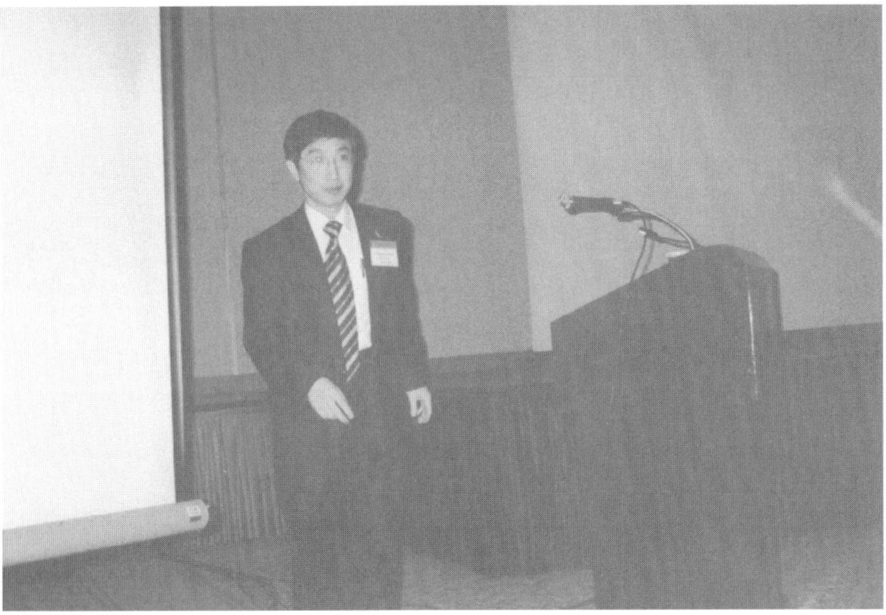

Dr. Myung Shik Lee.

List of contributors

Dr K.J. Ahn
Department of Medicine
Samsung Medical Center
50 Ilwon Dong
Kangnam-ku
Seoul, Korea

Dr Takayuki Asahina
Saiseikai Central Hospital
1-4-17 Mita, Minato-ku
Tokyo 108, Japan

Dr N. Babaya
Department of Geriatric Medicine
Osaka University Medical School
2-2 Yamakaoka, Suita
Osaka 565, Japan

Dr H.C. Bae
Department of Medicine
Chung-Ang University Hospital
Yong-San Hangang-Ro 3GA
Yongsan-Gu
Seoul, Korea

Dr B.S. Cha
Yonsei University
College of Medicine
134 Shinchon-dong
Sudaemon-ku
Seoul 120-752
Korea

Dr S.A. Chang
Department of Internal Medicine
Catholic University Medical College
#505 Banpo-Dong, Seocho-ku
Seoul 137-040
Korea

Dr N.H. Cho
Department of Preventive Medicine
Ajou University School of Medicine
#5 Wonchon-Dong
Paldal-Gu
Suwon 442-749
Korea

Dr Y.J. Cho
Department of Medicine
Hanyang University Hospital
249-1 Kyomun-dong, Kuri
Kyunggi-do
Seoul 471-020
Korea

Dr S.B. Choi
Department of Medicine
Kunkook University College of Medicine
Chungcheong Buk-Do
Asan City BaeBang-Meon
Seochul-Risan 29-1
Korea

Dr C.H. Chung
Department of Internal Medicine
Wonju College of Medicine
Yonsei University
162 Ilsan-Dong
Kangwon-do, Wonju-Si 220-701
Korea

Dr Y.E. Chung
Department of Internal Medicine
University of Ulsan, College of Medicine
#388-1 Pungnap-Dong
Songpa-Ku, Seoul 138-736
Korea

Dr Y.S. Chung
Department of Endocrinology and Metabolism
Ajou University School of Medicine
5 Wonchon-Dong
Paldal-Gu, Suwon 442-749
Korea

Dr Y. Goriya
Department of General Medicine
Kanazawa Medical University
Uchinada, Kahoku-gun
Ishikawa Prefecture 920-02
Japan

Dr T. Goto
Third Department of Internal Medicine
Hirosaki University School of Medicine
Zaifu-cho, Hirosaki-shi
Aomori-Ken 036
Japan

Dr S.W. Ha
Department of Medicine
Kyungpook National University College of Medicine
50 Samduck-Dong 2 Ga
Jung-Gu, Taegu 700-422
Korea

Dr Y. Hamada
Department of Geriatric Medicine
Osaka University Medical School
2-2 Yamadaoka, Suita
Osaka 565
Japan

Dr H. Hidaka
Shiga University of Medical Science
Seta-Tsukinowa-cho
Otsu, Shiga 520-21
Japan

Dr H. Hiroyuki
Department of Internal Medicine
1-1 Daigaku Uchinada
Ishikawa 920-02
Japan

Dr C. Ito
Hiroshima A-bomb Casualty Council Health Management Center
8-6, 3-chome, Senda-machi
Naka-ku, Hiroshima 730
Japan

Dr K. Iwashima
Osaka-Minaki National Hospital
Kawashinagano-city
Kidomachi, Osaka 677-2
Japan

Dr M.H. Kang
Department of Internal Medicine
Chung Ang Gil Hospital
1198 Kawol-dong, Nandong-ku
Inchon 405-220
Korea

Dr Y. Kang
Laboratory of Endocrinology
Institute for Medical Science
Ajou University
Woncheon-Dong San 5
Paldal-Gu, Suwon
Kyunggi-do 442-749
Korea

Dr Y. Kawabata
Department of Geriatric Medicine
Osaka University Medical School
2-2 Yamadaoka, Suita
Osaka 565
Japan

Dr B.W. Kim
Department of Internal Medicine
Kuyngpook National University
Taegu 700-721
Korea

Dr H.J. Kim
Department of Internal Medicine
Ewha Women's University
Mokdong Hospital
911-1 Mokdong
Yangcheon-ku, Seoul
Korea

Dr H.K. Kim
Department of Internal Medicine
University of Ulsan, College of Medicine
#388-1 Pujgnap-Dong
Songpa-Ku, Seoul 138-736
Korea

Dr H.M. Kim
Division of Endocrinology and Metabolism
Ajou University School of Medicine
San #5 Wonchon-Dong
Paldal-gu, Suwon 442-749
Korea

Dr H.S. Kim
Yonsei University College of Medicine
134 Shinchon-dong
Sudaemoon-ku
Seoul 120-752
Korea

Dr H.S. Kim
Department of Internal Medicine
Wonju College of Medicine
Yonsei Unversity
162 Ilsan-Dong
Kangwon-do, Wonju-Si 220-701
Korea

Dr J.B. Kim
Department of Medicine
Hanyang University Hospital
249-1 Kyomun-dong, Kuri
Kyunggi-do, Seoul 471-020
Korea

Dr J.G. Kim
Department of Medicine
Kyungpook National University College of Medicine
50 Sam-Duck Dong 2 Ga
Jung-Gu, Taegu 700-721
Korea

Dr J.S. Kim
Department of Internal Medicine
Seoul National University Hospital
28 Yungun-Dong, Chongno-Gu, Seoul 110-744
Korea

Dr J.Y. Kim
Division of Endocrinology and Metabolism
Department of Internal Medicine
Chonnam National University Medical School
8-Hakdong, Dong-ku
Kwangju City 501-757
Korea

Dr K.A. Kim
Division of Endocrinology and Metabolism
Department of Medicine
Samsung Medical Cente
50 Ilwon Dong, Kangnam-ku, Seoul
Korea

Dr K.-W. Kim
Department of Medicine
Samsung Medical Center
50 Ilwon-Dong, Kangnam-ku
Seoul 135-710, Korea

Dr S.G. Kim
Department of Internal Medicine
Korea Medical Center
Kuro Hospital
80 Kuro-dong, Kuro-gum, Seoul
Korea

Dr S.K. Kim
Department of Internal Medicine
Seoul National University Hospital
28 Yungun-Dong
Chongno-Gu, Seoul 110-744
Korea

Dr S.W. Kim
Department of Medicine
Kyung-hee University Hospital
#1 Hocki-dong
Dongdacmoon-ku
Seoul, Korea

Dr I.Y. Ko
Yu-Han Research Center
27-3 Dan-Jung Dong
Kun-Po Si
Kyungi-ki Do, Korea

Dr J.J. Koh
Department of Internal Medicine
Seoul National University Hospital
28 Yungun-Dong
Chongno-gu, Seoul 100-744
Korea

Dr H.C. Lee
Division of Endocrinology and Metabolism
Severance Hospital Yonsei University College of Medicine
134 Shinchon-dong
Seodaemun-ku, Seoul 120-752
Korea

Dr K.W. Lee
Hallyn University Department of Internal Medicine
Hankang Sacred Heart Hospital
Yeongdungpo-dong 92-300
Yeondungpo-ku
Seoul 150-020
Korea

Dr M.-K. Lee
Department of Medicine
Samsung Medical Center
50 Ilwon-dong, Kangnam-ku
Seoul 135-710, Korea

Dr M.-S. Lee
Department of Medicine
Samsung Medical Center
50 Ilwon-Dong, Kangnam-ku
Seoul 135-710, Korea

Dr S.H. Lee
Department of Medicine
Hanyang University Hospital
249-1 Kyomun-dong, Kuri,
Kyunggido, Seoul 471-020
Korea

Dr S.W. Lee
Department of Internal Medicine
Kangbuk Samsung Hospital
#108 Pyung-dong
Jongno-ku, Seoul 100-752
Korea

Dr T.H. Lee
Division of Endocrinology and Metabolism
Department of Internal Medicine
Chonnam National University Medical School
8-Hakdong, Dong-ku
Kwangju City 501-757
Korea

Dr H.R. Li
Department of Medicine
Yonsei University College of Medicine
134 Shinchon-dong, Sudaemoon-ku
Seoul 120-757
Korea

Dr S. Masashi
Department of Medicine
Osaka Kousei-Nenkin Hospital
Fukushima 4-2-78
Osaka, Japan

Dr T. Matsumura
Department of Metabolic Medicine
Kumamoto University School of Medicine
1-1-1 Honjo
Kumamoto 860
Japan

Dr K. Matsuoka
Department of Medicine
Saiseikai Diabetes Center
1-4-17 Mita
Minato-ku
Tokyo 108
Japan

Dr H.W. Moon
Department of Medicine
Ajou University School of Medicine
San #5 Wonchon-Dong
Paldal-gu, Suwon 442-749
Korea

Dr Y. Mori
Department of Internal Medicine
National East-Utsunomiya Hospital
Shmookamoto 2160
Kawachi-machi
Kawachi-Gun, Tochigi 329-11
Japan

Dr Y. Murakawa
Department of Internal Medicine
National East-Utsunomiya Hospital
Simookamoto 2160
Kawachi-machi
Kawachi-Gun, Tochigi 329-11
Japan

Dr J.H. Nam
Department of Medicine
Yonsei University College of Medicine
#134 Sinchon-Dong
Swodaemun-gu, Seoul 120-752
Korea

Dr K. Nojima
Department of Geriatric Medicine
Osaka University Medical School
2-2 Yamadaoka, Suita
Osaka 565
Japan

Dr M. Nomura
Center for Diabetes Mellitus
Osaka Rosai Hospital
1179-3 Nagasone-cho, Sakai
Osaka 591
Japan

Dr K.S. Oh
Department of Preventive Medicine
Ajou University Medical School
#5 Wonchon-Dong
Paldal-Gu, Suwon 442-749
Korea

Dr S. Okuya
Yamaguchi University School of Medicine
1144 Kogushi, Ube
Yamaguchi 755
Japan

Dr H.R. Park
Myong-Ji University
38-2 san, Namdong, Yongin City
Kyunggi-do 449-728
Korea

Dr H.Y. Park
Department of Medicine
Chung Ang Gil Hospital
1198 Kuwol-dong
Namdong-ku, Inchon
Korea

Dr J.H. Park
Division of Endocrinology and Metabolism
Department of Internal Medicine
Chonnam National University Medical School
8-Hakdong, Dong-ku
Kwangju City 501-757
Korea

Dr S.M. Park
Department of Food and Nutrition
Hoseo University
29-1 Sechulri Baebang-Mun
Asan City
Chungnam-Do 336-795
South Korea

Dr T.S. Park
Department of Medicine
Chonbuk National University Medical School
Chunju, Chonbuk 560-182
Korea

Dr Y.S. Park
Department of Medicine
Hanyang University Hospital
249-1 Kyomun-dong, Kuri
Kyunggi-do, Seoul 471-020
Korea

Dr Y.J. Pyun
Department of Internal Medicine
Kangbuk Samsung Hospital
#108 Pyung-Dong
Jongno-ku, Seoul 100-752
Korea

Dr J.H. Shin
Department of Medicine
Hanyang University Hospital
249-1 Kyomun-dong, Kuri
Kyunggi-do, Seoul 471-020
Korea

Dr S.H. Shhin
Department of Internal Medicine
Chung-Ang University College of Medicine
82-1 Pil-Dong 2-Ga
Chung-Gu, Seoul 100-272
Korea

Dr M. Shintani
Department of Geriatric Medicine
Osaka University Medical School
2-2 Yamadaoka, Suita, Osaka 565
Japan

Dr H.S. Son
Department of Medicine
Catholic University Medical College
St Mary's Hospital
65-1 Kum Oh Dong
Kyung Gi Do 480-130
UiJong Bu City
Korea

Dr Y.D. Song
Department of Internal Medicine
Yonsei University College of Medicine
#134, Shinchong-Dong
Swodaemun-gu, Seoul 120-752
Korea

Dr Y. Takahashi
Diabetes Center
Tokyo Women's Medical College
Shinjuku-ku
Tokyo 162
Japan

Dr S. Takayama
Diabetes Center
Tokyo Women's Medical College
Shinjuku-ku, Tokyo 162
Japan

Dr K. Takekawa
Higashiosaka Municipal Central Hospital
2-3-1 Mikuriaminami
Higashiosaka, Osaka 577
Japan

Dr K. Tanigawa
Department of Clinical Nutrition
Suzuka University of Medical Science and Technology
Kishioka-cho 1001-1
Suzuka, Mie 510-02
Japan

Dr H. Ueda
2nd Department of Internal Medicine
Kobe University School of Medicine
7-5-1 Kusunoki-cho, Chuo-ku
Kobe 650
Japan

Dr J.I. Yang
Department of Preventive Medicine
Ajou University Medical School
#5 Wonchon-Dong
Paldal-gu, Suwon
Korea

Dr J.H. Yoo
Department of Internal Medicine
Kangbuk Samsung Hospital
#108 Pyung-Dong
Jongno-ku
Seoul 100-752
Korea

Dr S.J. Yoo
Department of Medicine
Catholic University Medical College
Holy Family Hospital
2 Sosa-Dong
Wonmi-gu
Pucheon, Kyunggi-do
Korea

Dr T.W. Yoon
Biotechnology Research Center
Boryung Central Research Institute
Keum-Jeong Dong
Kunpo-City, Kyungki-Do 435-050
Korea

Dr Y. Yoshida
The Institute for Diabetes Care
and Research
Asahi Life Foundation
1-6-1 Marunouchi, Chiyoda-ku
Tokyo 100
Japan

Dr Y.S. Yun
Department of Internal Medicine
Yonsei University
College of Medicine
#134, Sinchon-Dong
Swodaemun-gu, Seoul 120-752
Korea

Dr Y.S. Yun
Department of Internal Medicine
Yonsei University
#134, Shinchong-Dong
Swodaemun-gu, Seoul
Korea

Contents

Etiology

Clinical diabetes

Immunology

Lipids and lipoproteins

Insulin synthesis and secretion

Treatment

Insulin action

Epidemiology

Diabetes education

Complications

Lectures

Recent Advances on the Pathogenesis and Management of Diabetes Mellitus.
S.H. Shinn, M. Shichiri and K.-W. Kim, editors.

PLENARY LECTURE

Oxidative stress and diabetic vascular complications in Korea

Soon Hyun Shinn
Department of Internal Medicine, College of Medicine, Chung-Ang University, Seoul, Korea

Introduction

Chronic vascular complications are the main causes of morbidity and mortality in diabetic patients. Although the precise mechanisms are not yet defined, hyperglycemia induces chronic vascular complications probably through multiple pathways.

Numerous evidence has accumulated indicating that increased oxidative stress might play an important role in the pathogenesis of diabetic vascular complications. In this lecture, I review the current evidence on oxidative stress and the link to chronic vascular complications in diabetes, and introduce several studies in Korean diabetic patients.

The prevalence of diabetes mellitus has been increasing progressively during the last 30 years reaching 7.2% in certain rural areas, making it the seventh leading cause of death in Korea, and the chronic vascular complications represent the main causes of premature morbidity and mortality in diabetic patients [1]. As a result, atherosclerosis occurs more extensively and earlier than in general population. Also, it has long been suggested that a strong relationship exists between cardiovascular diseases and diabetes.

The Diabetes Control and Complication Trial [2] confirmed that chronic hyperglycemia was an important cause of the late microvascular complications in diabetes. Thus, glycemic control in diabetes predicts not only microvascular complications but also macrovascular complications.

The mechanisms through which chronic hyperglycemia leads to vascular complications of diabetes are not yet clearly defined. Various mechanisms are proposed to explain the link between chronic hyperglycemia and vascular damages [3–7] (Table 1).

Increased oxidative stress in diabetes

For the cellular and molecular mechanisms through which hyperglycemia may

Address for correspondence: Soon Hyun Shinn, Department of Internal Medicine, College of Medicine, Chung-Ang University, 82-1, Pil-Dong 2 Ga, Chung-Gu, Seoul 100-272, Korea.

Table 1. Possible mechanisms of diabetic vascular complications.

Nonenzymatic glycations
Sorbitol – myoinositol changes
Redox potential alterations
Diacyglycerol – protein kinase C pathway activation
Glycoxidation
Insulin resistance and hyperinsulinemia
Platelet aggregation
Hyperlipidemia
Oxidative stress

exert its toxic effect on vasculature, Baynes [8] suggested that oxidative stress might be a common pathway linking diverse mechanisms for the pathogenesis of complications in diabetes.

Recently, evidence has accumulated that suggests that oxidative stress may play an important role in the etiology of diabetes and diabetic vascular complications. There are also many ways by which hyperglycemia may increase the generation of free radicals (Table 2).

Increased free radical generation such as reactive oxygen radicals (superoxide, hydrogen peroxide and lipid peroxide) causes chemical modifications of lipid and proteins through oxidation, fragmentation, cross-linking and fluorescence-resulting in damage in cell and tissue function leading to pathology.

Hyperglycemia increases the oxidative stress through the activated polyol pathway and increased glucose autoxidation and protein glycation.

Increased oxidative stress stimulates LDL oxidation and decreases heparan sulfate and endothelial function. Ultimately, diabetic vascular complications could be the outcome.

There is also evidence that hyperglycemia depresses natural antioxidant capacity. In general, antioxidant enzymes such as superoxide dismutase (SOD), catalase and glutathione peroxidase have been reported to be decreased and related to poor glycemic control [9]. In addition, there are numerous reports indicating increased oxidative stress in diabetic patients.

Increased production of malondialdehyde (MDA), a marker of lipid peroxidation in the erythrocyte membrane and depressed erythrocyte content of reduced gluthatione in diabetic patients was reported by Nagasaka et al. [10]. Higher circulating levels of malondialdehyde and lipid peroxide levels, conjugated dienes

Table 2. Potential sources of oxidative stress in diabetes.

Autoxidation
Advanced glycation endproducts
Increased nonenzymatic glycosylation
Activated polyol pathway
Prostanoid metabolism
Metabolic stress
Depressed natural antioxidant defenses

and decreased inhibition of lipid peroxidation by the glutathione-dependent system in erythrocytes were also reported in several studies [11].

Hyperglycemia also causes glycosylation of DNA and decreases the DNA repair process leading to higher DNA damage.

Oxidative stress affects endothelial functions leading to impaired relaxation, local hypoxia, metabolic derangement and eventually tissue damage. Tesfamariam and Cohen [12] reported that exposure to elevated glucose concentration for 6 h causes endothelial dysfunction, which could be prevented by free radical scavengers such as catalase and SOD. Endothelial dysfunction promotes atherosclerosis.

Cameron et al. [13] reported nerve dysfunction and 38% reduction of sciatic nerve glutathione concentration which was improved with free radical scavengers in animal studies.

Loss and decreased synthesis of heparan sulfate proteoglycans and reversal by catalase was reported by Kashihara et al. [14] in a diabetic animal with nephropathy. Also, a reduced glutathione level and glutathione peroxidase activity in the lens and retina, especially with proliferative retinopathy and correction by antioxidant vitamin, was reported in animal studies. The above data suggested that increased oxidative stress was involved in the pathogenesis of vascular complications in diabetes.

Oxidative stress in Korean diabetic patients

Studies on oxidative stress in diabetes and the relationship between oxidative stress and vascular complications were conducted in animals and diabetic patients a few years ago and therefore the data in Korea is not extensive.

Now I would like to introduce a few clinical studies on oxidative stress in Korean diabetic patients with and without microvascular complications.

Plasma NO_2/NO_3 concentrations in patients with diabetic retinopathy were studied by Chung et al. [15]. The objective was to assess the role of nitric oxide in the severity of diabetic retinopathy, and the subjects were 51 NIDDM patients and 20 normal controls. The plasma NO_2/NO_3 concentrations were significantly increased in NIDDM patients with background and proliferative retinopathy. They concluded that nitric oxide might be related to the presence and severity of diabetic retinopathy.

Levels of plasma lipid hydroperoxides in NIDDM patients were measured by Lee et al. [16]. The objective was to see whether NIDDM patients showed an increased plasma lipid peroxidation. The subjects were 60 NIDDM patients and 20 normal controls. The plasma lipid hydroperoxides were measured using the FOX 2 method. The plasma lipid hydroperoxide level was significantly higher in NIDDM patients compared to that in normal controls. But there was no correlation between the plasma lipid hydroperoxide level and the presence of diabetic retinopathy. They concluded that the increased plasma lipid hydroperoxides in NIDDM patients might be associated with oxidative stress.

However, similar studies done by Bae et al. reported conflicting results that the plasma lipid peroxide concentration was not different between patients with NIDDM and normal controls and also presence of diabetic retinopathy.

Studies on the increased membrane lipid peroxidation of erythrocyte in NIDDM were carried out by Jang et al. [17] to determine whether the membrane lipid peroxidation of erythrocyte increased in diabetic patients, and to observe the relationship between the level of lipid peroxidation and blood glucose. The subjects were 38 NIDDM patients and 16 normal controls and MDA was measured with the thiobarbituric acid reaction. The membrane MDA concentrations in erythrocytes were significantly increased in diabetic patients than those of normal controls, and a significant positive correlation was found between fasting plasma glucose levels, HbA1c levels, duration of diabetes and membrane MDA concentrations of erythrocyte in patients with NIDDM. The membrane MDA concentrations in erythrocytes decreased significantly after glycemic control for 40 days.

The study "Mononuclear cell manganese superoxide dismutase activity in patients with diabetes mellitus" was carried out by Koh et al. [18] to investigate the possible role of manganese SOD in the genesis of microangiopathy. The subjects were 13 patients with IDDM, 13 patients with NIDDM and 14 normal controls. The manganese SOD activity was measured at basal and after culture in different γ-interferon concentrations. There were no significant differences in basal γ-interferon stimulated mononuclear cell manganese SOD activities among patients with IDDM, NIDDM and normal controls.

But the mononuclear cell manganese SOD activities were significantly lower in diabetic patients with retinopathy than without retinopathy. They concluded that decreased mononuclear cell manganese SOD activity might be related to the development of diabetic retinopathy.

A similar study was carried out by Kim et al. [19] in 34 patients with NIDDM and 16 normal controls. Mononuclear cell manganese SOD activity was significantly lower in patients with NIDDM compared to that of normal controls, but there were no differences according to the severity of diabetic retinopathy. They concluded that mononuclear cell manganese SOD activity might play a role in the pathogenesis of NIDDM. The study on the antioxidant status in patients with NIDDM was carried out by Yu et al. [20].

The SOD activity of erythrocytes was significantly lower in patients with NIDDM than that in normal controls. The catalase and glutathione peroxidase activities in erythrocytes were significantly lower in diabetics with retinopathy than in those without retinopathy. The glutathione peroxidase activity and total glutathione levels were significantly lower in diabetic patients with nephropathy than in those without nephropathy. They concluded that the tissue antioxidant status might be an important factor in the etiology and complications of diabetes.

They also conducted a similar study [21] to assess the relationship between the degree of hyperglycemia and antioxidant enzyme activity after incubation in different glucose concentrations. The SOD activity of erythrocytes in normal controls and in patients with NIDDM were decreased in higher glucose concentrations and longer incubation period. They concluded that hyperglycemia might be an important factor for the decrease of erythrocyte SOD activities.

Similar studies were undertaken by others that showed the increased lipid peroxidation in IDDM patients with nephropathy [22]. In addition, there were several animal studies including increased oxidative stress in sciatic nerves and oxidatively modification of hepatic intracellular proteins and prevention by vitamin E administration and possibility of inhibition of insulitis by aminoguanidine administration [23].

Conclusion

Oxidative stress is increased in Korean diabetics, especially with vascular complications, although it is not clarified whether increased oxidative stress is a cause or an effect of vascular complications in diabetes.

Further studies are required to define the extent and the precise mechanisms through which increased oxidative stress results in vascular complications in diabetes and develop effective strategies for limiting the damage from oxidative stress.

References

1. Park YS et al. Prevalence of diabetes and IGT in Yonchon county, South Korea. Diabet Care 1995;18:545—548.
2. Diabetes Control and Complication Trial Research Group. The effect of intensive treatment of diabetes on the development and progression of long-term complications in insulin-dependent diabetes mellitus. N Engl J Med 1993;329:977—986.
3. Lyons TJ. Lipoprotein glycation and its metabolic consequences. Diabetes 1992;41(Suppl 2): 67—73.
4. Brownlee M et al. Advanced glycosylation end products in tissue and biochemical basis of diabetes complications. N Engl J Med 1988;318:1315—1321.
5. Byer DG et al. Accumulation of Millard reaction products in skin collagen in diabetes and aging. J Clin Invest 1993;91:2463—2469.
6. Williamson JR et al. Hyperglycemic pseudohypoxia and diabetic complications. Diabetes 1993; 42:801—813.
7. Oda A et al. Inactivation of Cu, Zn-superoxidedismutase by in vitro glycosylation and in erythrocytes of diabetic subjects. Horm Metab Res 1994;26:1—4.
8. Baynes JW. Role of oxidative stress in development of complications in diabetes. Diabetes 1991; 40:405—412.
9. Asayama K. Antioxidants in the serum of children with insulin-dependent diabetes mellitus. Free Rad Biol Med 1993;15:597—602.
10. Nagasaka Y et al. Effects of high glucose and sobitol pathway on lipid peroxidation of erythrocytes. Horm Metab Res 1989;21:275—276.
11. Altomare E et al. Increased lipid peroxidation in type 2 poorly controlled diabetic patients. Diabetes Metab 1992;18:264—271.
12. Tesfamariam B, Cohen RA. Free radicals mediate endothelial cell dysfunction caused by elevated glucose. Am J Physiol 1992;263:H321—H326.
13. Cameron NE et al. Anti-oxidant and pro-oxidant effects on nerve conduction velocity, endo-

neural blood flow and oxygen tension in non-diabetic and streptozotocin-diabetic rats. Diabetologia 1994;37:449–459.

14. Kashihara N et al. Selective decreased de novo synthesis of glomerular proteoglycans under the influence of reactive oxygen species. Proc Natl Acad Sci USA 1992;89:6309–6313.
15. Chung HK et al. Plasma NO_2^-/NO_3^- concentrations in patients with diabetic retinopathy (Abstract). In Abstracts of the 8th Japan-Korea Symposium on Diabetes Mellitus. Ube, Japan, October 5–6 1994;60A.
16. Lee MH et al. Level of plasma lipid hydroperoxidase in NIDDM patients. J Korean Diabetes Assoc 1996;20:124–133.
17. Jang HC et al. Increased membrane lipid peroxidation of erythrocytes in NIDDM. J Korean Diabetes Assoc 1992;16:309–316.
18. Koh JJ et al. Mononuclear cell manganese superoxide dismutase (Mn-SOD) activity in patient with diabetes mellitus. J Diabetes Assoc 1994;18:330–336.
19. Kim JT et al. Mononuclear cell, manganese superoxide dismutase (Mn-SOD) activities in non-insulin-dependant diabetic patients. In Abstracts of the 3rd International Diabetes Federation Western Pacific Regional Congress. Hong Kong, September 25–28, 1996;A75.
20. Yu BJ et al. The activity of erythrocyte antioxidant enzymes in diabetes mellitus. Korean J Int Med 1993;44:766–774.
21. Cho HC et al. The activity of erythrocyte antioxidant enzymes according to glucose concentration in non-insulin-dependent diabetes mellitus. J Korean Diabetes Assoc 1994;18:337–343.
22. Yu JM, Choi DS. Effects of aminoguanidine administration on pancreatic islet and glomerular lesions in multiple low dose streptozotocin induced diabetic (LDSD) mice. J Korean Diabetes Assoc 1995;19:266–278.
23. Jang-Yang YJ et al. The oxidative modification of hepatic intracellular proteins in the streptozotocin-induced diabetic rats. J Korean Diabetes Assoc 1993;17:175–182.

Recent Advances on the Pathogenesis and Management of Diabetes Mellitus.
S.H. Shinn, M. Shichiri and K.-W. Kim, editors.

LUNCHEON LECTURE

Artificial endocrine pancreas – past, present and future

Motoaki Shichiri
Department of Metabolic Medicine, Kumamoto University School of Medicine, Kumamoto, Japan

Keywords: bedside-type artificial endocrine pancreas, diabetes mellitus, glucose sensor, implantable-type artificial endocrine pancreas, microdialysis sampling method, vascular complications, wearable-type artificial endocrine pancreas.

The Diabetes Control and Complications Trial (DCCT) [1] with insulin-dependent diabetic patients (IDDM) and the Kumamoto Study [2] with non-insulin-dependent diabetic patients (NIDDM), were randomized clinical trials designed to compare intensive and conventional insulin therapy. When considering the effects on the development and/or progression of the early microvascular complications, the studies indicated that the microvascular complications associated with IDDM and NIDDM can be prevented or delayed by intensive therapy. Intensive insulin therapy, however, is usually associated with clinical problems, including severe hypoglycemia and inherent instability of glycemic control due to the open-loop control technique. The difficulty of achieving long-term effective glycemic control has stimulated us to develop the closed-loop control system, an artificial endocrine pancreas. In this article, the great progress that we have made in the development of an artificial endocrine pancreas is presented.

The artificial endocrine pancreas is a feedback control system, regulating insulin delivery on a minute-by-minute basis according to the measured blood glucose level. Pancreatic β cells recognize the changes in blood glucose, transmit the information within the cells, and then secrete enough insulin to regulate glucose levels. Therefore, in order to substitute the functions of a pancreatic β cell, it is necessary to artificially create the glucose sensing system (sensor), signal transduction system (processor) and insulin secretory system (effector).

In 1974, Albisser et al., and our team in 1975, developed the first generation of artificial endocrine pancreas composed of Technicon AutoAnalyzer, a minicomputer system and set of pumps for infusing insulin and glucose (Fig. 1) [3,4]. In order to make the system smaller, a glucose sensor was developed by combining a glucose oxidase membrane with an electrode that measured hydrogen peroxide, (one of the reaction products) polarographically. This bedside-type artificial

Address for correspondence: Motoaki Shichiri, MD, PhD, Department of Metabolic Medicine, Kumamoto University School of Medicine, 1-1-1 Honjo, Kumamoto 860, Japan. Tel.: +81-96-373-5169. Fax: +81-96-366-8397.

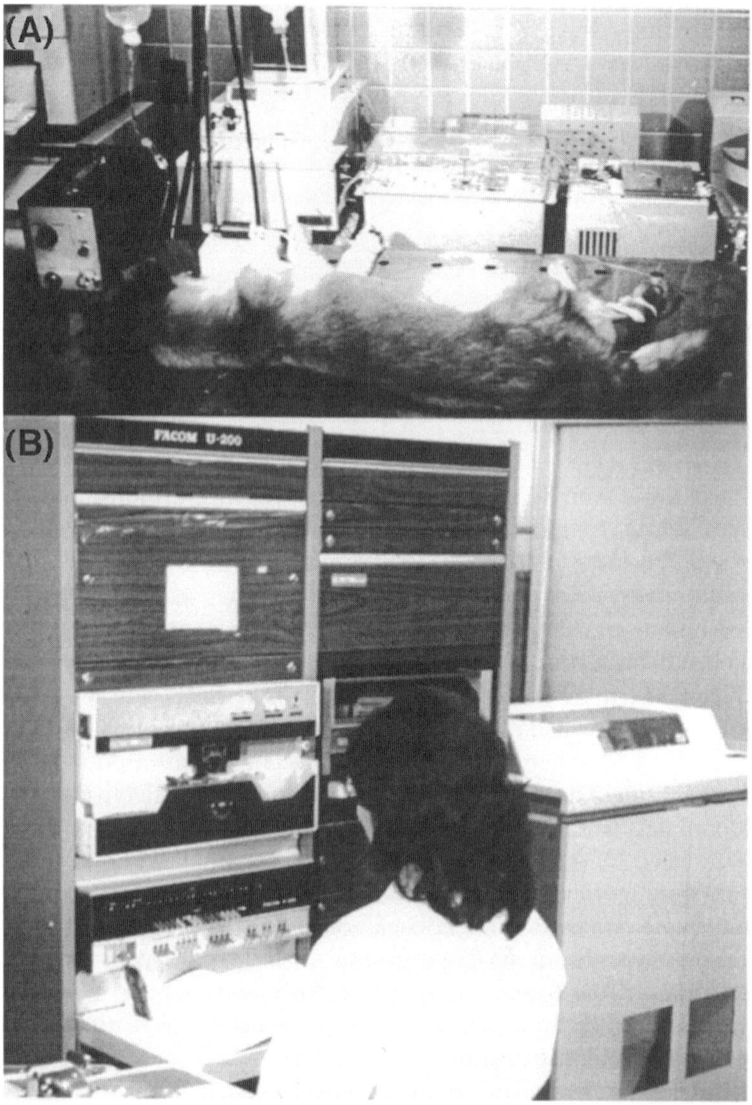

Fig. 1. Artificial endocrine pancreas which we developed in 1975. **A:** AutoAnalyzer system as glucose sensing unit. **B:** Minicomputer system (FACOM U-200).

endocrine pancreas has proven to be useful not only as a therapeutic tool, but also as an excellent research tool for investigating the pathophysiology of diabetes mellitus (Fig. 2).

The ultimate long-term goal in the development of an artificial endocrine pancreas is strict glycemic control and therefore, the trend in development has moved from bedside-type to wearable-type. In 1982, we succeeded in miniaturizing the glucose monitoring system into a needle-type (the first in the world) and

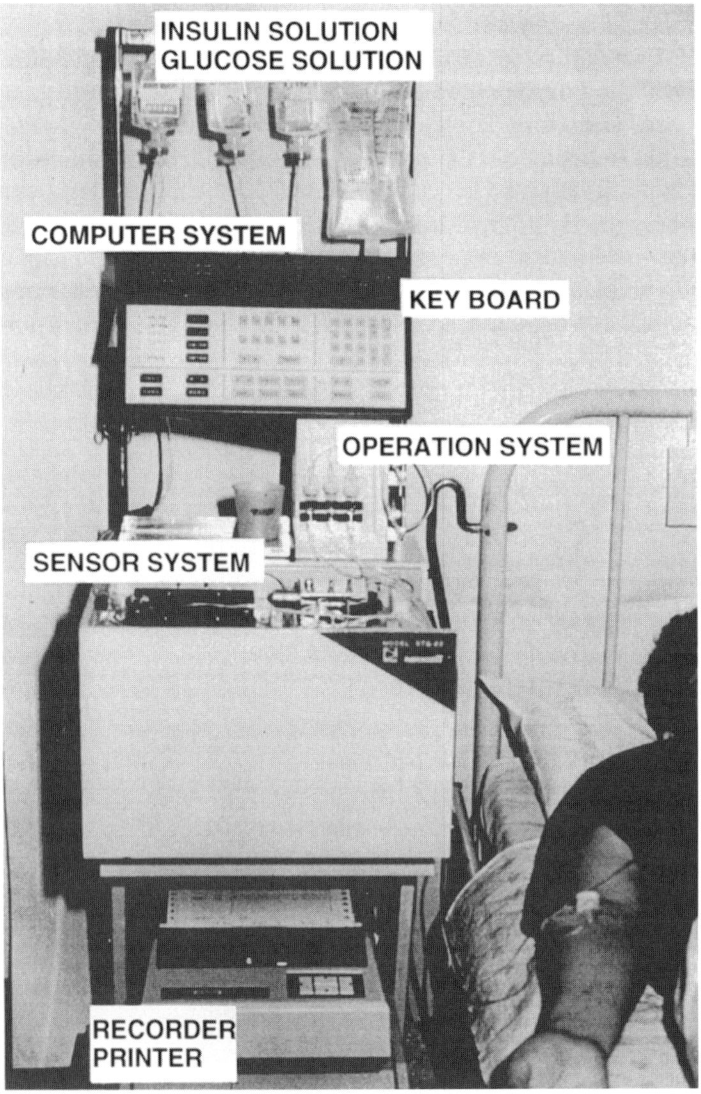

Fig. 2. Bedside-type artificial endocrine pancreas (STG-22A, Nikkiso Co. Ltd. Japan).

developed a wearable-type artificial endocrine pancreas [5—9]. With this system, it has been suggested that physiological glycemic regulation for longer periods could be established in ambulatory diabetic patients.

However, there still remain many problems to be solved. Among them, there are two major problems that should be solved before there can be long-term clinical application of wearable-type artificial endocrine pancreas in ambulatory diabetic patients. One problem is the development of a reliable and stable glucose monitoring system [10], and the other is the development of a subcutaneous insulin infusion algorithm [11,12].

For either problem, a miniaturized extracorporeal glucose monitoring system based on a microdialysis sampling method [13] or a ferrocene-mediated needle-type glucose sensor covered with highly biocompatible membrane (MPC) [14,15], would mean that subcutaneous tissue glucose concentrations could be monitored for 7 days without any in vivo calibrations, followed by 14 days with one-point calibration (Fig. 3) [16]. Then, taking into consideration the management and safety of the insulin delivery route, subcutaneous insulin infusion is obligatory. With the subcutaneous insulin infusion algorithm using a short-acting insulin analogue (Insulin Lispro, which is absorbed 2–3 times faster than nor-

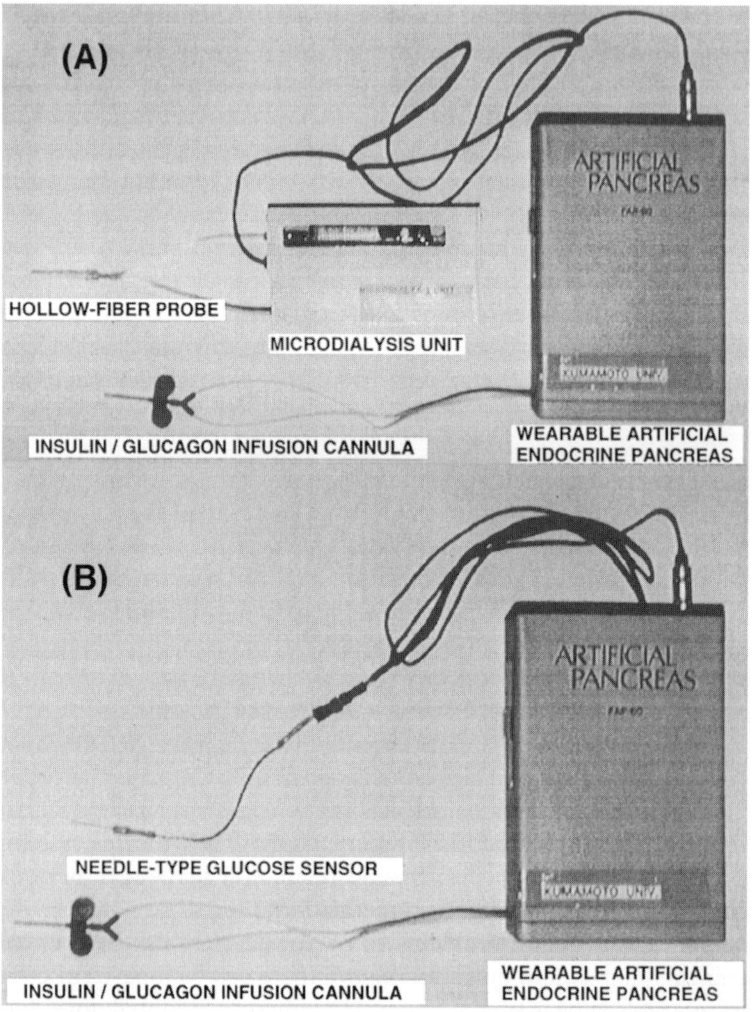

Fig. 3. Wearable-type artificial endocrine pancreas with (**A**) miniaturized extracorporeal glucose monitoring system based on microdialysis sampling method and (**B**) needle-type glucose sensor.

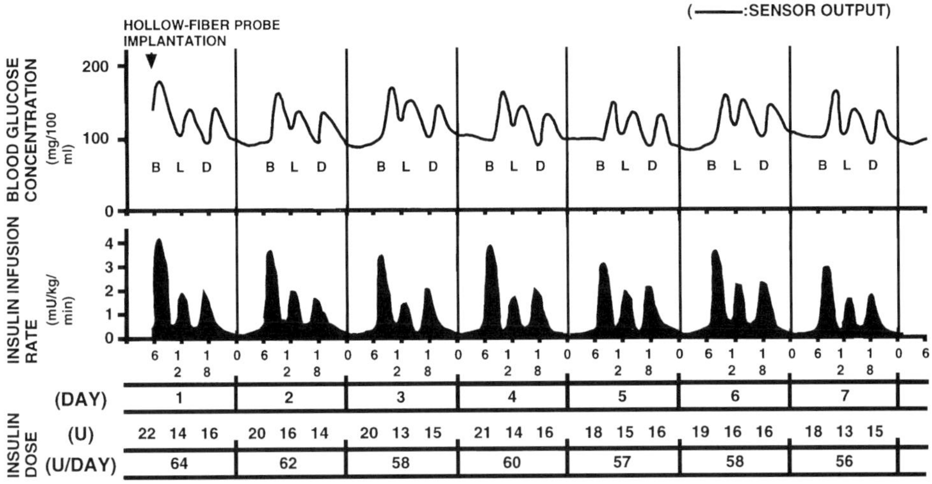

Fig. 4. Blood glucose regulation in an insulin-dependent diabetic patient with wearable-type artificial endocrine pancreas operating subcutaneous insulin Lispro infusion algorithm.

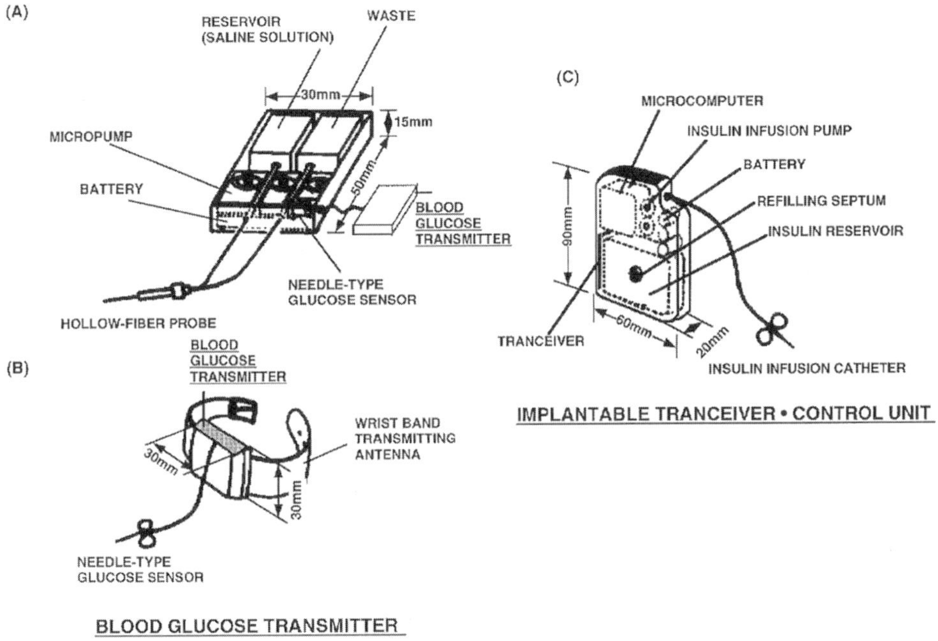

Fig. 5. Schematic diagram of implantable-type artificial endocrine pancreas with telecommunication system. **A**: Miniaturized extracorporeal glucose monitoring system based on microdialysis sampling method. **B**: Needle-type glucose sensor as blood glucose transmitter. **C**: Implantable transceiver-control unit.

mal insulin), near-physiological glycemic control could be established in diabetic patients without showing any delayed hyperinsulinemia or hypoglycemia [17]. Therefore, wearable-type artificial endocrine pancreas is now recognized as an excellent therapeutic tool for regulating blood glucose excursions physiologically in ambulatory diabetic patients on a long-term basis (Fig. 4).

The next step is the development of implantable-type artificial endocrine pancreas. Although the development of a sophisticated glucose monitoring system (either an amperometric glucose sensor, an electrocatalytic glucose sensor or a noninvasive blood glucose monitoring system) will be a key technology, an implantable-type artificial endocrine pancreas with telemetric maneuver will be available for the treatment of diabetes mellitus in the near future (Fig. 5).

References

1. The Diabetes Control and Complications Trial Research Group. The effect of intensive treatment of diabetes on the development and progression of long-term complications in insulin-dependent diabetes mellitus. N Engl J Med 1993;329:977–986.
2. Ohkubo Y, Kishikawa H, Araki E, Miyata T, Isami S, Motoyoshi S, Kojima Y, Furuyoshi N, Shichiri M. Intensive insulin therapy prevents the progression of diabetic microvascular complications in Japanese patients with non-insulin-dependent diabetes mellitus: a randomized prospective study. Diabet Res Clin Pact 1995;28:103–117.
3. Shichiri M, Kawamori R, Yamasaki Y. Computer algorithm of the artificial pancreatic beta cell. Artif Organs 1978;2(Suppl):247–250.
4. Goriya Y, Kawamori R, Shichiri M, Abe H. The development of an artificial beta cell system and its validation in pancreatectomized dogs – the physiological restoration of blood glucose homeostasis. Med Prog Technol 1979;6:99–108.
5. Shichiri M, Kawamori R, Yamasaki Y, Hakui N, Abe H. Wearable-type artificial endocrine pancreas with needle-type glucose sensor. Lancet 1982;ii:1129–1131.
6. Shichiri M, Kawamori R, Goriya Y, Yamasaki Y, Nomura M, Hakui N, Abe H. Glycemic control in pancreatectomized dogs with a wearable artificial endocrine pancreas. Diabetologia 1983;24:179–184.
7. Shichiri M, Kawamori R, Hakui N, Yamasaki Y, Abe H. Closed-loop glycemic control with a wearable-type artificial pancreas. Variations in daily insulin requirements to glycemic response. Diabetes 1984;33:1200–1202.
8. Nomura M, Shichiri M, Kawamori R, Yamasaki Y, Iwama N, Abe H. A mathematical insulin-secretion model and its validation in isolated rat pancreatic islets perifusion. Comput Biomed Res 1984;17:570–579.
9. Shichiri M, Kawamori R. Optimized algorithms for closed-loop glycemic control systems. In: Beyer J, Albissor M, Schrezenmeir J, Lehmann L (eds) Computer Systems for Insulin Adjustment in Diabetes Mellitus. Switzerland: Panscienta-Verlag, 1985;171–183.
10. Shichiri M, Fukushima H, Yamaguchi K, Kawamori R, Yamasaki Y, Ueda N, Kamada T. Membrane design for extending the long-life of an implantable glucose sensor. Diab Nutr Metab 1989;2:309–313.
11. Shichiri M, Kawamori R, Asakawa N, Yamasaki Y, Hakui N, Goriya Y. Blood glucose regulation in ambulant diabetics with the wearable artificial endocrine pancreas – closed-loop iv vs. sc insulin infusion. In: Nose Y, Kjellstrand C, Ivanovich P (eds) Progress in Artificial Organs. Cleveland: ISAO Press, 1986;695–699.
12. Asakawa N, Saito Y, Yamasaki Y, Kawamori R, Shichiri M. Validation of closed-loop subcutaneous insulin infusion algorithm – application of subcutaneous insulin absorption kinetics. Diabet Res 1987;5:193–198.

13. Hashiguchi Y, Sakakida M, Nishida K, Uemura T, Kajiwara K, Shichiri M. Development of a miniaturized glucose monitoring system by combining a needle-type glucose sensor with microdialysis sampling method; long-term subcutaneous tissue glucose monitoring in ambulatory diabetic patients. Diabet Care 1994;17:387–396.
14. Sakakida M, Ichinose K, Fukushima H, Nishida K, Kajiwara K, Hashiguchi Y, Taniguchi I, Shichiri M. Development of ferrocene-mediated needle-type glucose sensor as a measure of true subcutaneous tissue glucose concentrations. Artif Organs Today 1992;2:145–158.
15. Nishida K, Sakakida M, Ichinose K, Uemura T, Uehara M, Kajiwara K, Miyata T, Shichiri M, Ishihara K, Nakabayashi N. Development of a ferrocene-mediated needle-type glucose sensor covered with newly designed biocompatible membrane, 2-methacryloyloxyethyl phosphorylcholine -co-n-butyl methacrylate. Med Prog Technol 1995;21:91–103.
16. Shichiri M, Sakakida M, Nishida K, Shimoda S, Konno Y, Miyata T. Wearable-type artificial endocrine pancreas and optimal blood glucose regulation in diabetic patients. Diabet Rev Int 1995;4:10–14.
17. Shimoda S, Nishida K, Sakakida M, Konno Y, Ichinose K, Uehara M, Nowak T, Shichiri M. Closed-loop subcutaneous insulin infusion algorithm with short-acting insulin analogue for long-term clinical application of wearable artificial endocrine pancreas. Front Med Biol Eng 1997;(In press).

Recent advances in the pathogenesis of diabetes mellitus

Recent Advances on the Pathogenesis and Management of Diabetes Mellitus.
S.H. Shinn, M. Shichiri and K.-W. Kim, editors.

Approach to the pathogenesis of non-insulin-dependent diabetes mellitus using genetically engineered knockout animals

Takashi Kadowaki, Yasuo Terauchi, Hiroyuki Tamemoto, Kazuyuki Tobe and Yoshio Yazaki
Third Department of Internal Medicine, University of Tokyo, Tokyo, Japan

Abstract. Manipulation of the mouse germline through the genetic modification of embryonic stem cells is definitely a very useful and important tool for analyzing the pathogenesis of human diseases and creating models of the diseases. Non-insulin-dependent diabetes mellitus (NIDDM) is a polygenic disease requiring the interactions of multiple genetic factors and environmental factors for its development. The genetic manipulation of defects in human NIDDM genes in mice (via gene targeting) should give important insights into the molecular mechanism and actual biochemical pathways of human NIDDM.

Introduction

Non-insulin-dependent diabetes mellitus (NIDDM) is characterized by peripheral insulin resistance and insulin secretory dysfunction [1,2]. These abnormalities are either genetically defined or augmented by hyperglycemia itself, and may interact in a complex manner to cause and sustain hyperglycemia. Previous prospective studies have demonstrated that both insulin resistance/hyperinsulinemia and low insulin response to glucose are predictors of NIDDM [3–7]. Genetically engineered knockout models [8,9] are powerful tools to investigate the roles of diabetogenic genes and their interaction in the development of diabetes. This brief review attempts to summarize the recent application of developmental biology, especially gene targeting technology, to develop mouse models of human NIDDM. Table 1 presents the significance of gene targeting in the research for pathogenesis of NIDDM.

Gene targeting

The analysis of genes by inactivation or modification, and the study of the consequences of the mutation in the organism are central to an understanding of the function of genes in vivo. In mammals, before gene targeting, this approach was limited to the rare spontaneous mutations reflected in obvious phenotypes, as in

Address for correspondence: T. Kadowaki, Third Department of Internal Medicine, Faculty of Medicine, University of Tokyo, 7-3-1 Hongo, Bunkyo-ku, Tokyo 113, Japan. Tel.: +81-3-3815-5411 ext. 3111. Fax: +81-3-5689-7209. E-mail: kadowaki-3im@h.u-tokyo.ac.jp

Table 1. The significance of gene targeting in the research for pathogenesis of NIDDM.

1. Investigating molecular mechanism of diabetogenic genes in vivo.
2. Creating animal models of human NIDDM.
3. Characterizing the interplay between genetic factors and environmental factors on the development of NIDDM as a polygenic disease.

the case of inheritable diseases in the human. The targeted mutagenesis in the mouse germline was therefore a fundamental breakthrough in this area of research. Gene targeting involves the inactivation of a given gene in the genome of embryonic stem (ES) cells by homologous recombination [10,11]. ES cells derive from the inner cell mass of a mouse blastocyst and have retained their totipotency, thus they can participate in the generation of cell lineages of the mouse if transferred into an early mouse embryo. Transfer of mutant ES cells into mouse embryos thus allows the transmission of the mutation into the mouse germline. In the classical experiment, gene inactivation was achieved by replacing a predetermined gene segment with a mutant version of this segment, through homologous recombination [12]. Since the latter is infrequent in mammalian cells, the isolation of the mutant ES cells requires stringent selection. This was achieved by placing a selectable gene (neomycin resistance gene, in this case) into the targeted locus in a manner that allows its expression and hence cellular selection while inactivating the target gene (positive selection). On the other hand, inclusion of another selectable marker in the targeting vector just outside one of the regions of homology allows for concomitant negative selection. The herpes simplex thymidine kinase gene (tk) in conjunction with the drug ganciclovir or the diphtheria toxin A fragment gene (DTA) has been used successfully in this context. Most of the cells taking up the targeting vector randomly into their genomes retain and express the negative selection marker gene; they are consequently unable to survive (Fig. 1).

Furthermore, many researchers are achieving conditional, i.e., cell-type-specific and/or inducible, gene targeting for several reasons [13,9]. First, germline mutations may be lethal, in which case there is no mouse to study gene function. Second, genes may exert their function at several stages of ontogeny and in different cell types. Third, conditional gene targeting could allow one to generate models of somatically acquired genetic diseases rather than of inherited ones. The conditional gene targeting approach as well as the classical approach will be applied for creating animal models of NIDDM.

Manipulating insulin biosynthesis and secretion in the mouse: glucokinase gene

Glucokinase (GK), mainly expressed in pancreatic β cells and the liver, converts glucose to glucose-6-phosphate. It is thought to constitute a rate-limiting step in glucose metabolism in these tissues, and has been proposed to act as a glucose sensor in the pancreatic β cell [14]. Alternative splicing of a single GK gene gives

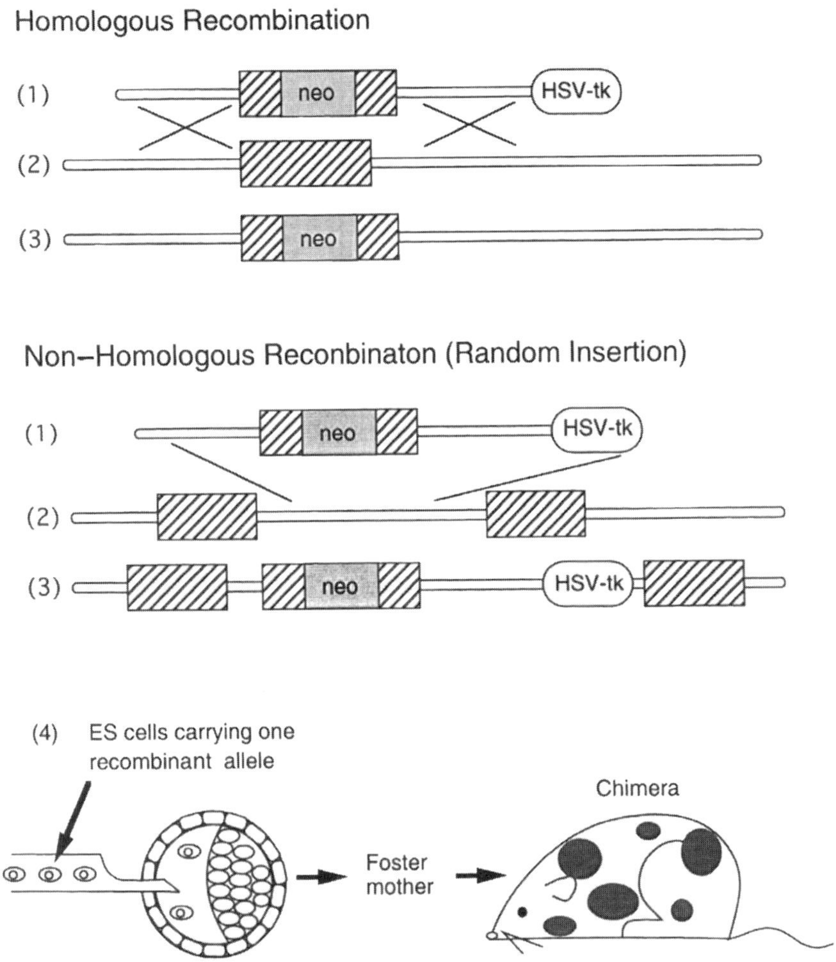

Fig. 1. Generation of mice carrying targeted gene. (1) Gene targeting vector containing neomycin resistance (neo) gene and the HSV-tk gene, which are used for positive and negative selection, respectively (exons drawn as filled boxes). (2) Target gene in the genome of ES cells. (3) Genomic locus modified by homologous recombination between vector and target gene. After electroporation into ES cells, G418-resistant clones that have undergone the adequate homologous recombination event are identified. In case of random insertion, transfected cell are unable to survive because of negative selection. (4) Recombinant ES cells are injected into blastocysts, which are reimplanted into foster mothers, and generate chimeras at term.

rise to two isoforms of GK, one expressed in the pancreatic β cells and the other in liver, which have a different first exon (exon 1β and exon 1L, respectively). By disrupting β cell specific exon, mice lacking the pancreatic β cell GK isoform were generated [15]. Heterozygous β cell glucokinase knockout mice ($GK^{+/-}$) showed early onset nonprogressive impaired glucose tolerance due to decreased insulin secretion to glucose. Despite normal morphology and β cell mass, insulin secretion from $GK^{+/-}$ islets was decreased in the perifusion experiments [16]. The clinical symptoms of the heterozygous mutant mice are very similar to those of Maturity Onset Diabetes of the Young (MODY) patients who possess a mutant form of GK in both pancreatic β cells and liver. It is suggested that a heterozygous mutation of GK in the pancreatic β cells, but not in liver, is sufficient to cause mild glucose intolerance. In this respect, Efrat et al. have generated mice in which pancreatic GK expression was attenuated by a ribozyme-mediated method [17]. Although the GK activity of these mice was only 30% compared to normal, and they showed an impaired insulin response to glucose in perfused pancreas experiments, the fasting and postprandial glucose levels were normal. It is possible that the different strategies used to attenuate GK expression may explain the apparent discrepancy between the ribozyme-mediated method and the gene knockout method. For example, the gene knockout method is likely to block the expression of GK more completely and in a more stable manner. It is also possible that the different strains of mice used (Efrat et al. (C3H), vs. Terauchi et al. (ICR)) [17,15] might account for the different results. In this respect, Ishihara et al. established GK antisense transgenic mice using the strains C3H or C57BL/6J as background. In both strains, GK activity in pancreatic islets was reduced by 50%. However, mice which were maintained in C3H as background showed normal glucose tolerance, while mice maintained in C57BL/6J as background developed mild glucose intolerance [18].

Homozygous mutant pups ($GK^{-/-}$) were normal in size, appearance, body weight, and blood glucose level at birth. Although they were able to suck, they showed no increase in body weight with age. They also showed marked glycosuria within a day and almost all animals died within 7 days of birth apparently due to dehydration. At 3–4 days of age, their blood glucose levels were markedly higher than those of wild-type or heterozygous animals, while serum insulin levels were low relative to the elevated blood glucose concentrations, suggesting the presence of relative insulin deficiency. Subcutaneous injection of insulin or oral administration of sulfonylurea enabled homozygous mutant mice to survive longer, indicating that neonatal death in untreated animals was presumably due to hyperglycemia resulting from β cell dysfunction. Histological examinations showed that both endocrine and exocrine pancreas formation seemed to be normal in homozygous mutant mice. Immunostaining for glucagon, insulin, and somatostatin and electron microscopy revealed that differentiation into pancreatic α, β, and δ cells also appeared to be unaffected. Thus, β cell GK is not absolutely required for normal development or differentiation of endocrine pancreas or insulin biosynthesis. $GK^{-/-}$ islets showed defective insulin secretion in response to glucose, but normal insulin secretion in response to other nutrient secretagogues and sulfonylureas.

In order to test the hypothesis that GK is the glucose sensor for insulin secretion, and to resolve the relative roles of liver cell GK in maintaining glucose levels, Grupe et al. have generated mice completely deficient in GK and transgenic knockout in which GK is expressed only in pancreatic β cells [19]. In mice with only one GK allele, blood glucose levels are elevated and insulin secretion is reduced. GK-deficient mice die perinatally with severe hyperglycemia. Expression of GK in the β cells in the absence of expression in the liver is sufficient for survival. Absence of GK in the liver resulted in reduced glycogen stores and steatosis, although they might be secondary to metabolic disorders.

Thus, GK-deficient mice provide the first direct proof that GK serves as a glucose-sensor molecule for insulin secretion and plays a pivotal role in glucose homeostasis. GK-deficient mice also serve as an animal model of the insulin-secretory defect in human NIDDM.

Manipulating insulin action in the mouse

IRS-1

Insulin receptor substrate-1 (IRS-1) is tyrosine phosphorylated in physiological target tissues of insulin such as liver, muscle, and adipocytes, and serves as an intracellular substrate for the insulin receptor or IGF-1 receptor [20,21]. In addition, tyrosine phosphorylation of IRS-1 is reported in response to several interleukins, interferons, angiotensin II, and growth hormone. Tyrosine phosphorylation of IRS-1 provides binding sites for several distinct Src homology 2 (SH2) proteins and mediate multiple signaling pathways. IRS-1 deficient mice were generated by two groups [22,23].

Growth of the homozygous IRS-1 knockout mice was retarded. At the age of 3, 8, and 15 weeks, the weight was about 30% less than that of normal littermates; the serum IGF-1, IGF-2 and growth hormone levels were normal in the mutant mice. The growth retardation of the embryos became apparent at 15.5 embryonic days and the weight of homozygous IRS-1 knockout embryos was about 80% compared to normal and heterozygous embryos at 18.5 embryonic days. The growth retardation of the IRS-1 knockout mice was milder than that of insulin receptor knockout mice [24,25], and leprechaunism, human insulin receptor deficient state, and also milder than that of IGF-1 receptor knockout mice [26], suggesting the existence of both IRS-1 dependent and IRS-1 independent pathways in signal transduction through insulin and IGF-1 receptor tyrosine kinases.

The drop in the blood glucose levels after injection of human insulin was significantly smaller in homozygous mutant mice than those of heterozygous mutant and wild-type mice. Similar results were observed with IGF-1 injection and also with IGF-2. Thus, homozygous mutant mice have resistance to IGF-1 and IGF-2 in addition to insulin. The stimulation of glucose transport activity of the isolated adipocytes with insulin [27] and soleus muscle with insulin and IGF-1 was significantly impaired in homozygous mutant mice compared with that of the wild-type mice. Although there was no significant difference in blood glucose among the three genotypes, the serum insulin levels before and after glucose load were significantly higher in the homozygous mutant mice. Thus, IRS-

1 knockout mice show mild to moderate postreceptor insulin resistance in the muscle [28] yet normal glucose tolerance by compensatory hyperinsulinemia from pancreatic β cells. Histologically, they exhibited β cell hyperplasia accompanied by partial differentiation of nonendocrine tissues into insulin-positive cells [29]. Insulin secretory profile and glucose sensitivity of insulin secretion were indistinguishable between wild-type and IRS-1 knockout mice when the same amounts of islets were compared. Therefore, moderate insulin resistance appeared to induce hyperplasia and neogenesis of pancreatic β cells rather than β cell hyperfunction leading to moderate increase in fasting and postprandial insulin levels in vivo. Since these mice were not associated with hyperglycemia, it seems possible that factor(s) related to insulin resistance other than glucose were also involved in these changes in the pancreatic β cells. Thus, IRS-1 deficient mice provide an excellent animal model for normoglycemic insulin resistance seen in the prediabetic stage of human NIDDM.

In addition to IRS-1, another weakly tyrosine phosphorylated protein of an Mr 190-kDa (pp190), which was not recognized by anti IRS-1 antibody, was observed in liver of insulin-injected wild-type mice. Insulin-stimulated tyrosine phosphorylation of pp190 was increased in IRS-1 deficient mice compared with that in wild-type mice, thus compensating the effects of IRS-1 deficiency [30]. In fact, pp190, cloned by Sun et al. and named IRS-2, has many structural homologies with IRS-1 [31].

Insulin resistance

Insulin resistance is a major predisposing factor in NIDDM, and is transmitted in a non-Mendelian fashion. It is not clear whether the complex genetics of insulin are due to heterogeneity, polygenic inheritance, or both. To dissect the genetics of insulin resistance, mice carrying a null mutation in the insulin receptor gene have been created [24,25]. Homozygous mutant mice were almost normal at birth, but rapidly developed metabolic disorders, such as hyperglycemia associated with hyperinsulinemia and elevated triglyceride levels, and died invariably within a few days of birth of diabetic ketoacidosis. In contrast, the metabolic status of mice heterozygous for a null insulin receptor allele varied considerably [32]. The expected reduction in insulin receptor number in these mice was associated with a horseshoe-shaped relationship between plasma glucose and insulin levels, recominiscent of NIDDM. Only 10% of heterozygotes developed hyperglycemia, suggesting that interactions between the null mutation of the insulin receptor gene and other predisposing alleles were required to develop diabetes.

Genetic reconstitution of NIDDM as a polygenic disease

Double knockout mouse with disruption of IRS-1 and β cell GK genes

Non-insulin-dependent diabetes mellitus (NIDDM) is considered a polygenic disorder in which insulin resistance and insulin secretory defect are the major etiologic factors. Homozygous mice with insulin receptor substrate-1 (IRS-1)

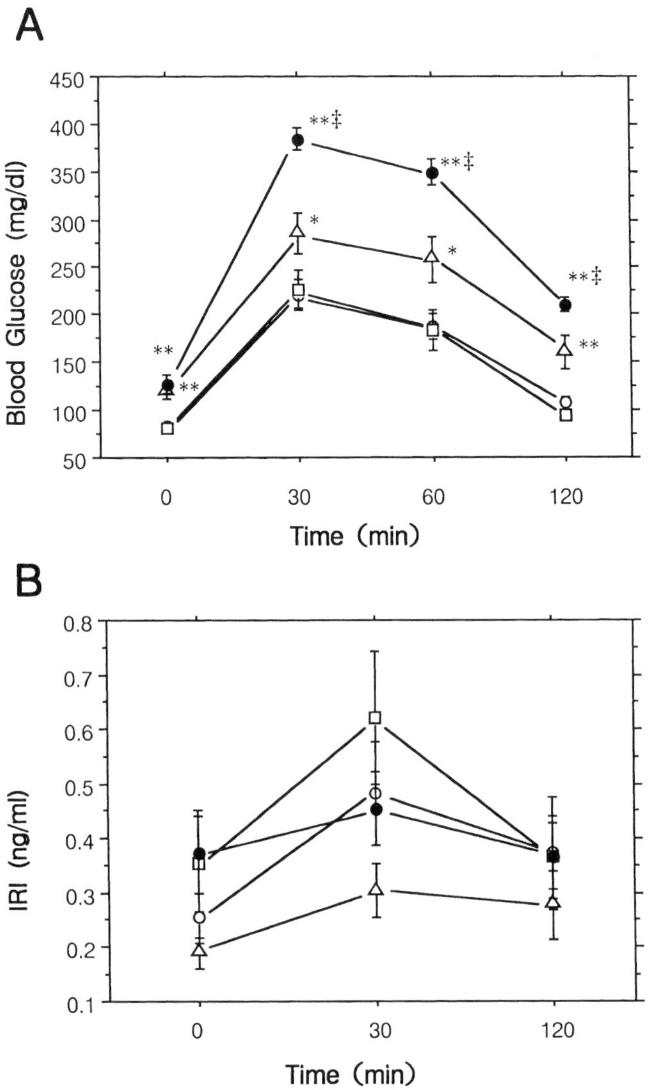

Fig. 2. The exacerbation of diabetes in the double knockout mice. The result of glucose tolerance test was adapted from Terauchi et al. 1997 [29]. Wild-type mice (open circles), $GK^{+}/^{+}IRS\text{-}1^{-/-}$ (open squares), $GK^{+}/^{-}IRS\text{-}1^{+/+}$ (open triangles) and $GK^{+}/^{-}IRS\text{-}1^{-/-}$ (filled circles) were fasted for more than 16 hours before the study. They were then loaded with 1.5 mg g^{-1} (body weight) glucose by intraperitoneal infusion. Profiles of blood glucose levels (**A**) and insulin levels (**B**) in 30–40 week-old mice are shown. Results are shown as mean ± SEM. *Indicates $p < 0.05$, **Indicates $p < 0.01$ compared with wild-type. ‡Indicates $p < 0.01$ compared with $GK^{+}/^{-}IRS\text{-}1^{+/+}$.

gene knockout showed normal glucose tolerance associated with insulin resistance and compensatory hyperinsulinemia. Heterozygous mice with β cell glucokinase (GK) gene knockout showed impaired glucose tolerance due to decreased insulin secretion to glucose. To elucidate the interplay between insulin resistance and insulin secretory defect for the development of NIDDM, Terauchi et al. generated a double-knockout mouse with disruption of IRS-1 and β cell GK genes by crossing the mice with each of the single gene knockout [29]. The double-knockout mice developed overt diabetes (Fig. 2). Blood glucose levels 120 min after intraperitoneal glucose load were significantly elevated compared with wild-type, IRS-$1^{-/-}$, or $GK^{+/-}$. The double-knockout mice showed fasting hyperinsulinemia and selective hyperplasia of the β cells as the IRS-1 knockout mice, but impaired insulin secretion to glucose. Thus, the genetic abnormalities, each of which is nondiabetogenic by itself, cause overt diabetes if they coexist. The exacerbation of diabetes in the double-knockout mice indicated that insulin resistance and insulin secretory defect played a cooperative role in the development and exacerbation of diabetes, even though neither was strong enough alone to cause overt diabetes. Development of diabetes in the double-knockout mice appears to be age-dependent, since this phenomenon was not observed at younger ages; $GK^{+/-}$ did not show any age-dependent exacerbation of glucose tolerance unlike the double-knockout mice even though they were similarly glucose intolerant at younger ages. Thus, β cell exhaustion by continuous exposure to insulin resistance rather than glucose toxicity might be involved in the development of diabetes in the double-knockout mice.

Double heterozygous knockout mice for IR and IRS-1 gene locus

NIDDM is a polygenic disease characterized by insulin resistance in muscle, fat, and liver, followed by a failure of pancreatic β cells to adequately compensate for this resistance despite increased insulin secretion. Mice double heterozygous for null alleles in the insulin receptor and insulin receptor substrate-1 genes exhibit the expected 50% reduction in expression of these two proteins, but a synergism at a level of insulin resistance with 5- to 50-fold elevated plasma insulin levels and comparable levels of cell hyperplasia [32]. Although the double heterozygotes showed normal glucose levels at 2 months of age, 40% of them become overtly diabetic at 4–6 months of age. This NIDDM mouse model in which diabetes arises in an age-dependent manner (from the interaction between two genetically determined, subclinical defects in the insulin-signaling cascade) demonstrates the role of epistatic interactions in the pathogenesis of common diseases with non-Mendelian genetics.

These two reports provide the first genetic reconstitution of NIDDM as a polygenic disorder in mice.

Conclusions

Human NIDDM is a polygenic disease requiring the interactions of multiple genetic factors and environmental factors for its development. In this respect, use of inbred animal models such as GK rat [33] and OLETF rat [34] that spontaneously reproduce the main features of NIDDM has been an important strategy for genetic investigations. The strategy as well as gene targeting approach shares advantages in that the interactions of genetic defects as well as those between genetic and environmental factors can be studied in multifactorial traits such as NIDDM [35,36]. Nevertheless, since actual genetic defects have not yet been identified in spontaneous NIDDM animal models, interpretations of crossing studies are much more straightforward in genetic manipulation and reconstitution of this disease. More importantly, since whole genome mapping and identification of human NIDDM genes are progressing rapidly [37,38], the genetic manipulation of defects in human NIDDM genes in mice via gene targeting should give important insights into the molecular mechanism and actual biochemical pathways of human NIDDM.

References

1. Taylor SI, Accili D, Imai Y. Insulin resistance or insulin deficiency: Which is the primary cause of NIDDM? Diabetes 1994;43:735–740.
2. Polonsky KS, Sturis J, Bell GI. Non-insulin-dependent diabetes mellitus – a genetically programmed failure of the beta cell to compensate for insulin resistance. N Engl J Med 1996;334: 777–783.
3. Lillioja S, Mott DM, Spraul M et al. Insulin resistance and insulin secretory dysfunction as precursors of non-insulin-dependent diabetes mellitus: prospective studies of Pima Indians. N Engl J Med 1993;329:1988–1992.
4. Martin BC, Warram JH, Krolewski AS. Role of glucose and insulin resistance in the development of type 2 diabetes mellitus: results of a 25-year follow-up study. Lancet 1992;340:925–929.
5. Kadowaki T, Miyake Y, Hagura R et al. Risk factors for worsening to diabetes in subjects with impaired glucose tolerance. Diabetologia 1994;26:44–49.
6. Johnston C, Ward WK, Beard JC et al. Islet function and insulin sensitivity in the nondiabetic offspring of conjugal type 2 diabetic patients. Diabet Med 1990;7:119–125.
7. Haffner SM, Miettinen H, Gaskill SP, Stern MP. Decreased insulin secretion and increased insulin resistance are independently related to the 7-year risk of NIDDM in Mexican-Americans. Diabetes 1995;44:1386–1391.
8. Bronson SK, Smithies O. Altering mice by homologous recombination using embryonic stem cells. J Biol Chem 1992;269:27155–27158.
9. Rajewsky K, Gu H, Kühn R et al. Conditional gene targeting. J Clin Invest 1996;98:600–603.
10. Robertson EJ. Teratocarcinomas and Embryonic Stem Cells, The Practical Approach Series. IRL Press, 1987.
11. Capecchi MR. The new mouse genetics: altering the genome by gene targeting. Trends Genet 1989;5:70–76.
12. Thomas KR, Capecchi MR. Site-directed mutagenesis by gene targeting in mouse embryo-derived stem cells. Cell 1987;51:503–512.
13. Kühn R, Schwenk F, Aguet M, Rajewsky K. Inducible gene targeting in mice. Science 1995; 269:1427–1429.

14. Matschinsky FM. Glucokinase as glucose sensor and metabolic signal generator in pancreatic beta cells and hepatocytes. Diabetes 1990;39:647—652.
15. Terauchi Y, Sakura H, Yasuda K et al. Pancreatic β cell specific targeted disruption of glucokinase gene: defective insulin secretion to glucose. J Biol Chem 1995;268:30253—30256.
16. Aizawa T, Asanuma N, Terauchi Y et al. Analysis of the pancreatic β cell in the mouse with targeted disruption of the pancreatic β cell-specific glucokinase gene. Biochem Biophys Res Commun 1996;229:460—465.
17. Efrat S, Leiser M, Wu Y et al. Ribozyme-mediated attenuation of pancreatic β cell glucokinase expression in transgenic mice results in impaired glucose-induced insulin secretion. Proc Natl Acad Sci USA 1994;91:2051—2055.
18. Ishihara H, Tashiro F, Ikuta K et al. Inhibition of pancreatic β cell glucokinase by antisense RNA expression in transgenic mice: mouse strain-dependent alteration of glucose tolerance. FEBS Lett 1995;371:329—332.
19. Grupe A, Hultgren B, Ryan A et al. Transgenic knockouts reveal a requirement for pancreatic beta cell glucokinase in maintaining glucose homeostasis. Cell 1995;83:69—78.
20. White MF, Maron R, Kahn CR. Insulin rapidly stimulates tyrosine phosphorylation of a Mr-185,000 protein in intact cells. Nature 1985;318:183—186.
21. Sun XJ, Rothenberg P, Kahn CR et al. The structure of the insulin receptor substrate IRS-1 defines a unique signal transduction protein. Nature 1991;352:73—77.
22. Tamemoto H, Kadowaki T, Tobe K et al. Insulin resistance and growth retardation in mice lacking insulin receptor substrate-1. Nature 1994;372:182—186.
23. Araki E, Lipes MA, Patti ME et al. Alternative pathway of insulin signaling in mice with targeted disruption of the IRS-1 gene. Nature 1994;372:186—190.
24. Accili D, Drago J, Lee EL et al. Early neonatal death in mice homozygous for a null allele of the insulin receptor gene. Nature Genet 1996;12:106—109.
25. Joshi RL, Lamothe B, Cordonnier N et al. Targeted disruption of the insulin receptor gene in the mouse results in neonatal lethality. EMBO J 1996;15:1542—1547.
26. Liu J-P, Baker J, Perkins AS et al. Mice carrying null mutations of the genes encoding insulin-like growth factor-1 (Igf-1) and type 1 Igf receptors (Igf1r). Cell 1993;75:59—72.
27. Kaburagi Y, Satoh S, Tamemoto H et al. Role of insulin receptor substrate-1 and pp60 in the regulation of insulin-induced glucose transport and GLUT4 translocation in primary adipocytes. J Biol Chem 1997;272:25839—25844.
28. Yamauchi T, Tobe K, Tamemoto H et al. Insulin signaling and insulin action in the muscles and livers of insulin-resistant, insulin receptor substrate-1 deficient mice. Molec Cell Biol 1996;16: 3074—3084.
29. Terauchi Y, Iwamoto K, Tamemoto H et al. Development of non-insulin-dependent diabetes mellitus in the double knockout mice with disruption of insulin receptor substrate-1 and β cell glucokinase genes. J Clin Invest 1997;99:861—866.
30. Tobe K, Tamemoto H, Yamauchi T et al. Identification of a 190-kDa protein as a novel substrate for the insulin receptor kinase functionally similar to insulin receptor substrate-1. J Biol Chem 1995;270:5698—5701.
31. Sun XJ, Wang LM, Zhang Y et al. Role of IRS-2 in insulin and cytokine signaling. Nature 1995;377:173—177.
32. Brüning JC, Winnay J, Bonner-Weir S et al. Development of a novel polygenic model of NIDDM in mice heterozygous for IR and IRS-1 null alleles. Cell 1997;88: 561—572.
33. Kimura K, Toyota T, Kakizaki M et al. Impaired insulin secretion in the spontaneous diabetic rats. Tohoku J Exp Med 1981;137:453—459.
34. Kawano K, Hirashima T, Mori S et al. Spontaneous long-term hyperglycemic rat with diabetic complications. Otsuka Long-Evans Tokushima Fatty (OLETF) strain. Diabetes 1992;41: 1422—1428.
35. Galli J, Li L-S, Glaser A et al. Genetic analysis of non-insulin-dependent diabetes mellitus in the GK rat. Nature Genet 1996;12:31—37.

36. Gauguier D, Froguel P, Parent V et al. Chromosomal mapping of genetic loci associated with non-insulin-dependent diabetes in the GK rat. Nature Genet 1996;12:38–43.
37. Hanis CL, Boerwinkle E, Chakraborty R et al. A genome-wide search for human non-insulin-dependent (type 2) diabetes genes reveals a major susceptibility locus on chromosome 2. Nature Genet 1996;13:161–166.
38. Melanie MM, Widen E, Lehto M et al. Mapping of a gene for type 2 diabetes associated with an insulin secretion defect by a genome scan in Finnish families. Nature Genet 1996;14:90–94.

Additional reading

1. Bali D, Svetlanov A, Lee HW et al. Animal model for maturity-onset diabetes of the young generated by disruption of the mouse glucokinase gene. J Biol Chem 270:21464–21467.
2. Sosa-Pineda B, Chowdhury K, Torres M et al. The Pax4 gene is essential for differentiation of insulin-producing beta cells in the mammalian pancreas. Nature 1997;386:399–403.

Recent Advances on the Pathogenesis and Management of Diabetes Mellitus.
S.H. Shinn, M. Shichiri and K.-W. Kim, editors.

Diabetic angiopathy and oxygen free radicals

Bo-Wan Kim
Department of Internal Medicine, Kyungpook University School of Medicine, Taegu, Korea

The mechanisms for development of vascular disease in patients with diabetes mellitus are poorly understood. There is increasing evidence that in diabetes mellitus the altered free radical-related process may play a crucial role in determining vascular tissue injury. Free radical-mediated oxidation of biological molecules, membranes and tissues may result from overproduction of precursors to reactive oxygen radicals and/or decreased efficiency of inhibitory and scavenger systems. Under physiological conditions, glucose is prone to oxidation and consequently generates hydrogen peroxide and reactive intermediates such as hydroxyl free radicals. Although the mechanism through which hyperglycemia may increase the generation of free radicals is not known, several studies support the theory that peroxide formation is increased in an elevated glucose solution. The sources of oxygen-derived free radicals are not known, but it is possible that the sources of free radicals may be from: 1) the autoxidation of glucose, 2) the polyol pathway, and 3) protein glycation. Several studies are summarized here which demonstrate that one possible mechanism lies in the fact that free radicals participate in the deleterious effects of diabetes on vascular endothelial cell function.

Free radicals and endothelial dysfunction

Vascular endothelial cells play an obligatory role in the vasodilating responses to several vasoactive agents. The endothelium-dependent relaxation is mediated by vasodilatory factors, including the endothelium-derived relaxing factor (EDRF) and the endothelium-derived hyperpolarizing factor (EDHF), that the endothelium produces and liberates in response to vasoactive substances such as acetylcholine (ACh) and bradykinin. A diminished response of morphologically unaltered blood vessels to endothelium-dependent vasodilators is called endothelial dysfunction. If endothelial dysfunction promotes atherosclerosis, it may be a link between hyperglycemia and alterations of large vessels [1].

In many experimental studies, isolated blood vessels from diabetic animals showed the selective impairment of endothelium-dependent relaxation. Our previous studies showed that these dysfunctions could be found early, even over a 3-

Address for correspondence: Bo-Wan Kim MD, Department of Internal Medicine, School of Medicine, Kyungpook National University, Taegu 700-721, South Korea. Tel.: +82-53-420-5565. Fax: +82-53-426-2046. E-mail: bwkim@kyungpook.ac.kr

week period after induction of diabetes, and the impairment would be greater in those with longer duration of the diabetic state [2] and that these impairments of endothelium-dependent relaxation were mainly due to EDRF, not to EDHF [3] (Fig. 1). Exposure of a diabetic rat aortic ring to an oxygen-free radical (e.g., hydrogen peroxide generated by mixing xanthine and xanthine oxidase), caused some increase in selective impairment of endothelium-dependent relaxation, but the sensitivity to free radical-induced endothelial dysfunction was not significantly different between diabetic and control rat aorta [2]. After treatment of diabetic rats with bacterial lipopolysaccharide as a potent free-radical generator, the endothelial dysfunction of their aortic rings was significantly aggravated but the degree of impairment of endothelium-dependent relaxation in diabetic rat aortas was also similar to that of control rats [4].

In human diabetes, endothelium-dependent relaxation may be impaired. A study of impotence associated with diabetes mellitus [5] showed that penile tissue from diabetics relaxed less to ACh, despite morphologically intact endothelium. Several clinical studies [6,7] have shown that endothelium-dependent vasodilation, as assessed by forearm venous plethysmography, is diminished in patients both with IDDM and NIDDM.

Endothelial dysfunction and radical scavengers

Recent studies have demonstrated that a number of free radical scavengers prevent endothelial dysfunction caused by hyperglycemia and exogenous free radicals. Experimentally the superoxide scavenger could reverse the abnormal endothelium-dependent relaxations in diabetic animals. We have also reported that in diabetic rat aorta free radicals, generated by mixing xanthine and xanthine oxidase, induced impairment of vascular relaxation can be prevented by superoxide dismutase and catalase [8] (Fig. 2) and this protective effect of the scavengers was greater in the EDRF-mediated relaxative response than in the

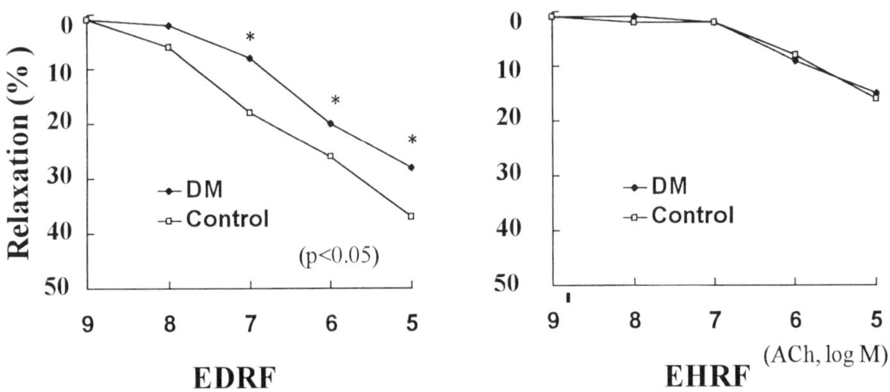

Fig. 1. EDRF-mediated (left panel) and EDHF-mediated (right panel) relaxative responses to acetylcholine (ACh) of diabetic and control rat aortas.

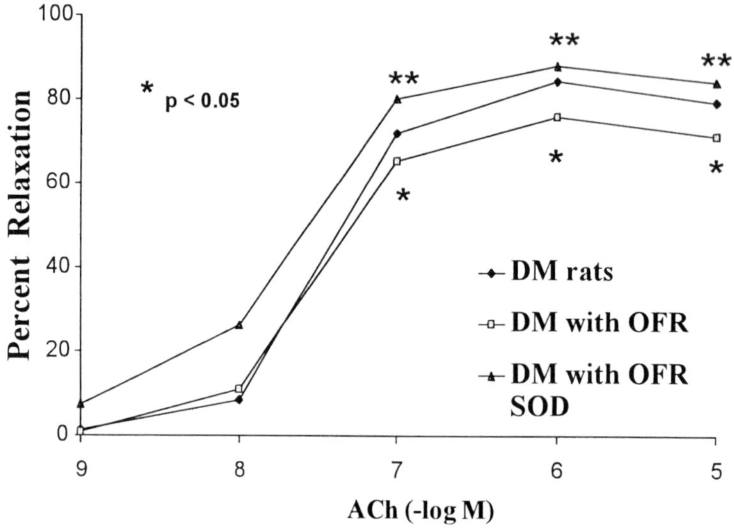

Fig. 2. Effects of superoxide dismutase (SOD) on the oxygen free radical (OFR)-induced impairment of endothelium-dependent relaxation to acetylcholine (ACh) in diabetic rat aortic rings.

EDHF-mediated one. It has also been found that pretreatment of the diabetic rat with radical scavengers protect the endothelium-dependent relaxation of aortic rings from bacterial lipopolysaccharide-induced vessel damage [4].

In conclusion, diabetic hyperglycemia can predict the endothelial dysfunction of the blood vessels and the generation of a reactive oxygen species may play an important role in the pathogenesis of diabetic vasculopathy. This oxidative stress-induced endothelial dysfunction may be prevented by free radical scavenger systems. But the possible link between the endothelial dysfunction caused by free radicals and long-term vascular diabetic complications has yet to be proven.

References

1. Giugliano D, Paolisso G, Ceriello A. Oxidative stress and diabetic vascular complications. Diabet Care 1996;19:257–267.
2. Kim JG, Kim SW, Kim SD, Seo YK, Ha SW, Kim BW. Influences of the duration of diabetes on the impairment in relaxative responses and on the sensitivity to oxygen free radical induced damage in streptozotocin-diabetic rat aortas. Korean J Med 1996;50:19–26.
3. Seo YK, Nam JH, Shin BH, Kim JG, Ha SW, Kim BW. Effect of superoxide dismutase on lipopolysaccharide-induced changes in vascular reactivity of diabetic rat aorta. Korean J Med 1995;47(suppl):63.
4. Kim JG, Nam JH, Shin BH, Seo YK, Kim SW, Ha SW, Kim BW. Comparisons between EDRF and EDHF-mediated relaxative responses in streptozotocin-diabetic rat aortas. Korean J Med 1994;46(suppl):72.
5. Saenz de Tejada I, Goldstein I, Azadzoi K, Krane RJ, Cohen RA. Impaired neurogenic and endothelium-dependent relaxation of human penile smooth muscle: the pathophysiological basis for impotence in diabetes mellitus. N Engl J Med 1989;320:1025–1030.

6. McVeigh GE, Brennan GM, Johnston GD, McDermott BJ, McGrath LT, Henry WR, Andrews JW. Impaired endothelium-dependent and independent vasodilation in patients with type 2 (non-insulin-dependent) diabetes mellitus. Diabetologia 1992;35:771–776.
7. Johnston MT, Creager SJ, Kathleen MS, Cusco JA, Lee BK, Creager MA. Impaired endothelium-dependent vasodilatation in patients with insulin-dependent diabetes mellitus. Circulation 1993;88:2510–2516.
8. Kim DH, Seo YK, Nam JH, Sin BH, Kim JG, Ha SW, Kim BW. Effects of superoxide dismutase on changes in EDRF- and EDHF-mediated relaxation of diabetic rat aortas exposed to oxygen free radicals. J Korean Soc Endocrinol 1997;12:265–274.

Recent Advances on the Pathogenesis and Management of Diabetes Mellitus.
S.H. Shinn, M. Shichiri and K.-W. Kim, editors.

Mutations of the IRS-1 gene and their impact on insulin resistance

Eiichi Araki, Ryohei Yoshimura, Sachiko Ura, Mikio Todaka, Kaku Tsuruzoe, Hiroyuki Motoshima, Kazuaki Yoshizato, Atsuhisa Shirakami and Motoaki Shichiri

Department of Metabolic Medicine, Kumamoto University School of Medicine, Kumamoto, Japan

Abstract. In order to determine the impact of the IRS-1 gene on the development of NIDDM, we screened the IRS-1 gene mutation and analyzed the function of the mutant IRS-1s. Through the screening of the IRS-1 gene, we identified four missense mutations [Pro^{170} to Arg (P170R), Met^{209} to Thr (M209T), Ser^{809} to Phe (S809F) and Gly^{971} to Arg (G971R)]. The prevalence of these mutations was significantly higher in NIDDM (23.4%) than in controls (8.5%). The glucose infusion rate during euglycemic clamps in subjects with the mutations tended to be lower than those without. Then we expressed wild-type (WT) and mutant IRS-1s (G971R, P170R, and M209T) in 32D-IR cells and analyzed their function. All the cells expressing mutant IRS-1s showed a significant reduction in DNA synthesis when compared with WT. Upon insulin stimulation, G971R showed a significant decrease (~40%) in both binding and activity of PI 3-kinase and a 22% decrease in MAP kinase activity. P170R and M209T showed slight decreases in binding and activity of PI 3-kinase, and greater decreases in MAP kinase activity. In addition, P170R and M209T showed significant decreases in tyrosine phosphorylation and binding to the insulin receptor, whereas G971R showed no difference compared to the WT. These data suggest that the impaired function of P170R and M209T was mainly due to reduced binding to the insulin receptor, whereas that of G971R was mainly due to reduced association with PI 3-kinase. This data implies that the mutations of IRS-1 gene could cause insulin resistance and contribute in part to the development of NIDDM.

Keywords: insulin receptor, insulin receptor substrate-1, MAP kinase, NIDDM, phosphatidylinositol 3 kinase, phosphotyorosine-binding domain.

Introduction

Following insulin stimulation, the insulin receptor undergoes autophosphorylation on tyrosine residues which in turn activates the tyrosine kinase activity of the receptor toward other substrates. Insulin receptor substrate-1 (IRS-1) is one of the major intracellular substrates for various receptors of insulin, IGF-1 (insulinlike growth factor-I), growth hormone and various cytokines including several interleukins and interferons [1—3]. After insulin stimulation, IRS-1 is immediately tyrosine phosphorylated by the insulin receptor tyrosine kinase. Recent

Address for correspondence: Eiichi Araki MD, PhD, Department of Metabolic Medicine, Kumamoto University School of Medicine, 1-1-1 Honjo, Kumamoto 860, Japan. Tel.: +81-96-373-5169. Fax: +81-96-366-8397.

studies have revealed that at least two regions of IRS-1 are important for interaction with the insulin receptor. One region, termed a pleckstrin homology (PH) domain is located at the N-terminus of IRS-1 (nt 14—144) and the other, a phosphotyrosine binding (PTB) domain is located near PH domain (nt 162—267) [3,4] (Fig. 1). Phosphorylated tyrosine residues of IRS-1 serve as docking sites for several src homology 2 (SH2) containing proteins, such as a 85 kDa regulatory subunit of phosphatidylinositol 3(PI-3)-kinase (PI 3-kinase p85), SH2 containing protein-tyrosine phosphatase (SHP-2) and growth factor-bound protein 2 (GRB2) (Fig. 1) [5]. The binding of these SH2 proteins to IRS-1 results in the activation of two major signaling pathways, MAP (mitogen activated protein) kinase and PI 3-kinase, which finally leads to the mitogenic and metabolic responses to insulin.

Recently, IRS-1 knockout mice were created by targeted disruption of the IRS-1 gene, and the function of IRS-1 in vivo was analyzed [6,7]. The IRS-1 knockout mice showed insulin resistance in the insulin tolerance test and impaired glucose tolerance in the intraperitoneal glucose loading test. In addition, decreased insulin-stimulated glucose uptake was observed in isolated adipocytes, and decreased insulin-stimulated PI 3-kinase activity was observed in skeletal muscle, suggesting the presence of impaired insulin signaling in major insulin-sensitive tissues in the mice. These data indicated a significant involvement of IRS-1 in insulin-

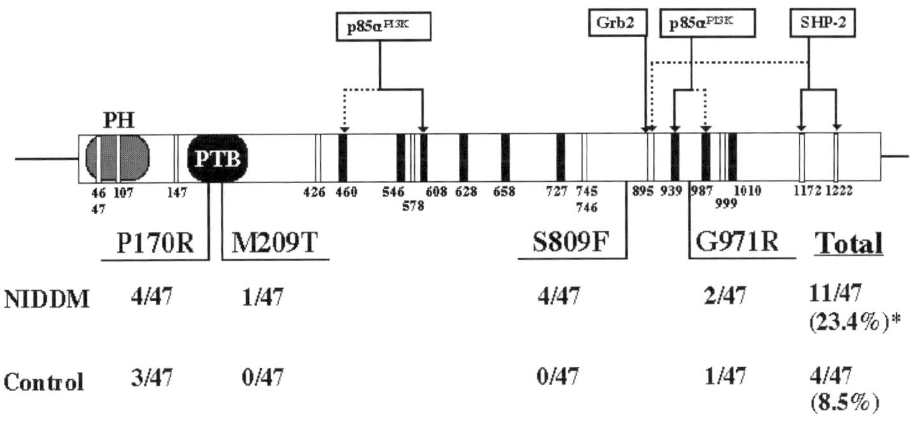

Fig. 1. Locations and frequencies of the IRS-1 missense mutations. Top: Schematic representation of human IRS-1 showing locations of mutations. PH and PTB indicate a pleckstrin homology domain and a phosphotyrosine binding domain, respectively. Solid bars indicate the YMXM or YXXM motifs, and open bars indicate other potential tyrosine phosphorylation sites. Amino acid numbers of the tyrosine residues are indicated below the bars. Reported binding sites for PI 3-kinase p85 ($p85\alpha^{PI3K}$), GRB2 and SHP-2 are indicated above. Solid arrows indicate the strong binding sites and dotted arrows indicate the weak binding sites. Locations of the four IRS-1 point mutations are indicated below. Bottom: Frequencies of the mutations in 47 NIDDM and 47 control subjects. *$p<0.05$ vs. control.

stimulated glucose uptake in vivo, and suggested that mutations in the IRS-1 gene may be involved in the development of NIDDM.

Recently, several groups have reported IRS-1 gene polymorphisms in patients with NIDDM [8–10]. However, some of these polymorphisms have also been found in nondiabetic patients, and therefore, the contribution of the IRS-1 gene mutation to the development of NIDDM has been unclear.

In this study, in order to clarify the impact of the IRS-1 gene on the development of NIDDM, we screened the mutations of the IRS-1 gene. We determined the function of mutant IRS-1s, identified (by expressing mutant IRS-1 proteins in 32D-IR cells) a myeloid progenitor cell line lacking endogenous IRS-1 and IRS-2, and stably expressing human insulin receptor.

Materials and Methods

Screening of the IRS-1 gene and clinical characterization of the subjects with IRS-1 gene missense mutations

Age- and BMI-matched 47 NIDDM and 47 control subjects were selected, and the mutation of the IRS-1 gene in the entire coding region was screened by PCR-SSCP (single-stranded conformation polymorphisms) analysis followed by sequencing. Selected subjects with or without missense mutations of the IRS-1 gene were analyzed by hyperinsulinemic euglycemic clamps.

In this paper, the numbers of amino acids of IRS-1 were used according to Araki et al. [11].

Cell line

The murine IL-3 dependent hematopoietic cell line, 32D-IR, which overexpresses the human insulin receptor, was grown and maintained in RPMI 1640 medium supplemented with 10% fetal bovine serum and 5% WEHI-conditioned medium.

Expression of various IRS-1s in 32D-IR cells

The expression vector containing the wild-type or three mutants (P170R, M209T and G971R) human IRS-1 cDNAs was transfected using electroporation methods. The cells were selected in the presence of 5 mM L-histidinol for 4 weeks. Each clone that survived was confirmed with the expression of IRS-1 protein by Western blotting with antirat IRS-1 C-terminus antibody.

Western blotting

After SDS-PAGE, proteins were transferred to nitrocellulose filters, probed with antirat IRS-1 antibody, anti-PI 3-kinase p85α antibody, anti-insulin receptor β

subunit antibody, or antiphosphotyrosine antibody, and detected with the incubation of [^{125}I]-protein A. Signals were visualized by autoradiography and quantified by the Bio Image Analyzer BA 100.

[^{3}H]thymidine incorporation assay

Cell lines in log phase growth were seeded in 1 ml of WEHI free medium into each of the 24-well plates and exposed to various concentrations of insulin (0, 0.1, 1, 10 and 100 nM) for 40 h. [^{3}H]thymidine (final concentration 0.5 μCi/ml) was added for the last 4 h of the incubation period, and cells were harvested and applied onto glass microfiber filters. After unincorporated nucleotide was washed out, the filters were dried and counted by liquid scintillation for 1 min.

MAP kinase assay

Cells were stimulated with 100 nM insulin for 5 min and lysed. The supernatants were immunoprecipitated with anti-MAP kinase antibody on a 96-well tissue culture plate pretreated with antirabbit IgG Fc antibody. The kinase reaction was carried out by the addition of 1 mg/ml myelin basic protein (MBP), 1 mg/ml ATP and 6 μCi [γ-^{32}P]-ATP at 30°C for 20 min, then terminated by addition of Laemmli sample buffer. The phosphorylated MBP were separated by 15% SDS-PAGE, visualized by autoradiography, and quantified by Bio Image Analyzer.

PI 3-kinase assays

For measurement of IRS-1 associated PI 3-kinase activity, cells were stimulated with 100 nM insulin for 5 min and lysed. The lysates were incubated with the anti-IRS-1 antibody, and the immunocomplexes were washed and resuspended in 36 μl kinase buffer consisting of 10 μl of 5 X reaction buffer (0.1 M Tris-HCl, pH7.4, 0.25 M NaCl, 50 mM $MgCl_2$, and 2.5 mM EGTA), 10 μl of 0.6 mM adenosine, 10 μl of 1 mg/ml PI-PS liposome prepared with phosphatidylinositol and phosphatidyl-L-serine, and 6 μl H_2O. The reaction was initiated by addition of 10 μl of 50 mM ATP and 4 μCi [γ-^{32}P]-ATP and was incubated at 30°C for 10 min. Phosphorylated phosphatidylinositol was separated in a thin layer chromatography, visualized by autoradiography, and quantified by Bio Image Analyzer.

Statistical analysis

Statistical analysis was performed using the nonpaired Student's t test. A p value < 0.05 was considered to be significant. Data in figures are expressed as mean ± SD.

Results

Screening of the IRS-1 gene and clinical characterization of the subjects with IRS-1 gene missense mutations

By screening the entire coding region of the IRS-1 gene, we identified seven point mutations in the IRS-1 gene (three silent mutations and four missense mutations). Four missense mutations resulted in substitutions of Pro^{170} to Arg (P170R), Met^{209} to Thr (M209T), Ser^{809} to Phe (S809F) and Gly^{971} to Arg (G971R) (Fig. 1). Although the prevalence of each individual missense mutation was not statistically different between NIDDM and control subjects, the overall prevalence of the four missense mutations was significantly higher ($p<0.05\%$) in NIDDM subjects (23.4%) than in control subjects (8.5%) (Fig. 1) [12]. In addition, although it was not statistically significant, the equilibrium glucose infusion rate during euglycemic clamps in NIDDM and control subjects with the IRS-1 missense mutations tended to be lower than those in comparable groups without these mutations [12].

Expression of mutant IRS-1s in 32D-IR cells

Expression of wild-type IRS-1 and mutant IRS-1s (G971R, P170R, and M209T) was monitored by Western blotting. In all IRS-1 transfected cell lines, comparable amounts of IRS-1 proteins were observed [13].

DNA synthesis in 32D-IR cells expressing various IRS-1s

To analyze the insulin-stimulated mitogenic response, [^{3}H]thymidine incorporation was measured at insulin concentrations ranging from 0 to 100 nM. There was no stimulation of thymidine incorporation by insulin in parental 32D-IR cells as expected. Expression of WT or mutant IRS-1s restored proliferative response to insulin. However, the three cell lines expressing mutant IRS-1s showed obvious reduction when compared with WT. Although cells expressing G971R, P170R and M209T showed significant response at 10 nM insulin, which were significantly reduced by 54% ($p<0.05$), 49% ($p<0.05$) and 34% ($p<0.05$) compared with WT, respectively. At 100 nM insulin, the cells expressing G971R, P170R and M209T also showed a reduced response, and reduced by 32% ($p<0.05$), 23%, and 35% ($p<0.05$) compared with WT, respectively [13].

MAP kinase activity

In order to study the cause of the reduced mitogenic response in cells expressing mutant IRS-1s, we first analyzed MAP kinase activities. When compared with WT, cells expressing G971R showed a decrease of 22% in insulin-stimulated

MAP kinase activity ($p<0.05$). Cells expressing P170R and M209T showed decreases of 41% ($p<0.01$) and 43% ($p<0.01$), respectively [13].

PI 3-kinase activity

Next, we measured the PI 3-kinase activities in IRS-1 immunoprecipitates from insulin-stimulated cells. After insulin stimulation, the IRS-1 associated PI 3-kinase activity was increased 4.1-fold in cells expressing WT. However, in cells expressing G971R, M209T and P170R, the insulin-stimulated PI 3-kinase activities were decreased by 39% ($p<0.005$), 17% ($p<0.05$) and 14% ($p<0.05$), respectively, compared with cells expressing WT [13].

Binding of PI 3-kinase p85 to IRS-1

In order to determine if the reduced PI 3-kinase activity in mutant IRS-1s resulted from a decreased binding of PI 3-kinase p85 to IRS-1, equal amounts of total protein were immunoprecipitated with anti-IRS-1 antibody, and probed with anti-PI 3-kinase p85a antibody. In cells expressing G971R, M209T and P170R, insulin-stimulated binding of PI 3-kinase p85 to IRS-1 was significantly decreased by 43% ($p<0.01$), 16% ($p<0.05$) and 22% ($p<0.05$), respectively, compared with WT [13].

Insulin-stimulated phosphorylation of insulin receptor β subunit and IRS-1

Equal amounts of total cell protein were subjected to immunoblot analysis using antiphosphotyrosine antibody. Upon insulin stimulation, the insulin receptor β subunit was phosphorylated in all cell lines, which was almost equal in each cell. G971R showed almost the same phosphorylation as WT IRS-1. However, phosphorylation in P170R and M209T was reduced by 37% ($p<0.05$) and 42% ($p<0.05$), respectively, when compared with WT [13].

Binding of IRS-1 to the insulin receptor

Equal amounts of total protein were immunoprecipitated with the anti-insulin receptor β subunit antibody, subjected to SDS-PAGE followed by immunoblotting with anti-IRS-1 antibody. In cells expressing G971R, binding of IRS-1 to the insulin receptor was almost equal to that observed in cells expressing WT. In cells expressing P170R and M209T, binding was significantly decreased by 48% ($p<0.01$) and 53% ($p<0.01$), respectively, when compared with WT [13].

Discussion

By the analysis of IRS-1 knockout mice, we and others have confirmed that IRS-1 played a significant role in insulin-stimulated glucose uptake, suggesting the

IRS-1 gene may be involved in the development of NIDDM [6,7]. Since 1993, several groups have reported IRS-1 gene polymorphisms in patients with NIDDM [8–10]. However, it is unclear whether these mutations in IRS-1 contribute to the development of NIDDM.

In this study, we screened the entire coding region of the IRS-1 gene in 47 NIDDM and 47 control subjects, and identified three novel mutations (P170R, M209T and S809F) and one reported (G971R) missense mutation [8]. The prevalence of the missense mutations (taken together) was significantly higher in NIDDM than in control, suggesting the possible contribution of these IRS-1 mutations to the development of NIDDM [12].

To further analyze the impact of IRS-1 mutations on the insulin signaling pathway, we expressed wild-type and three mutant (G971R, P170R and M209T) IRS-1s in suitable cells and analyzed their function (summarized in Table 1) [13].

According to the [^{3}H]thymidine incorporation assay, all the cell lines expressing mutant IRS-1s showed significant reduction in insulin-stimulated DNA synthesis, suggesting the presence of insulin resistance in the cells. However, the mechanism of impaired insulin signaling was different among the mutations. Cells expressing G971R showed a significant decrease both in MAP kinase and PI 3-kinase activities compared with WT, but the decrease in PI 3-kinase was greater than that in MAP kinase. This result paralleled the reduced binding of G971R with PI 3-kinase p85. Since Gly^{971} is located between two potential PI 3-kinase p85 binding sites, Y^{939}MKM and Y^{987}MTM, the substitution of Gly^{971} for Arg could result in a conformational change in these binding sites and may impair the association of IRS-1 with PI 3-kinase p85. These results are in accordance with the previous study of G971R mutation [14]. Cells expressing P170R and M209T also showed decreases both in MAP kinase and PI 3-kinase activities, however, the decrease in MAP kinase was greater than that in PI 3-kinase. This was due to the decreased binding of these mutant IRS-1s to the insulin receptor and decreased tyrosine phosphorylation of IRS-1. Pro^{170} and Met^{209} are located in the PTB domain of IRS-1, and the substitutions of Pro to Arg and Met to Thr could result in diminished binding of IRS-1 to the insulin receptor due to structural changes in the PTB domain of the IRS-1 protein [4]. Interestingly, both Pro^{170} and Met^{209} are conserved in every reported IRS-1s

Table 1. Comparison of insulin-stimulated activities in cells expressing mutant IRS-1s.

	Binding to insulin receptor	IRS-1 phosphorylation	Binding to p85	PI-3 kinase activity	MAP kinase activity	DNA synthesis
P170R	↓↓	↓↓	↓	↓	↓↓	↓ ~ ↓↓
M209T	↓↓	↓↓	↓	↓	↓↓	↓↓
G971R	→	→	↓↓	↓↓	↓	↓↓

Results are compared with WT, using Student's t test [→: no change, ↓: significant reduction ($<30\%$), ↓↓: significant reduction ($>30\%$) compared with insulin-stimulated WT].

[2,11,15] and are located at very important sites in the PTB domain. Met^{209} is located on the helical turn which connects with β4 and β5 and forms a binding site for a phosphotyrosine residue [4]. This amino acid substitution could, therefore, impair binding of IRS-1 to the NPXY motif of the insulin receptor. Pro^{170} is located on the "cap" which forms the bottom of β sheets, and it may play an important role in preserving the higher structure of the IRS-1 PTB domain [4]. These two amino acid substitutions could therefore result in conformational change of the IRS-1 PTB domain and impair its function at the level of binding to the insulin receptor, resulting in decreased phosphorylation of IRS-1. This decrease in phosphorylation of IRS-1 could lead to reduced binding sites for SH2 proteins such as GRB2, SHP-2, and PI 3-kinase, resulting in decreased MAP kinase and PI 3-kinase activities.

These results suggest that the two groups of mutant IRS-1(s), one in the PTB domain and one near the SH2 protein binding sites, have impaired insulin responses at different steps of the insulin signaling pathway. Therefore, the mutations of IRS-1 gene may cause insulin resistance in humans and contribute in part to the development of NIDDM.

Acknowledgements

The authors are grateful to Dr C. Ronald Kahn (Research Division, Joslin Diabetes Center, Department of Medicine, Brigham and Women's Hospital, and Harvard Medical School) for 32D-IR cells and helpful support. This work was supported in part by a grant from Otsuka Pharmaceutical Co. Ltd. for diabetes research and a grant for scientific research from the Ministry of Education, Science and Culture of Japan (No. 086807479).

References

1. Kahn CR. Banting lecture. Insulin action, diabetogenes, and the cause of type II diabetes. Diabetes 1995;43:1066–1084.
2. Sun XJ, Rothenberg PL, Kahn CR, Backer JM, Araki E, Wilden P, Cahill DA, Goldstin BJ, White MF. Structure of the insulin receptor substrate IRS-1 defines a unique signal transduction protein. Nature (Lond) 1991;352:73–77.
3. White MF. The insulin signalling system and the IRS proteins. Diabetologia 1997;40:S2–S17.
4. Eck MJ, Dhe-Paganon S, Trub T, Nolte RT, Shoelson ST. Structure of the IRS-1 PTB domain bound to the juxtamembrane region of the insulin receptor. Cell 1996;85:695–795.
5. Sun XJ, Crimmins DL, Myers MG Jr, Miralpeix M, White MF. Pleiotropic insulin signals are engaged by multisite phosphorylation of IRS-1. Molec Cell Biol 1993;13:7418–7428.
6. Araki E, Lipes MA, Patti ME, Bruening JC, Haag B III, Johnson RS, Kahn CR. Alternative pathway of insulin signaling in mice with targeted disruption of the IRS-1 gene. Nature (Lond) 1994;372:186–190.
7. Tamemoto H, Kadowaki T, Tobe K, Yagi T, Sakura H, Hayakawa T, Terauchi Y, Ueki K, Kaburagi Y, Satoh S. Insulin resistance and growth retardation in mice lacking insulin receptor substrate-1. Nature (Lond) 1994;372:182–186.
8. Almind K, Bjobaek C, Vestergaard H, Hansen T, Echwald S, Pedersen O. Amino acid poly-

morphisms of insulin receptor substrate-1 in non-insulin-dependent diabetes mellitus. Lancet 1993;342:828–832.

9. Laakso M, Malkki M, Kekalainen P, Kuusisto J, Deeb SS. Insulin receptor substrate-1 polymorphisms in non-insulin-dependent diabetes. J Clin Invest 1994;94:1141–1146.
10. Hitman GA, Hawrami K, McCarthy MI, Viswanathan M, Snehalatha C, Ramachandran A, Tuomilehto J, Tuomilehto-Wolf E, Nissinen A, Pedersen O. Insulin receptor substrate-1 gene mutations in NIDDM: implications for the study of polygenic disease. Diabetologia 1995; 38:481–486.
11. Araki E, Sun XJ, Haag BL, Chuang LM, Zhang Y, Yang-Feng TL, White MF, Kahn CR. Human skeletal muscle insulin receptor substrate-1: characterization of the cDNA, gene, and chromosomal localization. Diabetes 1993;42:1041–1054.
12. Ura S, Araki E, Kishikawa H, Shirotani T, Todaka M, Isami S, Shimoda S, Yoshimura R, Matsuda K, Motoyoshi S, Miyamura N, Kahn CR, Shichiri M. Molecular scanning of the IRS-1 gene in Japanese patients with non-insulin-dependent diabetes mellitus: identification of five novel mutations in IRS-1 gene. Diabetologia 1996;39:600–608.
13. Yoshimura R, Araki E, Ura S, Todaka M, Tsuruzoe K, Furukawa N, Motoshima H, Yoshizato K, Kaneko K, Matsuda K, Kishikawa H, Shichiri M. Impact of natural IRS-1 mutations on insulin signals; mutations of IRS-1 in the PTB domain and near SH2 protein binding sites results in impaired function at different steps of IRS-1 signaling. Diabetes 1997;46:929–936.
14. Almind K, Inoue G, Pedersen O, Kahn CR. A common amino acid polymorphism in insulin receptor substrate-1 causes impaired insulin signaling. J Clin Invest 1996;97:2569–2575.
15. Araki E, Haag BL III, Kahn CR. Cloning of the mouse insulin receptor substrate-1(IRS-1) gene and complete sequence of mouse IRS-1. Biochem Biophys Acta 1994;1221:353–356.

Recent Advances on the Pathogenesis and Management of Diabetes Mellitus.
S.H. Shinn, M. Shichiri and K.-W. Kim, editors.

Cytokine and autoimmune diabetes

Myung-Shik Lee[1] and Nora Sarvetnick[2]
[1]*Department of Medicine, Samsung Medical Center, Seoul, Korea; and* [2]*Department of Immunology, The Scripps Research Institute, La Jolla, California, USA*

Abstract. *Background.* Immunomodulation by localized expression of cytokines in pancreatic β-cells would be possible because even small changes in the autoimmune process could abrogate the disease phenotype.

Methods. Human insulin promoter was used to direct selective expression in pancreatic β-islet cells.

Results. Pancreatic IFN-γ led to specific sensitization to islet-specific antigens. Pancreatic IL-10 was sufficient and necessary for autoimmune diabetes in conjunction with NOD MHC homozygosity. Pancreatic IL-4 abrogated insulitis and autoimmune diabetes in NOD mice.

Conclusions. Modulation of (auto)immune response by localized expression of cytokines could be a useful therapeutic strategy in the clinical point of view in that it does not cause systemic toxicity.

Keywords: immunomodulation, pancreatic islets, transgenic mouse.

Introduction

The regulation of autoimmune diabetes by localized expression of cytokines in the pancreatic islets has been studied. Sensitization to self-antigens is genetically determined and environmentally modified. Theoretically, the site of initial sensitization appears to be lymphoid tissue where the chance of an encounter between autoantigens and potentially autoreactive cells is high. However, local modulation of (auto)immune responses would play some kind of role in the final outcome of the autoimmune diseases because autoreactive lymphocytes would then have the chance to encounter huge amounts of autoantigens and secondary immune responses would probably occur in the local environment. Local modification of autoimmune responses is probably not able to change fundamental aspects of immune responses; however, even minor changes in autoimmune responses might have important clinical significance. Autoimmune diseases occur only if a substantial amount of tissue is destroyed, and are different from autoimmunity in the immunological sense alone. For example, diabetes occurs only when more than 80–90% of pancreatic β-islet cells are destroyed. A reduction of pancreatic islet death from 80 to 70% might inhibit development of diabetes, although it does not change the basic nature of the autoimmune processes. These special

Address for correspondence: Myung-Shik Lee, Division of Endocrinology and Metabolism, Department of Medicine, Samsung Medical Center, Seoul 135-230, Korea.

aspects of autoimmune diseases are the underlying background of our cytokine transgenic mouse studies.

Materials and Methods

Cytokines were expressed transgenically using a human insulin promoter to direct their selective expression in pancreatic β cells. As a immunostimulatory cytokine, interferon-gamma (IFN-γ) was expressed. "Immunoinhibitory" cytokines such as IL-4, IL-10 and TGF-β were also ectopically expressed.

Results

Diabetes was observed in IFN-γ transgenic mice (Ins-IFN-γ) and apparent sensitization of islet tissue was noticed. Further, specific sensitization to well-characterized islet antigens was demonstrated in double-transgenic mice expressing both IFN-γ and a known viral antigen (lymphocytic choriomeningitis virus antigens), although the mechanism of antiself (virus) sensitization in them is not clearly understood [1]. Unexpectedly, differentiation of ductal cells into islet cells was observed in Ins-IFN-γ mice [2]. Ins-IL-10 mice showed peri-insulitis but no diabetes. Pancreatic expression of IL-10 did not inhibit allograft rejection or autoimmune diabetes after virus infection occurring as a result of cross-reactivity [3]. Contrary to expectations, pancreatic IL-10 expression accelerated diabetes in NOD backcross experiments [4]. Actually, it was not a simple acceleration. Pancreatic IL-10 overcame the absence of all non-MHC Idd alleles described in NOD mice. Anti-IL-10 antibody administration also inhibited development of insulitis in NOD mice almost completely [4].

TGF-β expression in pancreatic islets cells resulted in fibrosis mostly in the exocrine pancreas but did not induce islet destruction or diabetes [5]. It also did not inhibit allograft rejection or autoimmune diabetes after virus infection [6]. On the other hand, pancreatic expression of IL-4 inhibited insulitis and diabetes in NOD mice almost completely. Only peri-insulitis was observed in the pancreas of NOD-IL-4 mice [7]. Islet isograft from NOD mice to NOD-IL-4 mice did not have mononuclear cell infiltration and was functionally intact for more than 4 weeks after transplantation.

Discussion

These results suggest that IL-10 might be necessary and sufficient for autoimmune diabetes in conjunction with NOD MHC homozygosity. Immunological mechanisms of acceleration or induction of autoimmunity by IL-10 is being investigated. Our preliminary data suggest that IL-10 might be related to "epitope spreading" mediated by B lymphocytes. In contrast to IL-10, pancreatic IL-4 appears to help establish "functional tolerance" to islet antigens in NOD mice [6]. IL-4 might downregulate a TC1 response by preventing their proliferation in situ, thus resulting in the abrogation of their cytotoxic activity and blockade of the disease development at the peri-insulitis stage.

Together, the above results suggest that modulation of an (auto)immune response by localized expression of cytokines is possible and might be a useful therapeutic strategy in the clinical point of view in that it does not cause systemic toxicity. Also, they suggest that the "initial" sensitization event alone is not sufficient for the development of clinical autoimmune diseases and amplifying steps are also necessary that could be regulated by cytokines in the local environmental milieu. This approach-modulation of autoimmune responses by localized cytokine production will not only serve as a powerful tool for the treatment of clinical diseases but will give clues to the understanding of complex immunogenetic processes leading to autoimmune disorders.

References

1. Lee M-S, von Herrath M, Reiser H, Oldstone MBA, Sarvetnick N. Sensitization to self (virus) antigen by in situ expression of murine interferon-γ. J Clin Invest 1995;95:486–492.
2. Gu D, Lee M-S, Krahl T, Sarvetnick N. Transitional cells in the regenerating pancreas. Development 1994;120:1873–1881.
3. Lee M-S, Wogensen L, Shizuru J, Oldstone MBA, Sarvetnick N. Pancreatic islet production of murine interleukin-10 does not inhibit immune-mediated tissue destruction. J Clin Invest 1994;93:1332–1338.
4. Lee M-S, Peterson L, Wicker L, Sarvetnick N. IL-10 is necessary, and sufficient for autoimmune diabetes in the presence of NOD MHC homozygosity. J Exp Med 1996;183:2663–2668.
5. Lee M-S, Gu D, Feng L, Curriden S, Arnush M, Krahl T, Gurushanthaiah D, Wilson CB, Loskutoff DL, Fox H, Sarvetnick N. Accumulation of extracellular matrix and developmental regulation in the pancreas by transgenic expression of TGF-β1. Am J Pathol 1995;147:42–52.
6. Lee M-S, Sawyer S, Arnush M, Krahl T, von Herrath M, Oldstone MBA, Sarvetnick N. TGF-β fails to inhibit allograft rejection or virus-induce autoimmune diabetes in transgenic mice. Transplantation 1996;61:1112–1125.
7. Mueller R, Krahl T, Sarvetnick N. Pancreatic expression of interleukin-4 abrogates insulitis and autoimmune diabetes in nonobese diabetic (NOD) mice. J Exp Med 1996;184:1093–1099.

New therapeutic approaches in diabetes mellitus

Recent Advances on the Pathogenesis and Management of Diabetes Mellitus.
S.H. Shinn, M. Shichiri and K.-W. Kim, editors.

The efficacy of metformin monotherapy in patients with NIDDM in Korea

Yu Bae Ahn and Ho Young Son
Department of Internal Medicine, Catholic University Medical College, Seoul, Korea

Introduction

In the treatment of non-insulin-dependent diabetes mellitus (NIDDM), sulfonylureas have long been used in Korea. Sulfonylureas reduce hyperglycemia by enhancing insulin secretion and hence may promote hyperinsulinemia, being overweight, and hypoglycemia [1–3]. Metformin is readily distinguished from sulfonylurea. In addition to countering hyperglycemia without weight gain, metformin improves insulin sensitivity and thus decreases the insulin resistance that is prevalent in NIDDM [4]. It is also known that these actions of metformin are not effective in the absence of insulin, so metformin offers potential advantages for obese NIDDM patients with hyperinsulinemia [5]. But the clinical characteristics of Korean NIDDM patients may be different from those of Western countries. The obese form of NIDDM is by far the most common, accounting for the majority of cases in Caucasoids [6]. Several studies showed that the proportion of nonobese form of non-insulin-dependent diabetes mellitus is about up to 80% in Korea. Most patients with NIDDM in Korea are nonobese and insulin secretory capacity was found to be much lower for a given blood glucose level when compared to Caucasian subjects [7].

In these studies, we evaluated: 1) insulin response to oral glucose load; 2) insulin secretion and insulin sensitivity using minimal model analysis in NIDDM subjects; and 3) the efficacy of metformin monotherapy in Korean NIDDM patients.

Insulin response to oral glucose load in NIDDM and impaired glucose tolerance

For this study the insulin response to oral glucose load in a total of 450 subjects (male, n = 222; female, n = 228; mean age, 46.6 years) was studied. The studied subjects were divided into three groups: normal glucose tolerance (NGT, n = 119), impaired glucose tolerance (IGT, n = 118), and diabetes mellitus (n = 213), according to the results of the oral glucose tolerance test (OGTT) using a glucose dose of 75 g. In addition, subjects were then subdivided into two subgroups, obese and nonobese, according to their BMI values at examination. A BMI value of 25 kg/m^2 was defined as obese. With the data of OGTT, the area under the curve of glucose, insulin, and insulin/glucose ratio was calculated. Areas under the curve of glucose and insulin in nonobese diabetic subjects were also significantly lower than those values in obese diabetic subjects. Areas under the curve of insulin and the insulin/glucose ratio in diabetic subjects were significantly lower than those values in NGT and IGT subjects. These results illustrate that there is no evidence of increment of insulin secretion as an increasing area of glucose in nonobese IGT subjects, and subsequently declined in diabetic subjects. Accordingly, these data suggest that impairment of insulin secretion may play an important pathogenic role in nonobese IGT and NIDDM.

Minimal model analysis of insulin secretion and insulin sensitivity

In order to evaluate glucose tolerance in NIDDM, quantification of both insulin secretion and insulin action should be measured. Insulin secretion can be evaluated using glucose, glucagon, or arginine [8]. Also, insulin action can be assessed by using glucose clamp techniques. However, glucose clamp techniques have drawbacks that limit broad clinical application. Bergman developed the minimal model approach, based on analysis of a frequently sampled intravenous glucose tolerance test which can quantify both insulin secretion and insulin action [9–11]. In comparison to glucose clamp techniques [12,13], minimal model analysis is less labor intensive, and well correlated with the results of the glucose clamp technique during a single test. However, the clinical application of minimal model analysis has been limited by the need for endogenous insulin secretion [9]. Although it is known that administration of exogenous insulin permits minimal model analysis to be applied to diabetic as well as normal subjects, evaluating insulin secretion and insulin sensitivity [14]. In this study we evaluated insulin secretion and insulin sensitivity in Korean subjects with NIDDM using minimal model analysis of an insulin-modified, frequently sampled, intravenous glucose tolerance test (FSIVGTT). Fifteen non-insulin-dependent diabetic treated subjects (six male, nine female) with a mean age of 48 years old were studied; and 10 normal subjects were randomly recruited from medical staffs, nurses and sisters. Each subject underwent an FSIVGTT after overnight fasting. After baseline blood sampling for insulin and glucose, 300 mg/kg of glucose was injected over 2 min and subsequent blood was sampled. After 20 min a bolus of insulin (0.05 U/kg in diabetic subjects, 0.03 U/kg in normal subjects) was injected. Insulin sensitivity index and glucose effectiveness were determined by the MINMOD computer program (R.N. Bergman©). The insulin sensitivity index represents the increase in the net fractional glucose clearance rate per unit change in plasma insulin concentration after the intravenous glucose load. The glucose effectiveness represents the fractional glucose clearance rate due simply to the increase in glucose itself in the absence of any increase in serum insulin concentration above baseline. The results of this study show that the mean basal glucose levels in diabetic subjects were higher than the values in normal subjects (116.7 ± 4.8 mg/dl vs. 87.6 ± 2.0 mg/dl) (Table 1). But mean basal glucose levels in diabetic subjects

Table 1. Plasma glucose and insulin response to FSIVGTT in normal subjects.

Subjects	Fasting		Peak before insulin		K_G (%/min)	Insulin area (uU/ ml/min)	SI ($\times 10^4$)	SG ($\times 10^2$)
	Glucose (mg/dl)	Insulin (uU/m)	Glucose (mg/dl)	Insulin (uU/m)				
1	85	2.6	258	25.6	0.194	525.9	8.84	4.75
2	97	3.7	330	27.5	0.532	327.4	2.43	1.87
3	81	1.0	393	60.3	1.582	401.4	9.21	6.43
4	85	1.6	231	20.7	1.170	275.2	12.05	5.63
5	87	1.9	229	39.6	0.103	277.1	5.07	3.60
6	84	4.8	269	75.7	0.970	894.3	2.59	4.37
7	90	5.2	281	60.5	0.914	525.9	5.02	4.49
8	100	7.9	293	87.9	1.704	999.7	14.01	6.00
9	81	6.7	253	24.6	0.132	331.7	3.57	3.36
10	86	19.8	295	181.0	1.026	1969.6	2.34	4.00
Mean	116.7	5.9	364.5	16.8	0.519	239.0	1.66	1.97
SE	4.8	0.8	29.2	3.7	0.063	38.8	0.24	0.19

Note: K_G = Glucose disappearance rate. SI = Insulin sensitivity index. SG = Glucose effectiveness.

were all below 140 mg/dl except in two cases. This means that effects of glucose toxicity on insulin secretion and insulin action can be excluded.

During insulin-modified FSIVGTT, after glucose injection, mean peak serum glucose levels were higher in diabetic subjects than in normal subjects (364.5 ± 29.2 mg/dl vs. 283.2 ± 15.6 mg/dl). But mean peak insulin levels and mean values of area under the curve of insulin were significantly lower in diabetic subjects than those values in normal subjects (16.8 ± 3.7 uU/ml vs. 60.31 ± 5.3 uU/ml; 239.0 ± 38.8 uU/ml/min vs. 652.8 ± 166.7 uU/ml/min). A blunted first phase of insulin secretion was also observed in diabetic subjects. Glucose effectiveness was also lower in diabetic subjects ($1.97 \pm 0.19 \times 10^2$ vs. $4.45 \pm 0.24 \times 10^2$). After insulin injection, the calculated glucose disappearance rate and insulin sensitivity index were significantly lower in diabetic subjects compared to normal subjects (0.519 ± 0.063%/min vs. 0.833 ± 0.18%/min; $1.66 \pm 0.24 \times 10^4$ vs. $6.51 \pm 1.34 \times 10^4$) (Tables 1 and 2).

The effect of metformin on glycemia and insulin secretion

To investigate the effect of metformin on glycemia, insulin secretion and body weight in patients with NIDDM who could not achieve satisfactory glycemic control by sulfonylurea or diet therapy, the following studies were carried out. A total of 142 patients with NIDDM (60 male, 82 female; mean age, 48.4 years) were included in this study. By measuring the value of fasting blood sugar (FBS) and HbA1c in patients after 3 months of metformin treatment, the response to treatment could be determined. FBS, anthropometric changes and the 75-g OGTT were re-evaluated in the responder group after 6 months of metformin treatment. The overall response rate in the study population was 55.6% (79/

Table 2. Plasma glucose and insulin response to FSIVGTT in diabetic subjects.

Subjects	Fasting		Peak before insulin		K_G (%/min)	Insulin area (uU/ml/min)	SI ($\times 10^4$)	SG ($\times 10^2$)
	Glucose (mg/dl)	Insulin (uU/m)	Glucose (mg/dl)	Insulin (uU/m)				
1	116	1.0	294	3.3	0.270	71.3	1.77	0.89
2	156	7.5	323	10.0	0.427	243.1	1.26	2.62
3	151	4.0	328	9.6	0.608	122.2	0.88	1.50
4	98	0.6	337	9.6	0.215	211.1	2.56	1.26
5	91	3.9	698	6.4	0.860	108.3	3.04	2.63
6	120	0.1	265	49.4	0.553	174.1	1.12	3.18
7	106	6.4	476	10.0	0.766	198.9	3.82	2.55
8	97	5.4	487	14.5	0.449	194.5	0.40	1.57
9	100	10.3	309	44.9	0.360	583.9	0.59	1.44
10	135	6.3	378	14.2	0.444	167.7	2.05	2.05
11	116	9.2	380	36.7	0.462	577.1	1.41	1.59
12	112	5.7	303	14.9	1.110	229.7	2.22	2.25
13	122	7.5	298	15.9	0.644	300.5	0.90	3.07
14	112	10.1	275	10.6	0.195	242.6	1.43	1.07
15	118	6.7	316	8.4	0.482	159.8	1.39	1.81
Mean	116.7	5.9	364.5	16.8	0.519	239.0	1.66	1.97
SE	4.8	0.8	29.2	3.7	0.063	38.8	0.24	0.19

142). FBS and duration of diabetes played an independent role for predicting the outcome of treatment (O.R.= 4.2, 1.4). There were significant changes in body weight (64.4 ± 8.2 vs. 62.9 ± 8.4, $p < 0.01$) and body mass index (25.3 ± 2.3 vs. 24.6 ± 2.3, $p = 0.01$). The value of FBS in the responder group was reduced from 182.6 ± 51.3 mg/dl to 138.8 ± 29.8 mg/dl, but there were no significant changes in fasting insulin concentration and lipid levels (Table 3). The level of

Table 3. Changes in fasting insulin, body weight, lipid levels and blood pressure before and after 6 months of metformin treatment.

Item	Before	After	p value
Body mass index (kg/m^2)	25.3 ± 2.3	24.6 ± 2.3	<0.01
Weight (kg)	64.4 ± 8.2	62.9 ± 8.4	<0.01
Waist hip ratio	0.93 ± 0.06	0.93 ± 0.05	ns
Glucose (mmol/l)			
Fasting	10.1 ± 2.8	7.9 ± 1.6	<0.01
Postprandial 2 h	15.2 ± 5.0	12.2 ± 3.9	<0.01
Fasting insulin (pmol/l)	43.2 ± 27.6	36.6 ± 21.6	ns
Total cholesterol (mmol/l)	5.21 ± 1.62	4.67 ± 3.50	ns
Triglyceride (mmol/l)	2.12 ± 0.35	1.76 ± 0.82	ns
HDL cholesterol (mmol/l)	1.17 ± 0.31	1.21 ± 0.36	ns
Systolic blood pressure (mmHg)	131.7 ± 22.2	127.5 ± 32.1	ns
Diastolic blood pressure (mmHg)	92.7 ± 12.5	79.48 ± 12.2	ns

Note: values represent mean ± SD. ns = not significant.

area under the glucose concentration during follow-up OGTT was decreased significantly (1066.4 ± 278.9 vs 890.3 ± 169.7 mg/dl/min, $p<0.01$), but there were no significant changes in the level of area under the insulin concentration (93.4 ± 82.6 vs. 89.4 ± 62.4 uU/l/min, p = 0.624) (Fig. 1). The results of decrement in glucose area without significant changes of insulin area after OGTT were consistent with earlier studies [15]. The reduction of fasting blood sugar without fasting insulin may be explained by the decrement of hepatic glucose overproduction.

Summary

1. Most Korean NIDDM patients are nonobese and insulin deficiency rather than insulin resistance might be the major determinant in the pathogenesis of NIDDM.
2. The overall response rate to metformin monotherapy was 55.6% (79/142) in the study population.
3. There were significant changes in body weight (64.4 ± 8.2 vs. 62.9 ± 8.4 kg, $p<0.01$) and BMI (25.3 ± 2.3 kg/m^2 vs. 24.6 ± 2.3, $p<0.01$).
4. The FBS was decreased significantly without changes of fasting insulin concentration.
5. The level of FBS and duration of diabetes played an independent role in predicting the response to metformin monotherapy.

Conclusion

In view of the fact that metformin is useful in the treatment of Korean NIDDM patients, most of whom are nonobese and in the state of insulin deficiency when

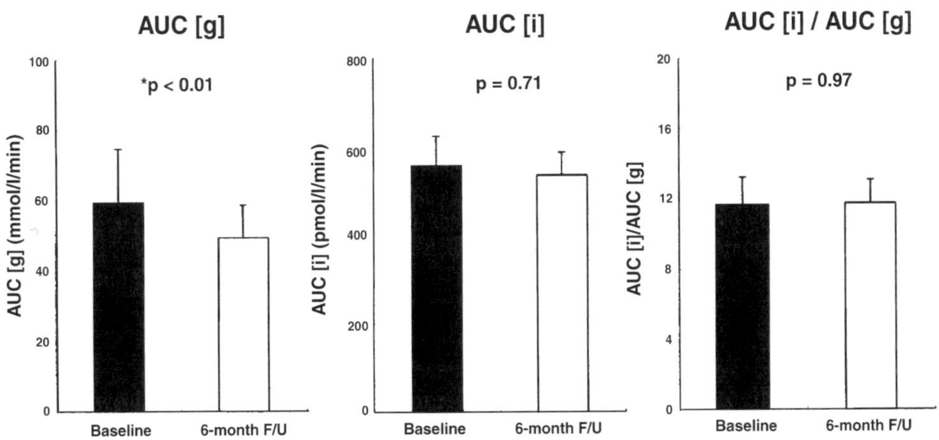

Fig. 1. The changes of glucose area under the curve (AUC[g]), insulin area under the curve (AUC[i]) and AUC[i]/AUC[g] levels in the responder group after metformin treatment. Values are mean ± SD for AUC[g], mean ± SE for AUC[i] and AUC[i]/AUC[g].

compared to Western diabetics, the main effects of metformin on glucose metabolism may be related to decreased hepatic glucose production.

References

1. Groop LC. Sulfonylurea in NIDDM. Diabet Care 1992;15:737–754.
2. Hosker JP, Burnett MA, Davies EG, Haris EA, Turner RC. Sulfonylurea therapy doubles cell response to glucose in type 2 diabetic patients. Diabetologia 1985;28:809–814.
3. Rains SGH, Wilson GA, Richmond W, Elkeles RS. The effect of glibenclamide and metformin on serum lipiprotein in type 2 diabetes. Diabetic Med 1988;5:653–658.
4. Bailey CJ. Biguanide and NIDDM. Diabet Care 1992;15:755–772.
5. Alberti KGMM, Gries FA. Management of non-insulin-dependent diabetes mellitus in Europe: a consensus view. Diabetic Med 1988;5:275–281.
6. Zimmet PZ. The pathogensis and prevention of diabetes in adults. Diabet Care 1995;18: 1050–1064.
7. Park YS, Yoo KY, Lee HG, Kim YK, Koh CS, Shin YS, Min HK. Prevalence of diabetes and IGT in Yonchon Country, South Korea. Diabet Care 1995;18:545–548.
8. Pfeifer MS, Holter JB, Porte D. Insulin secretion in diabetes mellitus. Am J Med 1981;70: 579–588.
9. Pacini G, Finegood DT, Bergman RN. A minimal model based glucose clamp yielding insulin sensitivity independent of glycemia. Diabetes 1982;31:432–441.
10. Bergman RN, Finegood DT, Ader M. Assessment of insulin sensitivity in vivo. Endocrine Rev 1985;6:45–86.
11. Bergman RN, Beard JC, Chen M. The minimal modelling method: assessment of insulin sensitivity and B-cell function in vivo. In: Clarke WL, Larner J, Pohl SL (eds) Methods in Diabetes Research. New York: Wiley and Sons Press, 1986.
12. Andres R, Swerloff R, Pozefsky T, Coleman D. Manual feedback technique for the control of blood glucose concentration. In: Skeggs JR (ed) Automation in Analytical Chemistry. New York: Mediad Press, 1966.
13. Insel PA, Liljenquest JE, Tobin JD. Insulin control of glucose metabolism in man: A new kinetic approach. J Clin Invest 1975;55:1057–1066.
14. Finegood DT, Hramiak IM, Dupre J. A modified protocol for estimation of insulin sensitivity with the minimal model of glucose kinetics in patients with insulin-dependent diabetes. J Clin Endocrinol Metab 1990:70:1538–1549.
15. Defronzo RA, Goodman AM, and The Multicenter Metformin Study Group. Efficacy of metformin in patients with non-insulin-dependent diabetes mellitus. N Engl J Med 1995;333: 541–549.

Recent Advances on the Pathogenesis and Management of Diabetes Mellitus.
S.H. Shinn, M. Shichiri and K.-W. Kim, editors.

Aldose reductase inhibitor and its therapeutic potential in diabetic complications

Nigishi Hotta, Naoki Koh, Jiro Nakamura, Yoji Hamada and Fumihiko Sakakibara
Third Department of Internal Medicine, Nagoya University School of Medicine, Japan

Abstract. Preventive or therapeutic approaches for diabetic complications based on the polyol pathway theory have been focused on the development of potential aldose reductase (AR) inhibitors although the exact mechanism is unknown. From the results obtained in animal models of diabetic complications, it is well-recognized at present that AR inhibitors have a positive inhibitory effect on neuropathy, retinopathy, cataract formation, keratopathy and possibly on infection and atherosclerosis.

However, clinically, there has been a massive concentration of effort on diabetic neuropathy, not all of the assessed studies support the polyol pathway theory. Among AR inhibitors, epalrestat was launched as a drug against diabetic neuropathy on the Japanese market in 1992. Other AR inhibitors, FK-366, SNK-860 and NZ-314 are under the clinical trial stage in Japan.

It is now clear that AR inhibitors may offer various benefits to patients with diabetic complications. However, more extensive efforts are needed for the evaluation of their effects.

Keywords: atherosclerosis, diabetic neuropathy, epalrestat, glycation, infection, polyol pathway.

Introduction

The etiology of late-onset diabetic complications is not yet clear but is probably multifactorial, and related to the quality of glycemic control [1] and genetic factors. Several general theories have emerged, each based on the premise that either hyperglycemia or some related metabolic abnormalities are the primary events which trigger tissue damage and result in the development of diabetic complications (Fig. 1). The polyol pathway is one of the possible biochemical mechanisms through which hyperglycemia can impair the function and structure of cells affected by diabetic complications [2–12].

If hyperglycemia-induced polyol pathway hyperactivity has an important role in the etiology of late-onset diabetic complications, the inhibition of aldose reductase (AR), a rate-limiting enzyme of the pathway, could become a key element in the prevention and reversal of diabetic complications [2,10–12].

Address for correspondence: Nigishi Hotta MD, Third Department of Internal Medicine, Nagoya University School of Medicine, 65 Tsuruma-cho, Showa-ku, Nagoya 466, Japan. Tel.: +81-52-741-2181. Fax: +81-52-744-2213.

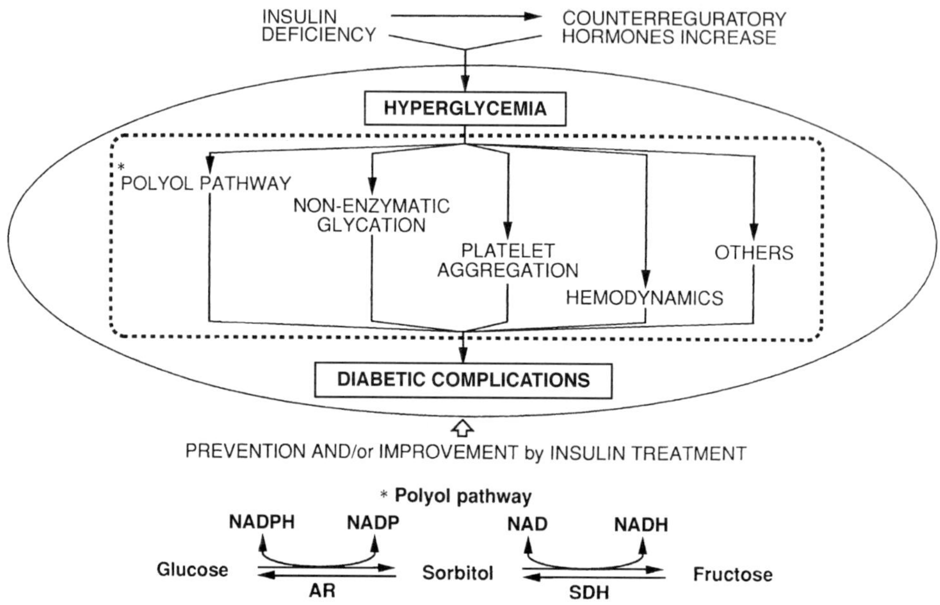

Fig. 1. Main hypotheses of pathogenesis on diabetic complications and its prevention and/or improvement by insulin treatment.

Polyol pathway and aldose reductase inhibitors

The polyol pathway

The polyol pathway consists of two steps: nonphosphorylated glucose is first reduced to sorbitol by the enzyme, aldose reductase (AR) and the resulting sorbitol is then changed to fructose by sorbitol dehyrogenase (Fig. 1). The activity of this pathway in relation to glucose metabolism is only about 3% under normal conditions. However, this activity increases 2–4 times in a concentration-dependent manner as the ambient glucose concentration rises above physiological levels. Thus, in response to hyperglycemia, sorbitol accumulates in complication-prone tissues that have a high capacity for polyol pathway enzymes and in which glucose entry is not rate limiting for glycolysis or mediated by insulin.

AR has been found in a number of tissues, including those affected by diabetes such as the nerve, retina, kidney, aorta, lens and cornea [5]. However, the physiological role of this pathway has remained unclear since its discovery by Hers [13] in sheep seminal vesicles. Recent findings suggest that this pathway may have an important role in the regulatory system of osmolar changes between the intracellular and extracellular milieu [14,15]. A progressive rise in AR activity and synthesis of sorbitol (in amounts related to the magnitude of the change in extracellular osmolarity) was induced by exposing cells derived from rabbit renal medulla to raised extracellular sodium and chloride ions [15].

Aldose reductase inhibitors

Although the exact mechanism is unknown, AR appears to be the possible link between increased polyol pathway activity and the development of some diabetic complications. Therefore, in recent years, preventive or therapeutic approaches to diabetic complications based on the polyol pathway theory have focused on the development of potent AR inhibitors.

A large number of AR inhibitors have been generated and studied in experimental animal models, but only a limited number of the drugs have reached the clinical trial stage [7]. All of the compounds listed in Table 1 are now either available for clinical use (such as epalrestat for neuropathy) or in the clinical trial stage. However, AD-5467 and tolrestat were dropped due to minimal efficacy for neuropathy in diabetic patients. In addition to the AR inhibitors listed in Table 1, zopolrestat is now at the clinical trial stage in the USA [16]. The developed AR inhibitors can be roughly classified into four groups: carboxylic acids, flavonoids, hydantoins, and other compounds [7]. Among the AR inhibitors in Table 1, epalrestat, FK-366, AD-5467, tolrestat, TAT and NZ-314 belong to the

Table 1. Chemical structure and activity of aldose reductase inhibitors which have reached the clinical evaluation for "triopathy" complications (neuropathy, retinopathy and nephropathy) in Japan.

Name	Structure	Company	Inhibitory activity of ARI ($IC_{50} \times 10^{-6}$M)		Pharmacokinetics of ARI[a]	
			HPAR	RLAR	Tmax (h)	T 1/2 (h)
Epalrest (ONO-2235)	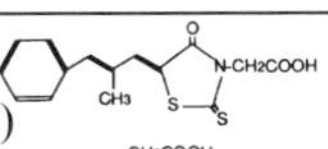	Ono	0.026	0.01	2	0.76
FK-366	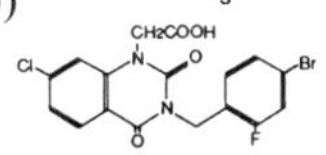	Fujisawa	—	0.044	0.9 ± 0.2	7.7 ± 0.5
AD-5467	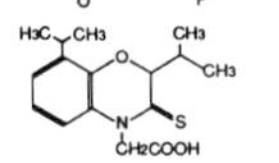	Takeda	0.051	0.129	1.3 ± 1.2	0.5–3.0
SNK-860	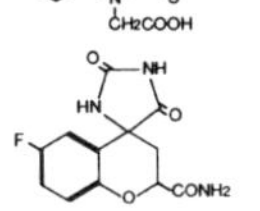	Sanwa		0.022	1.3	1.71
Tolrestat (AY-27773)	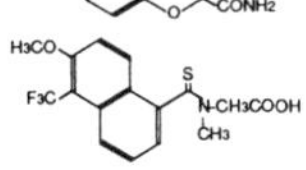	Ayerst		0.04	1.3 ± 0.1	9.2
TAT	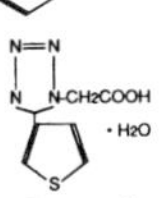	Wakamoto	0.028	0.021	1.0	1.49
NZ-314	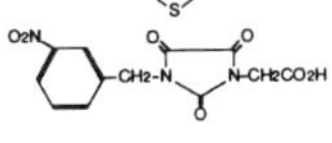	Nihonzoki		0.062	1.4 ± 0.6	1.8 ± 0.4

Note: HPAR = human placenta aldose reductase; RLAR = rat lens aldose reductase. [a]Single administration in healthy subjects: ONO-2235, AD-5467 → 200 mg p.o., FK-366 → 150 mg p.o., NZ-314 → 50 mg p.o., TAT → 20 mg p.o., SNK-860 → 15 mg p.o.

carboxylic acid group, as does zopolrestat. On the other hand, SNK-860 is classified into the hydantoin group. However, none of the flavonoid compounds has reached the clinical trial stage.

New insights of polyol pathway and its role in the pathogenesis of diabetic complications

Current concepts of the mechanisms involved in the development of polyol-pathway-associated diabetic complications

The polyol osmotic theory, alterations in myo-inositol and sodium metabolism, intermediary metabolites, abnormal changes of the redox state (NADH/NAD^+ ratio) and an abnormality of kinase C dependent protein phosphorylation have all been proposed as possible hypotheses for the pathogenesis of diabetic complications [2–9]. Williamson et al. [9] have proposed the role of hypoxia and hyperglycemia-induced pseudohypoxia, whereby an increase in NADH/NAD^+ and associated metabolic imbalances contribute to vascular changes. The proposal is attractive because the hyperglycemia-induced redox imbalance is largely the result of increased oxidation of sorbitol to fructose being coupled to the reduction of NAD^+ to NADH in the second step of the polyol pathway. It is suggested that hypoxia and hyperglycemia-induced pseudohypoxia may play an important role in the pathogenesis of diabetic complications. Recent findings in experimental models suggest that hyperglycemia-induced polyol pathway hyperactivity may play a role in the neurovascular dysfunction that is accompanied by impaired nerve conduction velocity [10,17,18]. In addition to metabolic factors, it is likely that vascular disorders caused by polyol pathway hyperactivity may contribute to the development of some complications of diabetes that involve nerves and the retina.

New insights of polyol pathway in the pathogenesis of diabetic complications

Recently, increasing evidence suggests that glycation [19,20] and oxidative stress [10,21] may have a cross-link with polyol pathway, contributing to the development of diabetic complications. In addition to this, it is an interesting possibility that increased synthesis of methylglyoxal modifying nucleic acid and protein [22] may be partially related to hyperglycemia-induced polyol pathway hyperactivity, resulting in diabetic complications (Fig. 2). More recently, Ishii et al. [23]. reported that the PKCβ inhibitor ameliorated the glomerular filtration rate, albumin excretion rate, and retinal circulation in diabetic rats in a dose-dependent manner, in parallel with its inhibition of PKC activity. The theory that hyperglycemia-induced PKC hyperactivity may contribute to the development of diabetic complications is attractive, but the relationship between polyol pathway hyperactivity and abnormal PKC activity remains partially unclear.

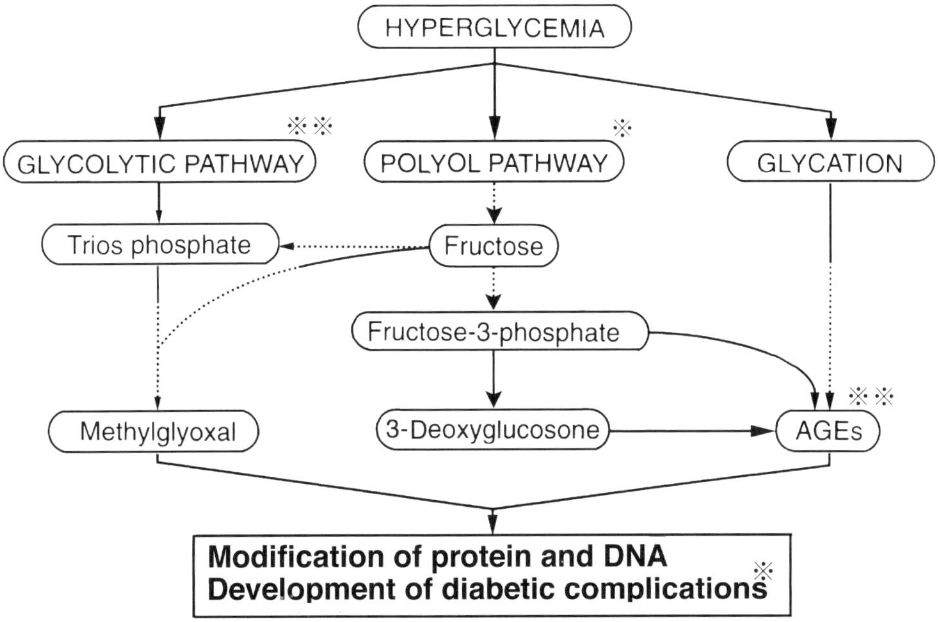

Fig. 2. Relationship between glycolytic pathway, polyol pathway and glycation in the development of diabetic complications.

Current and future therapeutic potential of AR inhibitors in diabetic complications

Current therapeutic potential of AR inhibitors

From the results obtained mainly in animal models of diabetic complications, it is well-recognized at present that AR inhibitors have a positive inhibitory effect on neuropathy, retinopathy, nephropathy, keratopathy, and cataract formation.

Although, clinically, there has been a massive concentration of efforts on diabetic neuropathy [5—7], not all of the assessed studies support the polyol pathway theory [5—7]. A double-blind study in patients with diabetic neuropathy by Sima et al. [24] gave exciting evidence of the efficacy of sorbinil, an aldose reductase inhibitor, against morphological signs of degeneration in sural nerve biopsies, accompanied by a decrease in the nerve sorbitol level and an increase in the nerve conduction velocity. A similar observation was reported by Greene et al. [25] using another aldose reductase inhibitor, FK-366 (zenarestat).

Since epalrestat was launched into the Japanese market in 1992, a clinical study for diabetic neuropathy has been started all over Japan to confirm the efficacy and safety of epalrestat in a large number of patients. In this study, 5,249 patients with diabetic neuropathy were treated with epalrestat for 3—12 months [26]. The improvement rates of subjective symptoms (i.e., spontaneous pain, numbness, coldness, and hypoesthesia) were 75% (slightly improved or better) and those of nerve function tests (i.e., motor nerve conduction velocity, sensory nerve conduction velocity, and vibration threshold) were 36%. Adverse drug reactions were encountered in 129 cases (2.5%) out of 5,249 patients (none of which were severe).

The possible mechanisms of AR inhibitors in diabetic neuropathy are summarized in Fig. 3.

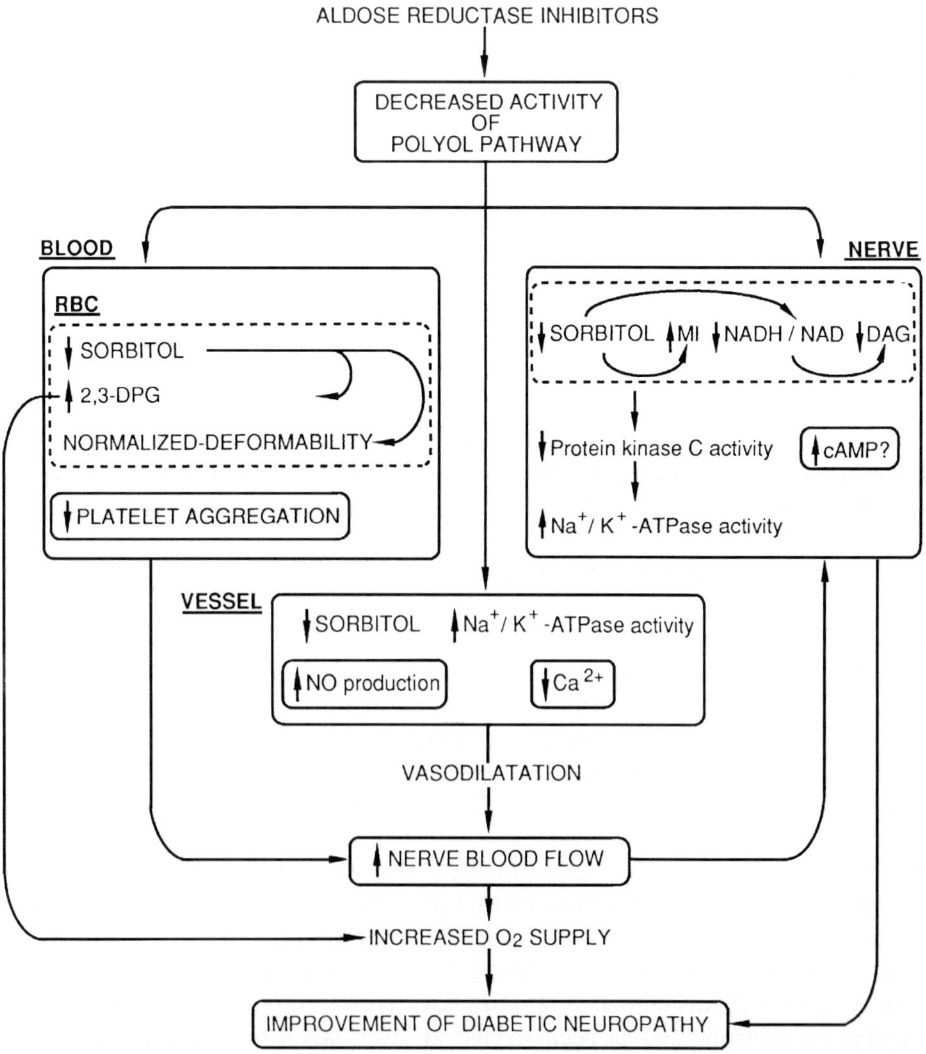

Fig. 3. Possible mechanisms of aldose reductase inhibitors in the improvement of diabetic neuropathy.

Future therapeutic possibility of AR inhibitors

It has been hypothesized that a reduction in Na^+/K^+-ATPase activity is the major pathogenic step in the development of hypertension [27]. This results in the accumulation of intracellular Na^+ and ultimately leads to significant increases in cytosolic-free Ca^{2+} concentrations $[Ca^{2+}]i$ in vascular smooth muscle cells. In diabetes, low Na^+/K^+ -ATPase activity in tissues is observed, which may be linked to the polyol pathway. Glucose-induced changes of sorbitol increasing, myo-inositol decreasing [28] and cytosolic-free Ca^{2+} increasing [29] were significantly prevented by epalrestat, using cultured rabbit aortic smooth muscle cells. It is suggested that this observation may be important for pathogenic factors in the development of hypertension and atherosclerosis in diabetes, and that AR inhibitors may be useful for their prevention. Its possibility may be supported by other findings that a strong cross-linking between polyol pathway and glycation is observed [19,20] and that an AR inhibitor can prevent the production of advanced glycation end products [20].

Diabetic patients have increased susceptibility to infection because of an impaired host defense mechanism. Although many factors may contribute to impaired host defense, in particular, the polymorphonuclear leukocyte (hereafter referred to as neutrophil) function plays an important role. Neutrophil function in well-controlled diabetic patients differs little from that in normal subjects [30], suggesting that dysfunction is in part related to poor metabolic control, induced by high glucose concentrations.

Wilson [31] reported that neutrophils have an active polyol pathway, which may be the cause of the decreased killing ability of neutrophils observed in diabetes. However, the mechanisms of altered cell function in diabetes are not fully understood. As bactericidal function is partially mediated by oxidative killing, the biochemical events necessary for causing the oxidative burst are those most susceptible to impaired glucose metabolism. These abnormalities may, therefore, be associated with the induction of the polyol pathway, which competes for supplies of nicotinamide adenine dinucleotide phosphate (NADPH). Boland et al. [32] demonstrated that the impaired killing of *Escherichia coli* in diabetic patients was improved by treatment with an AR inhibitor, ponalrestat. More recently, Kawamura et al. [33] measured lucigenin-enhanced chemiluminescence stimulated by phorbol myristate acetate as a function of neutrophils in high glucose concentration. The peak value of lucigenin-enhanced luminescence in human neutrophils was decreased by 86% by exposure to 40 mM glucose. This reduction was reversed by 91% with the addition of 10 μM SNK-860. In the in vivo study, using neutrophils from poorly controlled diabetic patients, epalrestat, an aldose reductase inhibitor, significantly improved the impaired *Cypridina* luciferin-analog-dependent chemiluminescence and L-dependent chemiluminescence in patients with diabetes mellitus [34]. The results obtained in human neutrophils suggest that in diabetic patients, the increase of the polyol pathway activity by high glucose concentrations may reduce the depletion of superoxide anion on the membrane of human neutrophils, resulting in the dysfunction of the oxidative killing. Therefore, it appears that AR inhibitors may also be capable of preventing the aggravation of various infections in diabetic patients.

Conclusion

It is now clear that AR inhibitors may offer various benefits to patients with diabetic complications. However, more extensive efforts are needed for the evaluation of their effects. Time will tell whether the hopes for these drugs are to be fulfilled.

References

1. The Diabetes Control and Complications Trial Research Group. The effect of intensive treatment of diabetes on the development and progression of long-term complications in insulin-dependent-diabetes mellitus. N Engl J Med 1993;329:977–986.
2. Gabbay KH. The sorbitol pathway and the complications of diabetes. N Engl J Med 1973;288:832–836.
3. Greene DA, Lattimer SA, Ulbrecht JS, Carroll P. Glucose-induced alterations in nerve metabolism: current perspective on the pathogenesis of diabetic neuropathy and future direction for research and therapy. Diabet Care 1985;8:290–299.
4. Kador PF, Kinoshita JH, Sharpless NE. Aldose reductase inhibitors: a potential new class of agents for the pharmacological control of certain diabetic complications. J Med Chem 1985; 28:841–849.
5. Dvornik D. Aldose Reductase Inhibition: An Approach to the Prevention of Diabetic Complications. New York: McGraw-Hill, 1987.
6. Sakamoto N, Kinoshita JH, Kador PF, Hotta N. Polyol Pathway and its Role in Diabetic Complications. Amsterdam: Excerpta Medica, 1988.
7. Hotta N, Sakamoto N. Aldose Reductase Inhibitors. In: Alberti KGMM, Krall LP (eds) The Diabetes Annual/5. Amsterdam: Elsevier Science Publishers BV, 1990;330–361.
8. Tomlinson DR. Aldose reductase inhibitors and the complications of diabetes mellitus. Diabet Med 1993;10:214–230.
9. Williamson JR, Chang K, Frangos M et al. Hyperglycemic pseudohypoxia and diabetic complications. Diabetes 1993;42:801–813.
10. Cameron NE, Cotter MA. The relationship of vascular changes to metabolic factors in diabetes mellitus and their role in the development of peripheral nerve complications. Diabet Metab Rev 1994;10:189–224.
11. Nathan DM. Long-term complications of diabetes mellitus. N Engl J Med 1993;328: 1676–1685.
12. Stevens MJ, Feldman EL, Greene DA. The aetiology of diabetic neuropathy: the combined roles of metabolic and vascular defects. Diabet Med 1995;12:566–579.
13. Hers HG. Le mechanisme de la transformation de glucose en fructose par les vesicules seminales. Biochim Biophys Acta 1956:22;202–203.
14. Bagnasco SM, Balaban R, Fales HM, Yang Y-M, Burg M. Predominant osmotically active solues in rat and rabbit renal medullas. J Biol Chem 1986;261:5872–5877.
15. Bagnasco SM, Murphy HR, Bedford JJ, Burg MB. Osmoregulation by slow changes in aldose reductase and rapid changes in sorbitol flux. Am J Physiol 1988;254:C788–C792.
16. Inskeep PB, Ronfeld RA, Peterson MJ, Gerber N. Pharmacokinetics of the aldose reductase inhibitor, zopolrestat, in humans. J Clin Pharm 1994;34:760–766.

17. Hotta N, Kakuta H, Fukasawa H et al. Effects of a potent new aldose reductase inhibitor, (5-(3-thienyl)tetrazol-1-yl) acetic acid (TAT), on diabetic neuropathy in rats. Diabet Res Clin Pact 1995;27:107–117.
18. Hotta N, Koh N, Sakakibara F et al. Effect of propionyl-L-carnitine on motor nerve conduction, autonomic cardiac function, and nerve blood flow in rats with streptozotocin-induced diabetes: comparison with an aldose reductase inhibitors. J Pharmacol Exp Ther 1996;276: 49–55.
19. Hamada Y, Araki N, Koh N, Nakamura J, Horiuchi S, Hotta N. Rapid formation of advanced glycation end products by intermediate metabolities of glycolytic pathway and polyol pathway. Biochem Biophys Res Commun 1996;228:539–543.
20. Hamada Y, Araki N, Horiuchi S, Hotta N. Role of polyol pathway in nonenzymatic glycation. Nephrol Dial Transplant 1996;11(Suppl 5):95–98.
21. Giugliano D, Paolisso G, Geriello A. Oxidative stress and diabetic vascular complications. Diabet Care 1996;19:257–267.
22. Thornalley PJ. Pharmacology of methylglyoxal: formation, modification of proteins and nucleic acids, and enzymatic detoxification: a role in pathogenesis and antiproliferative chemotherapy. Gen Pharmacol 1996;27:565–573.
23. Ishii H, Jirousek MR, Koya D et al. Amelioration of vascular dysfunctions in diabetic rats by an oral PKCß inhibitor. Science 1996;272:728–731.
24. Sima AAF, Bril V, Nathaniel V et al. Regeneration and repair of myelinated fibers in sural-nerve biopsy specimens from patients with diabetic neuropathy treated with sorbinil. N Engl J Med 1988;319:548–555.
25. Greene DA, Arrezo J, Brown M, the Zenarestat Study Group. Dose-related effects of the aldose reductase inhibitor Zenarestat on nerve sorbitol levels, nerve conduction velocity and nerve fiber density in human diabetic neuropathy. Diabetes 1996;45(Suppl 2):5A.
26. Hotta N, Sakamoto N, Shigeta Y, Kikkawa, R, Goto Y, Diabetic Neuropathy Study Group in Japan. Clinical investigation of epalrestat, an aldose reductase inhibitor, on diabetic neuropathy in Japan: multicenter study. J Diab Comp 1996;10:168–172.
27. Ohara T, Sussman KE, Draznin B. Effect of diabetes on cytosolic free Ca^{2+} and Na^{+}/K^{+}-ATPase in rat aorta. Diabetes 1991;40:1560–1563.
28. Sakakibara F, Hotta N, Koh N, Sakamoto N. Effects of high glucose concentrations and epalrestat on sorbitol and myo-inositol metabolism in cultured rabbit aortic smooth muscle cells. Diabetes 1993;42:1594–1660.
29. Sakakibara F, Hotta N, Koh N et al. Effect of high glucose concentrations and epalrestat on cytosolic free Ca^{2+} in cultured rabbit smooth muscle cells. In: Sakamoto N, Alberti KGMM, Hotta N (eds) Pathogenesis and Treatment of NIDDM and its Related Problems. Amsterdam: Excerpta Medica, 1994;437–440.
30. Bagdade JD, Root RK, Bulger RJ. Impaired leukocyte function in patients with poorly controlled diabetes. Diabetes 1974;23:9–15.
31. Wilson RM. Neutrophils function in diabetes. Diabet Med 1986;3:509–512.
32. Boland OM, Blackwell CC, Clarke BF, Ewing DJ. Effects of ponalrestat, an aldose reductase inhibitor, on neutrophil killing of *Escherichia coli* and autonomic function in patients with diabetes mellitus. Diabetes 1993;42:336–340.
33. Kawamura T, Suzuki K, Matsumae H, Sano T, Sakamoto N, Hotta N. Effect of glucose and SNK-860, an aldose reductase inhibitor, on the polyol pathway and chemiluminescence response of human neutrophils in vitro. Diabet Med 1995;12: 392–396.
34. Sato N, Kashima K, Uehara Y, Ohtani K, Shimizu H, Mori M. Epalrestat, an aldose reductase inhibitor, improves an impaired generation of oxygen-derived free radicals by neutrophils from poorly controlled NIDDM patients. Diabet Care 1997;20:995–998.

Obesity/insulin resistance

Recent Advances on the Pathogenesis and Management of Diabetes Mellitus.
S.H. Shinn, M. Shichiri and K.-W. Kim, editors.

Insulin resistance, visceral fat and hypertension

K. Tanigawa[1], S. Nakanishi[2], T. Miura[1], E. Ishihara[1], M. Usami[1] and H. Yano[1]
Departments of [1]Clinical Nutrition and [2]Radiology, Suzuka University of Medical Science and Technology, Suzuka, Mie, Japan

Abstract. The present study was undertaken to assess the relationship between insulin resistance and visceral fat volume and hypertension in genetically obese diabetic rats (Otsuka Long-Evans Tokushima Fatty (OLETF)) and control rats (Long-Evans Tokushima Otsuka (LETO)). Euglycemic hyperinsulinemic clamp and abdominal computed tomography were performed at the age of 15 and 29 weeks in the rats. Body weight was significantly greater in OLETF than in LETO rats at both ages. A significant relationship ($p < 0.05$) between glucose infusion rate (GIR) and visceral fat volume was obtained in the 15-week-old rats. Although we failed to find a difference in GIR between OLETF and controls in the 15-week-old rats, there was a significant difference in GIR in the 29-week-old rats. There was a significant negative correlation between GIR and systolic blood pressure at the age of 15 weeks, but such a relationship disappeared in the 29-week-old rats. The same phenomenon was also obtained regarding diastolic blood pressure. Thus, insulin resistance may be an important factor in regulating blood pressure, but an unknown factor may also be involved in the development of hypertension.

Keywords: blood pressure, genetic obese animal, insulin clamp, visceral fat.

Background

Visceral fat syndrome has been proposed recently by Matsuzawa et al. [1]. They summarized visceral fat syndrome as follows: 1) visceral fat accumulation; 2) glucose intolerance, possibly resulting from insulin resistance, in addition to hyperlipidemia and hypertension. Reaven and DeFronzo have previously proposed syndrome X and insulin resistance syndrome. Visceral fat accumulation may be presented first, and this gives rise to insulin resistance. In the present study, we examined the relationship between visceral fat accumulation, insulin resistance, glucose intolerance and hypertension in genetically obese diabetic animals.

To this end, we used Otsuka Long-Evans Tokushima Fatty (OLETF) rats, a genetically obese animal [2]. As a control, Long-Evans Tokushima Otsuka (LETO) rats were employed.

Methods

Both OLETF and LETO rats were examined at the age of 15 and 29 weeks. Their

Address for correspondence: Keiichiro Tanigawa MD, Department of Clinical Nutrition, Suzuka University of Medical Science and Technology, Suzuka, Mie 510-02, Japan.

visceral fat volume was determined by abdominal computed tomography (CT). We traced CT films from the diaphragm to the pelvis to determine both visceral and subcutaneous fat volumes. These procedures were carried out by a specific radiologist. Some of the animals were sacrificed after insulin clamp and visceral fat was removed and weighed. Euglycemic insulin clamp was performed after 20 h fasting. The rats were anesthetized with pentobarbital, and then insulin solution was infused at the rate of 10 mU/kg/min. Blood glucose was measured every 10 min to maintain euglycemia, and then glucose infusion rate (GIR) and metabolic clearance rate of glucose (MCR) were calculated. Blood pressure was measured using the tail-cuff method.

Results and Discussion

Body weight in the OLETF rats was already heavier than in the LETO rats at the age of 15 weeks. The difference in body weight between OLETF and LETO rats was more apparent at the age of 29 weeks (621 ± 19 vs. 489 ± 19 g, $p<0.001$). Fasting blood glucose was significantly higher in the OLETF rats than in the LETO rats at both ages. However, plasma insulin levels were not different between OLETF and LETO rats, suggesting insulin resistance in the OLETF rats. Systolic blood pressure was slightly higher in OLETF rats than in LETO rats, but statistical significance was only obtained in 29-week-old rats (155 ± 10 vs. 138 ± 3 mmHg, $p<0.05$). Diastolic blood pressure was also higher in the OLETF rats than in the LETO rats and statistical significance was obtained in the 15-week-old rats but not in the 29-week-old rats.

Steady-state blood glucose levels were significantly higher in the OLETF rats than in the LETO rats at both 15 and 29 weeks, but plasma insulin levels in the steady-state during insulin clamp were not different between OLETF and LETO rats. GIR was not significantly different among the four groups. However, the metabolic clearance rate of glucose was significantly lower in the OLETF rats than that in LETO rats at the age of both 15 and 29 weeks.

Computed tomography was very effective in determining visceral fat volume and subcutaneous fat volume. It was obvious that visceral fat accumulated very heavily in the OLETF rats compared with the LETO rats. Although subcutaneous fat accumulation at the age of 15 weeks was not different between OLETF and LETO rats, it was greater in OLETF rats than in LETO rats at the age of 29 weeks (16.0 ± 3.1 vs. 5.1 ± 0.8 g, $p<0.005$). On the other hand, visceral fat volume was obviously greater in the OLETF rats than in the LETO rats. Subcutaneous fat volume was not changed in the 29-week-old LETO rats, but was significantly increased in the OLETF rats. While visceral fat volume was only slightly increased in the LETO rats, it was increased 3-fold in the OLETF rats from 15 to 29 weeks. Visceral fat volume removed from the abdomen was significantly greater in the OLETF rats than in LETO rats at the age of 15 weeks (27.1 ± 2.2 vs. 16.5 ± 0.7 g, $p<0.05$). Visceral fat doubled from the 15th week to the 29th week in the OLETF rats, but there was only a marginal increase in the LETO rats. These results strongly suggest that there is a profound accumulation of visceral fat in genetically obese diabetic rats and that we can determine visceral fat volume by computed tomography without sacrificing animals. Based on these results, we are now going to study the long-term effects of some drugs on visceral fat accumulation in these animals.

We found a significant negative correlation ($p < 0.05$) between glucose infusion rate and systolic blood pressure. There is also a negative correlation ($p < 0.005$) between glucose infusion rate and diastolic blood pressure in these animals. Significance was greater in the relationship between GIR and diastolic blood pressure than in the relationship between GIR and systolic blood pressure. These results may suggest a relationship between insulin resistance and hypertension.

In conclusion, visceral fat accumulation may play an important role in the pathogenesis of glucose intolerance, insulin resistance and hypertension in obese diabetic patients. However, further studies are necessary to explain molecular events in visceral fat syndrome.

References

1. Fujioka S et al. Contribution of intra-abdominal visceral fat accumulation to the impairment of glucose and lipid metabolism in human obesity. Metabolism 1987;36:54.
2. Kawano K et al. Spontaneous long-term hyperglycemic rat with diabetic complications. Otsula Long-Evans Tokushima Fatty (OLETF) strains. Diabetes 1992;41:1422.

Recent Advances on the Pathogenesis and Management of Diabetes Mellitus.
S.H. Shinn, M. Shichiri and K.-W. Kim, editors.

Improvement of β-cell function with long-term treatment of acarbose or metformin in NIDDM

Y. Mori[1], Y. Murakawa[1], K. Okada[1], J. Yokoyama[2], N. Tajima[2] and Y. Ikeda[3]
[1]Department of Internal Medicine, National East-Utsunomiya Hospital, Utsunomiya; Departments of [2]Internal Medicine (III) and [3]Preventive Medicine, the Jikei University School of Medicine, Tokyo, Japan

Abstract. We investigated the effects of long-term administration of an α-glucosidase inhibitor and a biguanide agent on endogenous insulin secretion in NIDDM patients. Twenty-four NIDDM patients whose blood glucose levels had not satisfactorily been controlled by dietary or exercise therapy were divided into the α-glucosidase inhibitor group (n = 13) and the biguanide group (n = 11) and followed-up for 12 months. Prior to the study, there were no significant differences between the two groups in terms of age, BMI fasting blood glucose, HbA1c, serum lipids, blood pressure and body fat distribution. After the 12-month drug therapy, the HbA1c values of both groups were significantly lower than the corresponding pretreatment values. BMI values at 12 months were also significantly lower in the α-glucosidase inhibitor group. The area under the blood glucose-time curve/IRI-time curve ratio during a 75-g oral glucose tolerance test (OGTT) showed a significant increase after the treatment in both groups. The ΔIRI/Δglucose ratio from 0 to 30 min after the 12-month treatment was significantly higher in the biguanide group compared with the pretreatment values. In conclusion, long-term treatments with acarbose and metformin, both of which show hypoglycemic effects without stimulating insulin secretion, restored the endogenous insulin secretion in NIDDM patients. It is likely that the reversal of glucose toxicity may have improved the β-cell function of the pancreas.

Keywords: α-glucosidase inhibitor, biguanide, body fat distribution, endogenous insulin secretion.

Introduction

Sulfonylureas (SUs), which have been the mainstream of drug therapies for NIDDM, decrease blood glucose mainly by stimulating insulin secretion. Due to this obesity-promoting mechanism of action, we have posed a question about the long-term administration of SUs for the treatment of NIDDM patients [1,2]. By contrast, non-β-cell-stimulating oral hypoglycemic agents including metformin and troglitazone have been shown to improve β cell functions in animal experiments [3]. In the present clinical study, we investigated the effects of long-term administration of an α-glucosidase inhibitor and a biguanide agent on endogenous insulin secretion in NIDDM patients.

Address for correspondence: Y. Mori, 2160 Shimookamoto, National East-Utsunomiya Hospital, Kawachi-machi Kawachi-gun, Tochigi 329-11, Japan.

Subjects and Methods

The subjects were 24 NIDDM patients whose blood glucose levels had not satisfactorily been controlled by dietary or exercise therapy. (Extremely poorly controlled patients who showed 200 ml/dl or higher fasting blood glucose levels were excluded.) They were divided into the α-glucosidase inhibitor group (n = 13) and the biguanide group (n = 11). The patients were treated for 12 months with 150–300 mg acarbose/day in the former group and with 500–1,000 mg metformin/day in the latter. In both groups, the dose was appropriately changed within these respective ranges. Before and 12 months after the beginning of treatment, the two groups were compared in terms of BMI, HbA1c, insulin-secreting response after oral loading of 75-g glucose (oral glucose tolerance test (OGTT)), serum lipids, blood pressure, and body fat distribution measured using CT scanning at the umbilical level [4].

The values were expressed as the mean ± SD. The significance of the differences was tested by the paired t test for the pre- and posttreatment comparison and by the unpaired t test for the group comparison. Differences of $p<0.05$ were considered significant.

Results

Prior to the study, there were no significant differences between the two groups in terms of age, BMI, fasting blood glucose, HbA1c, serum lipids, blood pressure, visceral fat (V) area, subcutaneous fat (S) area and V/S ratio (Table 1). After the 12-month drug therapy, the HbA1c values of both groups were significantly low-

Table 1. Clinical profiles of patients before the treatment.

	α-glucosidase inhibitor group	Biguanide group
No. of subjects	13	11
Gender		
Male	9	5
Female	4	6
Age (year)	69.5 ± 8.5	62.7 ± 10.9
Body weight (kg)	60.3 ± 12.4	60.1 ± 10.2
BMI (kg/m^2)	24.0 ± 3.5	24.2 ± 2.8
FPG (mg/dl)	135.3 ± 17.6	152.3 ± 22.6
HbA1c (%)	7.4 ± 0.9	8.1 ± 1.0
Serum TC (mg/dl)	211 ± 28	210 ± 28
Serum TG (mg/dl)	129 ± 61	121 ± 61
Serum HDL-C (mg/dl)	51 ± 18	49 ± 9
BP max (mmHg)	132 ± 12	136 ± 16
BP min (mmHg)	80 ± 5	78 ± 8
Visceral fat (V) area (cm^2)	85.2 ± 53.8	70.8 ± 30.8
Subcutaneous fat (S) area (cm^2)	122.3 ± 80.0	141.3 ± 70.2
V/S ratio	0.70 ± 0.54	0.64 ± 0.42

Table 2. Changes in HbA1C, BMI, insulin secretion during a 75-g OGTT and body fat distribution.

	α-glucosidase inhibitor group		Biguanide group	
	0 month	12 months	0 month	12 months
HbA1C (%)	7.43 ± 0.92	6.73 ± 0.40[a]	8.11 ± 0.96	7.03 ± 0.74[b]
BMI	24.0 ± 3.5	23.4 ± 3.5[a]	24.2 ± 2.8	23.8 ± 2.9
75-g OGTT				
AUC glucose (mg min/dl)	28662 ± 6409	25767 ± 6612[a]	30034 ± 9353	29291 ± 5119
IRI (μU/ml)				
0 s	5.11 ± 3.59	4.78 ± 2.49	7.95 ± 3.91	7.05 ± 4.63
30 s	18.70 ± 9.97	24.15 ± 13.26	22.27 ± 9.54	28.92 ± 9.75
60 s	27.25 ± 15.05	47.27 ± 26.79	31.65 ± 18.26	51.56 ± 38.87
90 s	38.35 ± 19.01	59.30 ± 38.02	45.54 ± 15.70	59.55 ± 28.26
120 s	41.45 ± 23.51	59.01 ± 37.09	45.25 ± 13.20	52.43 ± 21.24
AUC_{IRI} (μU min/ml)	3227.1 ± 1508.8	4879.6 ± 2648.7	3781.4 ± 1369.3	5106.3 ± 2408.0[a]
$AUC_{IRI}/AUC_{glucose}$	0.112 ± 0.063	0.183 ± 0.107[a]	0.127 ± 0.062	0.182 ± 0.116[a]
ΔIRI/Δglucose (30 s) (10^2 μU/mg)	0.21 ± 0.30	0.23 ± 0.19	0.14 ± 0.11	0.24 ± 0.10[b]
Body fat distribution				
Visceral fat area (cm^2)	85.2 ± 53.8	79.5 ± 61.5	70.8 ± 30.8	69.9 ± 33.0
Subcutaneous fat area (cm^2)	122.3 ± 80.0	128.0 ± 88.0	141.3 ± 70.2	152.5 ± 77.9
V/S ratio	0.70 ± 0.54	0.62 ± 0.49	0.64 ± 0.42	0.60 ± 0.42

[a]$p<0.05$; [b]$p<0.01$ vs. value of 0 month.

er than the corresponding pretreatment values (Table 2). BMI values at 12 months were also significantly ($p<0.05$) lower in the α-glucosidase inhibitor group, but not in the biguanide group (Table 2). The area under the blood glucose-time curve ($AUC_{glucose}$) during a 75-g OGTT decreased significantly ($p<0.05$) from the pretreatment value in the α-glucosidase inhibitor group, and tended to decrease in the biguanide group. The area under the IRI-time curve (AUC_{IRI}) during a 75-g OGTT tended to increase from the pretreatment values in the α-glucosidase inhibitor group, and increased significantly ($p<0.05$) in the biguanide group (Table 2). The $AUC_{IRI}/AUC_{glucose}$ ratio showed a significant ($p<0.05$) increase after the treatment in both groups (Table 2). As a parameter reflecting the initial insulin-secreting response, the ΔIRI/Δ glucose ratio from 0 to 30 min was calculated. This ratio after the 12-month treatment tended to be higher in the α-glucosidase inhibitor group, and was significantly ($p<0.01$) higher in the biguanide group as compared with the corresponding pretreatment values. Serum lipids and blood pressure showed no significant differences between the pre- and posttreatment measurements in either group. Body fat distribution was not significantly changed by either treatment in terms of V area, S area, or V/S ratio (Table 2).

Discussion

Long-term treatments with acarbose and metformin, both of which show hypoglycemic effects without stimulating insulin secretion, restored endogenous insulin secretion in NIDDM patients. Sreenan et al. [4] treated Zucker diabetic fatty (ZDF) rats at 6 weeks of age with metformin and troglitazone until the animals reached the age of 12 weeks, and studied the effects on the pancreatic β-cell function. Sreenan et al. reported that metformin and troglitazone not only inhibited the development of hyperglycemia and decreased triglycerides and free fatty acids, but also decreased basal insulin secretion and improved their insulin-secreting responses to glucose stimulation. In more detail, metformin and troglitazone decreased basal insulin secretion from the perfused pancreas under the basal stimulation with 2 mM glucose, but its insulin-secreting response to 10-mM glucose stimulation was increased 22 times by metformin and 10 times by troglitazone. From these findings, Sreenan et al. concluded that these drugs corrected hyperglycemia, and thereby may have preserved or restored endogenous insulin secretion. These results from animal experiments are supported by our observation that the $AUC_{IRI}/AUC_{glucose}$ ratio during a 75-g OGTT was significantly increased by the 12-month treatments. It is likely that the reversal of glucose toxicity may have improved the β-cell function of the pancreas.

References

1. Katoh S. Long-term effects of oral hypoglycemic agents on fat distribution and glucose tolerance in OLETF rats. Tokyo Jikeikai Med J 1996;111:919–926 (in Japanese).
2. Katoh S, Mori Y, Yokoyama et al. Effect of long-term acarbose and glibenclamide treatment on visceral fat accumulation in patients with NIDDM. Diabetologia 1996;39(Suppl 1):A44.
3. Fujioka S, Matsuzawa Y, Tokunaga K et al. Contribution of intra-abdominal fat accumulation to the impairment of glucose and lipid metabolism in human obesity. Metabolism 1987;36:54–59.
4. Sreenan S, Sturis J, Pugh W et al. Preservation of beta-cell function with metformin or troglitazone in the Zucker diabetic fatty rat. Diabetologia 1996;39(Suppl 1):A69.

Recent Advances on the Pathogenesis and Management of Diabetes Mellitus.
S.H. Shinn, M. Shichiri and K.-W. Kim, editors.

The correlation between insulin resistance and the visceral fat vs. skeletal muscle ratio (VMR) in middle-aged women

B.S. Cha[1], Y.J. Won[1], J.H. Lee[1], S.Y. Nam[1], Y.D. Song[1], E.J. Lee[1], M.J. Shin[2], J.H. Lee[2], S.K. Lim[1], K.R. Kim[1], H.C. Lee[1] and K.B. Huh[1]

Departments of [1]Internal Medicine, College of Medicine and [2]Food and Nutrition, College of Human Ecology, Yonsei University, Seoul, Korea

Abstract. In humans, skeletal muscle comprises 35 to 40% of body weight, and major site of glucose disposal at high insulin concentration or after an oral glucose load, and bulk of skeletal muscle mass may influence insulin sensitivity via its capacity to uptake glucose load. The relative amount of visceral fat area in the umbilical level to skeletal muscle area in the midthigh, measured by computed tomogram (CT) scan, may represent an important anthropometric parameter to determine insulin resistance. We investigated the relationships among the metabolic variables, the ratio of visceral fat area vs. skeletal muscle area (VMR), percent of ideal body weight (PIBW), body mass index (BMI), waist-to-hip circumference ratio (WHR) and visceral fat vs. subcutaneous fat ratio (VSR) in 129 nondiabetic middle-aged women. From the results of this study, VMR may be a better anthropometric parameter indicative of insulin resistance than VSR, and the latter was better parameter representing serum lipid levels than the former in nondiabetic middle-aged women.

Keywords: insulin resistance, skeletal muscle, visceral fat vs. skeletal muscle ratio (VMR), visceral fat vs. subcutaneous fat ratio (VSR), visceral fat.

Introduction

Central-type obesity with visceral fat accumulation is known to be an important contributing factor to increased insulin resistance. In the 1950s, Vague et al. [1] divided obesity into android type and gynecoid type, with the android type of obesity being more related to diabetes, atherosclerosis and gout than the gynecoid type of obesity. In the 1980s, Kissebach et al. [2] said that WHR was correlated with metabolic complications related with obesity. Further, Tarui et al. [3] classified obesity into visceral type and subcutaneous type, using a CT-scan cross-sectional picture of the umbilical region, and a VSR of more than 0.4, suggesting that visceral type obesity showed significant risk factors for coronary artery disease, such as increased blood pressure, plasma glucose area, triglyceride (TG) and total cholesterol (TC) levels.

In humans, skeletal muscle comprises 35—40% of body weight, and is a major site of glucosal disposal at high insulin concentrations or after an oral glucose load, and the bulk of skeletal muscle mass may influence insulin sensitivity via

Address for correspondence: Prof Kap Bum Huh, 134 Shinchon-Dong, Seodaemun-Ku, Seoul 120-752, Korea. Tel.: +82-2-361-5410. Fax: +82-2-393-6884.

its capacity to uptake glucose load. The relative amount of visceral fat area in the umbilical level to skeletal muscle area in the midthigh, measured by CT scan, may represent an important anthropometric parameter for determining insulin resistance. Therefore, we investigated the relationships among the metabolic variables VMR, PIBW, BMI, WHR and VSR in healthy nondiabetic middle-aged women.

Subjects and Methods

Subjects comprised 114 females aged 49.7 ± 5.3 (range 40 ~ 60) years with overweight and obesity who were attending the Division of Endocrinology, Severance Hospital, Yonsei University, for the purpose of health checking. Their mean body weight was 63.2 ± 7.3 kg and BMI was 26.1 ± 2.5 kg/m^2. Ten subjects had the impaired glucose tolerance pattern in the 75-g oral glucose tolerance test (OGTT), but other subjects had no metabolic and endocrinologic disorders. The body fat distribution and muscle area were determined by means of CT scan according to the procedure of Tokunaga et al. [4], by which the cross-sectional area, subcutaneous and visceral fat area (Hounsfield number, −150 to −50) at the level of the umbilicus, and subcutaneous fat area and muscle area (Hounsfield number, −49 to 100) of the midportion between the greater trochanter and upper portion of the patella, were measured (Fig. 1). The VSR and VMR were calculated from the value of the visceral fat area divided by the abdominal subcutaneous fat area and thigh muscle area, respectively. Blood was drawn after an overnight fast for measuring TC, TG, HDL-cholesterol (HDL-C) and sex hormone-binding globulin (SHBG) levels. The 75-g OGTT was performed, and blood samples were collected at 0, 30, 60 and 120 min to determine glucose, free fatty acid (FFA) and insulin levels. The area under the curve of glucose

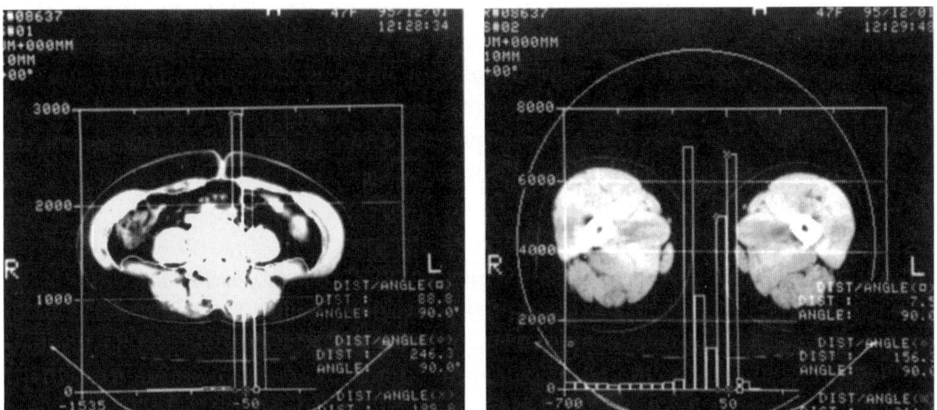

Fig. 1. CT scan at the umbilical level (**A**) and midthigh level (**B**).

(Glu-AUC), insulin (Ins-AUC), free fatty acid (FFA-AUC) and glucose/insulin ratio (GIR = Glu-AUC/Ins-AUC) were also calculated.

Results

Mean values of WHR, VSR and VMR in a total of 114 subjects were 0.93 ± 0.05 (0.79 ∼ 10.7), 0.40 ± 0.17 (0.15 ∼ 0.95) and 0.61 ± 0.27 (0.17 ∼ 1.40), respectively. Mean fasting levels of glucose, insulin, FFA, TC, HDL-C, TG, and SHBG were 5.1 ± 1.0 mmol/l, 68 ± 86 pmol/l, 623 ± 201 mmol/l, 5.41 ± 1.03 mmol/l, 1.19 ± 0.25 mmol/l, 1.65 ± 0.87 mmol/l, and 80 ± 37 nmol/l, respectively. According to Pearson's correlation coefficienct among the metabolic variables, the TG level was more significantly correlated with VSR than VMR (r = 0.3349, p < 0.001 vs. r = 2589, p = 0.006), but Ins-AUC, GIR and SHBG levels were more significantly correlated with VMR than VSR (r = 0.4487, p < 0.001 vs. r = 0.3124, p = 0.002; r = −0.4386, p < 0.001 vs. r = −0.2840, p = 0.004; r = −0.4281, p < 0.001 vs. r = −0.3050, p = 0.015, respectively). After multiple linear regression analysis with adjustment for age and BMI, the most important anthropometric parameters of each metabolic variables were: VMR in Ins-AUC, GIR and SHBG levels, WHR in Glu-AUC and TC levels, and VSR in the TG level (Table 1).

In subjects with a VMR more than 0.6, age (53.0 ± 4.2 vs. 47.0 ± 4.6 years, p < 0.001), Ins-AUC (925 ± 403 vs. 600 ± 297 pmol/l × h, p < 0.001), and TG (1.85 ± 1.00 vs. 1.49 ± 0.73 mmol/l, p < 0.05) levels were significantly elevated, and GIR (1.85 ± 0.78 vs. 2.74 ± 1.23, p < 0.001) and SHBG (73.4 ± 34.6 vs. 97.5 ± 37.8 pmol/l, p < 0.05) levels decreased more than in subjects with lower VMR. Regardless of the magnitude of VSR, subjects with VMR more than 0.6 were older and showed higher Ins-AUC and lower GIR than in subjects with lower VMR (Table 2). To exclude the compound factors, we compared the metabolic variables of 72 subjects who were matched for age, BMI and WHR. But, Ins-AUC was still significantly increased and GIR and SHBG levels decreased more in subjects with higher VMR than those with lower VMR (Table 3). There were no remarkable differences in anthropometric and metabolic variables between premenopausal and postmenopausal women except age (45.2 ± 3.1 vs. 52.5 ± 3.6 years, p < 0.001) and TG (1.27 ± 0.16 vs. 1.92 ± 0.27 mmol/l, p < 0.001) levels (data not shown).

Table 1. The most important independent anthropometric parameters for metabolic variables after multiple linear regression analysis in 114 middle-aged women.

Dependent variables	Glu-AUC	Ins-AUC	GIR	SHBG	TC	HDL-C	TG
Independent variable	WHR	VMR	VMR	VMR	WHR	–	VSR
Adjusted R square	0.73	0.161	0.160	0.152	0.127	–	0.094
β	0.288	0.412	−0.413	−0.411	0.370	–	0.323
p value	0.004	<0.001	<0.000	0.003	<0.000	–	0.01

Table 2. Comparisons of anthropometric parameters and metabolic variables according to the VMR in both subjects with higher and lower VSR in 114 middle-aged women.

	VSR < 0.4		VSR ⩾ 0.4	
	VMR < 0.6	VMR ⩾ 0.6	VMR < 0.6	VSR ⩾ 0.6
n	49	19	14	32
Age (years)	47.2 ± 4.8	55.1 ± 4.2[c]	46.3 ± 4.2	51.7 ± 3.6[e]
PIBW (%)	127 ± 13	134 ± 14	125 ± 9	124 ± 10
WHR	0.94 ± 0.05	0.92 ± 0.05	0.93 ± 0.06	0.93 ± 0.04
Glu-AUC (mmol/l × h)	14.1 ± 3.7	14.2 ± 2.9	16.0 ± 5.2	14.9 ± 2.0
Ins-AUC (pmol/l × h)	586 ± 308	790 ± 435[a]	652 ± 265	997 ± 374[d]
GIR	2.76 ± 1.18	2.13 ± 0.90[a]	2.70 ± 1.45	1.70 ± 0.68[d]
SHBG (nmol/l)	105.1 ± 32.6	76.6 ± 33.2[a]	88.2 ± 42.2	71.5 ± 35.9
TC (mmol/l)	5.31 ± 1.09	5.03 ± 1.25	5.74 ± 0.80	5.62 ± 0.78
HDL-C (mmol/l)	1.19 ± 0.24	1.30 ± 0.31	1.11 ± 0.23	1.16 ± 0.24
TG (mmol/l)	1.37 ± 0.64	1.82 ± 1.29[b]	1.94 ± 0.87	1.96 ± 0.80

[a]$p < 0.05$; [b]$p < 0.01$; [c]$p < 0.001$ compared to subjects with VSR < 0.4 and VMR < 0.6; [d]$p < 0.01$; [e]$p < 0.001$ compared to subjects with VSR ⩾ 0.4 and VMR < 0.6.

Discussion

Several recent studies have focused on the relation of body-fat distribution to the prevalence of metabolic complications of obesity [5,6]. It is now clear that the accumulation of fat at the abdomen and the upper segment of the body is a better predictor for an increased risk of reduced glucose tolerance, hyperlipoproteinemia, hyperuricemia and hypertension than the degree of overweight, in both males and females. Recently Tokunaga et al. [4] used a CT method that permits an accurate analysis of subcutaneous fat and intra-abdominal visceral fat. Based upon this method, they proposed a novel classification of obesity: visceral fat

Table 3. Comparisons of anthropometric parameters and metabolic variables according to the VMR after adjustment of age in 72 middle-aged women.

	VMR < 0.6	VMR ⩾ 0.6
n	36	36
Age (years)	50.1 ± 2.6	50.9 ± 2.6
PIBW (%)	124 ± 10	126 ± 11
WHR	0.95 ± 0.04	0.93 ± 0.36
Glu-AUC (mmol/l × h)	14.7 ± 3.9	14.6 ± 2.26
Ins-AUC (pmol/l × h)	590 ± 792	956 ± 380[b]
GIR	2.77 ± 1.26	1.78 ± 0.81[b]
SHBG (nmol/l)	106 ± 37	68 ± 30[a]
TC (mmol/l)	5.66 ± 1.10	5.45 ± 1.04
HDL-C (mmol/l)	1.14 ± 0.19	1.19 ± 0.28
TG (mmol/l)	1.65 ± 70	1.98 ± 1.08

Note: values are means ± SD. [a]$p < 0.01$, [b]$p < 0.001$.

vs. subcutaneous fat obesity [7].

We would now like to propose another novel anthropometric parameter, VMR [5]. The relative amount of visceral fat per skeletal mass might represent glucose and insulin metabolism and correlate peripheral insulin resistance. In this study, VSR was a good parameter indicative of plasma lipid levels such as TC, FFA and TG levels than VMR. But VMR was more closely correlated with the levels of Ins-AUC, GIR and SHBG than VSR.

VMR may be a better anthropometric parameter indicative of insulin resistance than VSR, and the latter was a better parameter for representing serum lipid levels than formerly in nondiabetic middle-aged women, and further prospective studies for diabetic patients are warranted to re-evaluate these results.

References

1. Vague J et al. The degree of masculine differentiation of obesities, a factor determining predisposition to diabetes, atherosclerosis, gout and uric calculous disease. Am J Clin Nutr 1956;4:20–34.
2. Kissebach AH, Uydelingum N et al. Relation of body fat distribution to metabolic complication to obesity. J Clin Endocrinol Metab 1982;54:254–260.
3. Tarui S, Fujioka S et al. Comparison of pathophysiology between subcutaneous-type and visceral-type obesity. In: Bray GA, LeBlanc J, Inoue S, Suzuki M (eds) Diet and Obesity. Tokyo: Japan Scientific Societies Press, 1988;143–152.
4. Tokugana K, Matsuzawa Y et al. A novel technique for the determination of the body fat by computed tomography. Int J Obes 1983;7:437–445.
5. Huh KB. The role of insulin resistance in Korean patients with metabolic and cardiovascular diseases. In: Huh KB, Shinn SH, Kaneko T (eds) Insulin Resistance in Human Disease. Amsterdam: Elsevier Science Publishers, 1993;7–12.
6. Bouchard C, Despres JP et al. Genetic and nongenetic determinants of regional fat distribution. Endocrine Rev 1993;14:72–93.
7. Fujioka S, Matsuzawa Y et al. Contribution of intra-abdominal fat accumulation to the impairment of glucose and lipid metabolism in human obesity. Metabolism 1087;36:54–59.

Recent Advances on the Pathogenesis and Management of Diabetes Mellitus.
S.H. Shinn, M. Shichiri and K.-W. Kim, editors.

The difference of SHBG concentration in patients with NIDDM

Yu Jang Pyun, Ki Chul Sung, Yoon Sang Choi and Sang Jong Lee
Department of Internal Medicine, Kangbuk Samsung Hospital, Sungkynunkwan University College of Medicine, Seoul, Korea

Abstract. *Background.* We measured serum sex hormone and sex hormone binding hormone (SHBG) levels in both men and postmenopausal women, and then tried to investigate the relationships between their serum levels and insulin resistance and NIDDM.

Methods. We conducted the study on the reports mentioned, and comparatively analyzed the SHBG, testosterone, which includes both the total and free forms, and estrone in 41 female patients with NIDDM and 40 female controls. The same study was also carried out in 24 male NIDDM patients and seven male controls.

Results. We compared the serum levels of SHBG, testosterone (free form and total form) and estrone in both 24 male patients with NIDDM and the seven male control group. In the female NIDDM group, SHBG showed statistically significant lower serum levels than the control group ($p < 0.002$). Other findings did not show any statistical differences between the two groups. In the male group, our study did not show any significant differences in free testosterone and SHBG levels between the diabetic and control groups.

Conclusions. Increased androgenesity and a low SHBG level seem to be of significance in the mechanism of NIDDM development in postmenopausal women.

Keywords: NIDDM, sex hormone, SHBG.

Introduction

Recently, insulin resistance has been reported as one of the major factors for NIDDM development [1]. The insulin sensitivity is known to be associated with androgen concentration [2], and some studies suggest that the adrenal or sex steroid hormones seem to control the insulin sensitivity of the glycogen synthesis system [3].

The serum sex hormone binding globulin (SHBG) level, thought to be a marker for androgenesity, acts as an important factor in NIDDM development [4]. In our study, we measured serum sex hormone and SHBG levels in both men and postmenopausal women, and then tried to investigate the relationships between their serum levels and insulin resistance and NIDDM.

Methods

We conducted the study on the reports mentioned, and comparatively analyzed the SHBG, testosterone, which includes both the total and free forms, and

Address for correspondence: Yu Jang Pyun MD, Department of Internal Medicine, Kangbuk Samsung Hospital, Sungkynunkwan University College of Medicine, 108 Pyung-Dong Jongro-Ku, Seoul 100-752, Korea.

estrone in 41 female patients with NIDDM and 40 control females. Also, the same study was carried out in 24 male NIDDM patients and seven control males. The subjects were NIDDM-diagnosed patients who had visited the Kangbuk Samsung Hospital. Patients who presented with severe liver disease, or heart and renal problems were excluded from the study. Subjects included in the control group were people who visited our hospital for their health check up. Also, any subjects in the control group who presented with severe liver disease, or heart and renal problems were excluded from the study. We compared the serum levels of SHBG, testosterone and estrone in 24 NIDDM patients with the normal control group. SHBG, testosterone (free form testosterone and total form testosterone) and estrone levels are detected with radioimmunoassay. The patients need not be fasting, and no special preparations are necessary. Blood was collected by venipuncture into plain (without anticoagulant) tubes, and then the serum was separated from the cells by centrifugation. The results were obtained using the IRMA-count SHBG assay, Coat-A-Count Total testosterone procedure, Coat-A-Count Free testosterone procedure and DSL-8700 Estrone Radioimmunoassay Kit.

Results

We compared the serum levels of SHBG, testosterone (free and total forms) and estrone for both 24 male patients with NIDDM and seven males in the control group (Table 1). Detailed information on the general comparison between the two groups is shown in Table 2. Age, BMI, serum total protein level, serum albumin level, serum triglyceride level, and serum total cholesterol level between the two groups did not show any significant difference statistically. In males, the serum SHBG level, serum free testosterone level, serum total testosterone level and serum estrone level did not show any significant difference statistically. The same method was applied for females and the results are shown in Tables 3 and 4. Also, in females, age, BMI, the serum total protein level, the serum albumin level, the serum triglyceride level and the serum total cholesterol level between the two groups did not show any significant difference statistically. However, in the female NIDDM group, SHBG showed a statistically significant lower serum level than the control group ($p < 0.002$). Other findings did not show any statistical differences between the two groups.

Table 1. Differences in SHBG, testosterone and estrone in males.

	NIDDM patients	Control group	p values
SHBG (mmol/l)	46.3 ± 25.3	61.09 ± 27.96	ns
Total testosterone (ng/dl)	412.03 ± 164.03	485.73 ± 186.13	ns
Free testosterone (ng/dl)	16.54 ± 7.8	13.28 ± 5.95	ns
Estrone (pg/ml)	19.55 ± 14.19	27.59 ± 25.39	ns

Note: ns = not significant.

Table 2. Difference between male NIDDM patients and the male control group.

	NIDDM patients	Control group	p values
Numbers	24	7	
Age (years)	53 ± 11	55 ± 6	ns
BMI (kg/m^2)	23.1 ± 3.9	21.5 ± 3.1	ns
Total protein (g/dl)	6.7 ± 0.9	6.5 ± 1.0	ns
Serum albumin (g/dl)	3.9 ± 0.7	4.0 ± 0.7	ns
Triglyceride (mg/dl)	178.3 ± 181.5	131.29 ± 86.17	ns
Total cholesterol (mg/dl)	188.65 ± 60.07	185.71 ± 56.96	ns

Note: ns = not significant.

Discussion

The SHBG level reflects the elevated free testosterone level and this in turn causes an impairment in insulin sensitivity. In postmenopausal women, it is reported that a low SHBG level was associated with impaired glucose tolerance and NIDDM [5]. Other studies report that hyperinsulinemia is suggested to cause increased androgen production [8]. In studies of animals it is reported that anabolic steroid administration induces insulin resistance in female rats, administration of small dose testosterone induced dramatic insulin resistance and this finding suggests the important role of hyperandrogenicity in NIDDM development [3,5,6]. In our study, a significant difference in the free testosterone level between the two female groups was not observed. However, this result is suggested to be due to the small number of cases and should be verified by further study. In the male group, some studies report that hypogonadism is related to insulin resistance and diabetic male patients show lower testosterone and SHBG levels than the normal group [7]. But the evidence that hypoandrogenicity contributes to NIDDM in males is not clear. In the male group, our study did not show any significant difference in free testosterone and SHBG levels between the diabetic group and control group. The above results demonstrate that increased androgenesity and a low SHBG level seem to be of significance in the mechanism of NIDDM development in postmenopausal women.

Table 3. Difference between female NIDDM patients and the female control group.

	NIDDM patients	Control group	p values
Numbers	41	40	
Age (years)	58 ± 8.1	59 ± 7.2	ns
BMI (kg/m^2)	24 ± 3.5	23 ± 3.1	ns
Total protein (g/dl)	6.95 ± 0.48	6.96 ± 0.56	ns
Serum albumin (g/dl)	4.2 ± 0.32	4.2 ± 0.32	ns
Triglyceride (mg/dl)	140 ± 76	174 ± 302	ns
Total cholesterol (mg/dl)	185 ± 34	178 ± 48	ns

Note: ns = not significant.

Table 4. Differences in SHBG, testosterone and estrone in females.

	NIDDM patients	Control group	p values
SHBG (mmol/l)	45.26 ± 23.10	74.12 ± 38.17	$p < 0.01$
Total testosterone (ng/dl)	21.83 ± 16	32.84 ± 89	ns
Free testosterone (ng/dl)	1.66 ± 3.22	0.55 ± 0.34	ns
Estrone (pg/ml)	20.27 ± 16	19.16 ± 23	ns

Note: ns = not significant.

References

1. DeFronzo R, Diebert D, Hendler RM, Felig P, Soman V. Insulin sensitivity and insulin binding to monocytes in maturity onset diabetes. J Clin Invest 1979;63:939—946.
2. Rebuffe-Scrive M, Cullberg G, Lundberg P, Lindstedt G, Bjomtrop P. Anthropometric variables and metabolism in polycystic ovarian disease. Horm Metab Res 1989;21:391—397.
3. Holmang A, Svedberg J, Jennische E, Bjomtrop P. Effect of testosterone on muscle insulin sensitivity and morphology in female rats. Am J Physiol 1990;259:E555—E560.
4. Lindstedt G, Lindberg PA, Lapidus L, Lundgren H, Benggison C, Bjomtorp P. Low sex-hormone binding globulin concentration as independent risk factor for development of NIDDM; 12-year follow-up of population study of women in Gothenburg, Sweden. Diabetes 1991;40: 123—128.
5. Landon JC, Wynn V, Samols E. The effects of anabolic steroids on blood sugar and plasma insulin levels in men. Metabolism 1963;12:924—930.
6. Holmang A, Larsson BM, Brzezinska Z, Bjorntorp P. The effects of short-term testosterone exposure on insulin sensitivity in female rats. Am J Physiol 1992;262:E851—E855.
7. Andersson B, Vermeulen A, Marin P, Bjorntorp P, Lissner L. Testosterone concentrations in women and men with NIDDM. Diabet Care 1994;17:405—411.
8. Poretsky L, Kalin ML. The gonadotropic function of insulin. Endocrine Rev 1987;8: 132—141.

Recent Advances on the Pathogenesis and Management of Diabetes Mellitus.
S.H. Shinn, M. Shichiri and K.-W. Kim, editors.

Correlation between serum leptin level and abdominal fat distribution in Korean adults

Seung-Won Lee, Yoon-Sang Choi and Sang-Jong Lee
Division of Endocrinology, Department of Internal Medicine, Kangbuk Samsung Hospital, College of Medicine, Sungkyunkwan University, Seoul, Korea

Abstract. *Background.* To investigate the relationship between the serum leptin level and abdominal wall fat distribution using ultrasonography.

Method. The population included in the study were 193 randomized Korean subjects (133 males and 60 females) who visited Kangbuk Samsung Hospital Mediscreen Center for health checkups from 1996 to 1997. Radioimmunoassay was employed to measure the serum levels of serum leptin, insulin and C-peptide. Ultrasonography was employed to measure the various preperitoneal fat layers and subcutaneous fat layers.

Results. Our study shows that the serum leptin level shows positive correlation with BMI ($r = 0.318$, $p < 0.005$). Among the various fat distribution indices, leptin showed the highest correlation with minimal thickness of the subcutaneous fat layer ($r = 0.494$, $p < 0.005$). Maximal thickness of the preperitoneal fat layer/minimal thickness of subcutaneous fat layer (abdominal fat wall index (AFI)) showed highest correlation with abnormal metabolic profiles.

Conclusion. Plasma leptin levels might be attributed mainly to the thickness of the subcutaneous fat layer in human adiposity. Also it is unlikely that leptin is directly associated with metabolic disorders, yet further studies are required for establishment of the relationship between leptin and metabolic disorders.

Keywords: abdominal fat distribution, leptin, subcutaneous fat.

Introduction

Leptin, a 16-kDa protein expressed primarily in adipose tissue, has been known to correlate with the BMI in both humans and mice. Also, studies have revealed its possible correlation with the fasting insulin level. Although it has not been fully elucidated if the mutated obesity (OB) gene is the culprit of obesity in humans, for the mice study at least, the mutated OB gene is suggested to play a major role in the development of obesity.

Regarding obesity, visceral fat mass rather than subcutaneous fat mass is reported to show a stronger correlation with many metabolic derangements, including abnormal glucose intolerance, lipid metabolism derangement, etc.

In this study, by measuring the serum leptin level and abdominal fat distribution and lipid profiles, we aimed to establish a correlation between the following:

Address for correspondence: Seung-Won Lee, Division of Endocrinology, Department of Internal Medicine, Kangbuk Samsung Hospital, College of Medicine, Sungkyunkwan University, 108 Pyung-dong Jongrogu, Seoul, Korea.

1) the serum leptin level and fat distribution indices measured by ultrasonography; and 2) the serum leptin level and the metabolic profile.

Subjects and Methods

The population included in the study were 193 randomized Korean subjects (133 males and 60 females) who visited Kangbuk Samsung Hospital Mediscreen Center for health checkups from 1996 to 1997. The subjects, from whom informed consent was obtained, were divided into obese (157 subjects) and nonobese groups (36 subjects) according to the definition of obesity (BMI over 26). Radioimmunoassay was employed to measure the serum levels of serum leptin, insulin and C-peptide level. Ultrasonography was employed to measure the various preperitoneal fat layers and subcutaneous fat layers.

Results

Our study shows that the serum leptin level shows a positive correlation with the BMI ($r = 0.318$, $p < 0.005$) as shown in Table 1. Among the many fat distribution indices, leptin showed the highest correlation with minimal thickness of subcutaneous fat layer ($r = 0.494$, $p < 0.005$), as shown in Table 1.

On the whole, the thickness of the subcutaneous fat layers is more likely to be correlated with the serum leptin level than with the thickness of the preperitoneal fat layer. Maximal thickness of the preperitoneal fat layer/minimal thickness of the subcutaneous fat layer (abdominal fat wall index (AFI)) showed the highest correlation with abnormal metabolic profiles, as shown in Table 2.

Table 1.

A: Correlation between leptin and various fat distribution indices.

	AFI	Pmax	Pmin	Smax	Smin	BMI	Pav	Sav
Leptin (r value)	−0.317	0.278[a]	0.278	0.475[a]	0.494[a]	0.318[a]	0.149[b]	0.391[a]

B: Correlation between leptin and metabolic profiles.

	Insulin	C-Peptide	FBS	HDL-Chol	T-Chol	TG
Leptin (r value)	0.20	0.063	−0.080	0.254[a]	0.089	−0.104

[a]$p < 0.005$, [b]$p < 0.05$.

Note: AFI = Maximum thickness of preperitoneal fat/minimum thickness of subcutaneous fat. Pmax = Maximum thickness of preperitoneal fat. Pmin = Minimum thickness of preperitoneal fat. Smax = Maximum thikness of subcutaneous fat. Smin = Minimum thickness of subcutaneous fat. Pav = Average thickness of preperitoneal fat. Sav = Average thickness of subcutaneous fat.

Table 2. Correlation between various fat distributions and metabolic profiles.

	FBS	C-Pep	Insulin	Leptin	T-Chol	TG	HDL-Chol
AFI	0.64	−0.037	0.078	−0.137	−0.023	0.225[a]	−0.200[a]
Pmax	0.085	−0.002	0.015	0.278[a]	0.079	0.155[b]	−0.101
Pmin	−0.156[b]	0.007	−0.131	0.018	−0.033	0.027	−0.075
Pav	0.040	−0.014	−0.014	0.149[b]	0.113	0.137	−0.069
BMI	−0.018	0.063	0.070	0.318[a]	0.140	0.140	−0.163[b]
Smax	−0.085	0.026	−0.024	0.475[a]	0.082	−0.078	0.126
Smin	−0.029	0.045	−0.092	0.494[a]	0.088	−0.194[b]	0.243[b]
Sav	−0.021	0.018	−0.036	0.391[a]	0.146[b]	−0.103	0.190[b]

[a]$p < 0.005$, [b]$p < 0.05$.

Discussion

Leptin, the protein product of the OB gene has recently been discovered in mice [1]. In humans, unlike mice, mutation in the OB gene is rare [2] and the serum leptin level is correlated with the percentage of body fat, suggesting that most obese people are insensitive to endogenous leptin production [3]. Intra-abdominal visceral fat mass is known to be closely correlated with diabetes mellitus, hyperlipidemia and hypertension.

Previous studies have reported on OB genes, and their products are more abundantly detected in subcutaneous fat mass compared with the same amount of visceral fat mass [4].

Also, Takahashi et al. have reported that the plasma leptin level might be attributed mainly to the extent of the subcutaneous fat mass in human obesity, however, a significant correlation between its plasma levels and visceral fat area was not found [5]. In our study, we investigated the relationship between regional fat distribution of the abdominal wall and serum leptin level, and instead of employing CT, a new method using ultrasonography [6] was employed. Serum leptin levels show a positive correlation with the thickness of the subcutaneous fat layer. This observation supports the conclusions of previous studies that plasma leptin levels might be attributed mainly to the extent of subcutaneous adiposity. Suzuki et al. [6] mentioned that preperitoneal fat reflects the amount of visceral fat. A correlation between the serum leptin level and thickness of preperitoneal fat was not observed and this finding might, in part, support the previous studies. However, further developmental analysis is required since the preperitoneal fat layer only partly shares the common property of the visceral fat layer. Contrary to the peritoneal fat layer, visceral fat is chained to a portal vein, however, anatomically the preperitoneal fat is covered by the peritoneum, like omental fat, which is part of the visceral fat.

Among the components of metabolic disorders, HDL-cholesterol seems to have a positive correlation with the serum leptin level. However, it is not known whether leptin affects directly.

References

1. Zhang Y, Proenca R, Maffei M, Barone M, Leopold L, Friedman JM. Positional cloning of the mouse obese gene and its human homologue. Nature 1994;372:425–432.
2. Carlsson B, Lindell K, Gabrielsson B, Karlsson C et al. Obese gene defects are rare in human obesity. Obes Res 1997;5(1):30–35.
3. Saladin R, De Vos P, Guerre-Millo M, Leturque A, Girard J, Staels B, Auwerx J. Transient increase in obese gene expression after food intake or insulin administration. Nature 1995;377: 6549.
4. Masuzaki H, Ogawa Y, Isse N, Satoh N, Okazaki T, Shigemoto M et al. Human obese gene expression. Adipocyte-specific expression and regional differences in the adipose tissue. Diabetes 1995;44(7):855–858.
5. Takahashi M, Funahashi M, Shimomura I, Miyaoka K, Matsuzawa Y. Plasma leptin levels and body fat distribution. Horm Metab Res 1996;28:751–752.
6. Suzuki R, Watanabe S, Hirai Y et al. Abdominal fat wall index, estimated by ultrasonography, for assessment of the ratio of visceral fat to subcutaneous fat in the abdomen. Am J Med 1993; 95:309–314.

Recent Advances on the Pathogenesis and Management of Diabetes Mellitus.
S.H. Shinn, M. Shichiri and K.-W. Kim, editors.

An interview-based assessment of eating behavior in nonobese and obese subjects

M. Shintani[1], H. Ikegami[1], E. Yamato[1], Y. Kawaguchi[1], T. Fujisawa[1], Y. Hamada[1], M. Hotta[1], H. Ueda[1], K. Nojima[1], Y. Kawabata[1], N. Babaya[1], G.Q. Shen[1], A. Kinashi[2], T. Sakata[3] and T. Ogihara[1]

[1]*Department of Geriatric Medicine, Osaka University Medical School, Osaka;* [2]*Uehara Scientific Research Institute, Osaka; and* [3]*Department of Internal Medicine I, Oita Medical University, Hasama, Oita, Japan*

Abstract. Overeating is one of the major predisposing factors for the development of NIDDM. To assess the contribution of overeating to body weight, eating behavior was estimated by interview-based assessment in 684 healthy control subjects. Questionnaires consist of seven categories: recognition, hunger, compensation, satiety, patterns, contents and rhythm. Total scores and scores of each category were examined, and the effects of age, sex and body mass index (BMI) on these scores were studied. The total scores toward overeating were significantly higher in the obese group than in nonobese group. Furthermore, age and sex affected the total score and/or scores in each category differently. These results suggest that eating behavior contributes to the development of obesity and that age and sex affect the relationship between eating behavior and obesity.

Keywords: body mass index, diabetes mellitus, obesity, overeating, questionnaire.

Background

Eating behaviors are a complex mixture of physiological and psychological phenomena. In the 1950s, Mayer classified obesity into three models: genetic, environmental and traumatic. The genetic model implies that the tendency towards obesity is inherited, whereas the environmental model states that obesity is caused by lifestyle and dietary intake. It is a biological fact that when more energy is consumed than is required, the results will be obesity.

NIDDM is associated with two major characteristics: 1) decreased sensitivity to insulin, which is more commonly known as insulin resistance; and 2) the decreased ability to secrete insulin, especially in response to glucose stimulation. It is still unclear which of these two characteristics is the primary defect in NIDDM, but both characteristics appear to contribute to the development of NIDDM. Since obesity is one of the major causes of insulin resistance, resulting in glucose intolerance and diabetes mellitus, overeating could be one of the major predisposing factors for the development of NIDDM. However, the contribution

Address for correspondence: Dr Hiroshi Ikegami, Department of Geriatric Medicine, Osaka University Medical School, 2-2 Yamadaoka, Suita, Osaka 565, Japan. Tel.: +81-6-879-3852. Fax: +81-6-879-3859.

of eating behavior to the development of obesity and/or diabetes mellitus is largely unknown due to the lack of measures for quantitating eating behavior and appetite. In this study an interview-based assessment was performed to assess the contribution of eating behavior to the development of obesity.

Methods

The subjects studied were 600 subjects (500 men and 100 women) who underwent an annual health checkup. Mean (±SD) age was 37.0 (±11.0) years and the mean body mass index (BMI) was 22.8 (±3.2) with the range of 17.2 to 35.6.

The measurement of the features of eating behavior is based on the method of Sakata et al. in Oita Medical University. Fifty questions were asked to the subjects and the eating behavior reflected by the answers to each question was scored. The questions were divided into seven categories: recognition, hunger, compensation, satiety, patterns, contents and rhythm. Recognition means that he or she easily develops obesity. Hunger means conscious sensation of hunger. Compensation means compensatory behaviors for eating. Satiety means lack of sensation of full stomach. Patterns means eating rapidly. Contents means addiction for greasy food. Rhythm means irregularity of dietary habits. The higher scores correspond to the abnormal eating behaviors.

Unpaired, two-tailed Student's t tests were used to compare scores among groups for static analysis. Date are expressed by mean ± SEM.

Results

Significant positive correlations were found between the total score and BMI ($r = 0.34$, $p < 0.0001$).

To elucidate the influence of eating behaviors on obesity, we divided subjects into three groups according to their BMI: 1) lean (BMI < 20), 2) normal (20 ⩽ BMI < 24), and 3) obese (BMI ⩾ 24). The total score for eating behavior in the obese group was highest, followed by normal ($p = 0.003$ vs. lean), and lean groups ($p < 0.0001$ vs. lean and normal). To investigate factors in eating behavior which contribute to the development of obesity, scores of individual categories were compared among lean, normal and obese groups. In the obese group, the scores for recognition ($p < 0.01$), hunger ($p < 0.01$), compensation ($p = 0.002$), satiety ($p = 0.0003$), patterns ($p < 0.05$), contents ($p < 0.05$) and rhythm ($p < 0.05$) were significantly higher than those of the lean group. In the obese group, the scores for recognition ($p < 0.01$), hunger ($p < 0.05$), compensation ($p < 0.05$), satiety ($p < 0.01$), patterns ($p < 0.0001$), contents ($p < 0.05$) and rhythm ($p < 0.05$) were significantly higher than those of the normal group.

Age is expected to be a factor that contributes to overeating. Therefore we examined the relationship between scores and age by dividing the subjects into age tertile. The total score was significantly lower in the older group than in intermediate and younger groups (older vs. younger, $p < 0.005$; intermediate vs. older,

$p<0.005$). To clarify which factors of eating behavior contribute to the development of obesity, scores from the individual categories were compared among the three groups. No significant difference was found in the categories of recognition, hunger and satiety. However, scores for compensation, contents and rhythm tended to be higher in the younger group and the score for patterns tended to be higher in the intermediate and older groups.

To study the sex difference in eating behavior, the total score and scores for each category were compared between males and females. No significant difference was found in total score between males and females. However, in the analysis of the scores from each category, scores for compensation ($p<0.0001$) and satiety ($p<0.001$) were higher in females and those for patterns ($p<0.0001$) and contents ($p<0.0001$) were higher in males.

Conclusions

In this study, we analysed eating behavior in subjects who underwent an annual health checkup by the interview-based questionnaires.

Previous reports showed that eating disturbances are common in young women with IDDM and are associated with impaired metabolic control, noncompliance to diabetes management, and more severe long-term medical complications of IDDM [1]. Recently, Justin et al. showed that prevalence of binge eating is higher in newly diagnosed NIDDM patients than in age-, sex- and weight-matched control subjects [2]. However, the questionnaires in these studies were based on the binge eating scale and designed to assess the psychiatric disorder, bulimia. In contrast, questionnaires used in this study for eating behavior were designed to assess the eating attitude and appetite which are more common than bulimia.

Positive correlation was found between total score for eating behavior and BMI, indicating that abnormality in eating behavior is significantly associated with obesity. Furthermore, detailed analysis of each category revealed that scores in obese subjects were significantly higher than those in lean and normal subjects in all categories. These data suggest that an improvement in eating behaviors in these categories will result in a reduction of body weight. Age and sex are considered to affect eating behavior and obesity. Our results suggest that the younger group tended to eat more under stress conditions and to eat greasy food and to have irregularity of dietary habits, and that intermediate and older groups tended to eat rapidly. Sex differences in scores for compensation, satiety, patterns and contents suggest that females eat more under stress conditions and that males prefer to eat more greasy food and eat more rapidly than females.

These data suggest that eating behavior contributes to the development of obesity and that eating behavior is affected by age and sex. These factors should be considered in the dietary education of obese subjects for successful therapy of obesity.

Acknowledgements

This study was supported in part by a grant for diabetes research from the Ministry of Health and Welfare, Grants-in-Aid for Scientific Research from the Ministry of Education, Science, Sports and Culture; a grant from the SANDOZ Foundation for Gerontological Research; and a grant from the Kato Memorial Trust for Nambyo Research.

References

1. Gary MR, Denis D. Eating disorders and IDDM. Diabet Care 1992;15:1402–1412.
2. Justin K et al. A comparison of eating behaviors in newly diagnosed NIDDM patients and case-matched control subjects. Diabet Care 1994;17:1197–1199.

Recent Advances on the Pathogenesis and Management of Diabetes Mellitus.
S.H. Shinn, M. Shichiri and K.-W. Kim, editors.

Mononuclear cell manganese superoxide dismutase (Mn-SOD) activity in non-insulin-dependent diabetic patients

Hyun-Chul Bae, Byoung-Ho Kong, Sung-Nam Choi, Kwang-Suk Kim, Yeon-Sahng Oh and Soon-Hyun Shinn

Department of Endocrinology and Metabolism, School of Medicine, Chung-Ang University, Seoul, Korea

Abstract. *Background.* There is some evidence that oxidative stress may play a role in the initiation and progression of diabetic complications. Superoxide dismutase (SOD) is an essential enzyme for dismutation of the superoxide (O_2^-) radical, and the activity is changed in some pathologic conditions such as diabetes. The aim of this study is to evaluate the association of SOD activity and severity of diabetic complication.

Methods. The Mn-SOD activities were measured in 34 patients with NIDDM and 16 normal controls using the spectrophotometric method, as described by Ross in 1979. The Mn-SOD activities were compared according to the severity of diabetic retinopathy, and were evaluated by correlation with various biochemical and clinical parameters.

Results. The Mn-SOD activity (U/mg protein) was significantly lower in diabetes patients than in normal controls (10.4 ± 1.8 and 12.9 ± 7.5 ($p < 0.05$), respectively). According to the severity of diabetic retinopathy, there was no statistical significance, but a decreasing tendency in Mn-SOD activity was observed. In diabetic patients, there was no correlation between Mn-SOD activity and various clinical and biochemical parameters.

Conclusion. With respect to our data, we observed low Mn-SOD activity in diabetic patients. However, we could not prove that the more severe the retinopathy, the lower the Mn-SOD; as it may only be related to a small number of patients with proliferative retinopathy.

Keywords: diabetic retinopathy, Mn-SOD, NIDDM.

Introduction

Reactive oxygen radicals such as superoxide anion (O_2^-) possess potent oxygen toxicity to cells [1–3]. Superoxide dismutase (SOD) is a essential enzyme for dismutation of O_2^- to H_2O_2 and O_2, so it is one of the most important initial components in the cellular defense mechanism against oxygen toxicity [4–6]. On the other hand, some previous reports have pointed out that this oxidative stress might be involved in the initiation and progression mechanisms of diabetic complications [7,8]. The aim of this study is to elucidate the association between burden of oxidative stress and severity of diabetic complications, especially diabetic retinopathy.

Address for correspondence: Hyun-Chul Bae MD, Chung-Ang University Medical Center, 82-1, Pil-Dong 2 Ga, Chung-Gu, Seoul, Korea. Tel.: +82-02-260-2184. Fax: +82-02-790-2068.

Material and Methods/Patients

Thirty-four patients with NIDDM and 16 normal controls were included. There were no significant differences in age, sex and BMI between control and diabetic patients groups (Table 1). In all diabetic patients, fundoscopic examinations were done separately by two ophthalmologists and the fluorescence angiography was checked. The results were then divided into three groups [8]: 1) no retinopathy (n = 20); 2) background retinopathy (n = 11); and 3) proliferative retinopathy (n = 3). IDDM, inflammatory or infectious disease, severe lung or liver disease and history of vitamin E medication were excluded because these conditions are prone to changes in SOD activity. For measurement of Mn-SOD activity, we used the method of Ross; mononuclear cells were separated with histopaque from whole blood and plasma membrane was disrupted by ultrasonic sonification method. Then, all three intracellular components of SOD were released. The Cu/Zn-SOD activity was excluded by precipitation with cyanide. The spectrophotometric method using cytochrome C and xanthine measured Mn-SOD activities. The stronger the SOD activity the more reduced form cytochrome C was induced from oxidized cytochrome C.

Results

The Mn-SOD activity (U/mg protein) was significantly lower in diabetics than in normal controls (10.4 ± 1.8 and 12.9 ± 7.5 ($p<0.05$), respectively). According to severity of diabetic retinopathy, there was no statistical significance, but a decreasing tendency in Mn-SOD activity was observed (Table 2). In diabetic patients there was no correlation between Mn-SOD activity and various clinical and biochemical parameters (Table 3).

Discussion

The Mn-SOD locates in the mitochondrial fraction of a cell. Therefore, we postu-

Table 1. Characteristics of the diabetes and controls group.

	Diabetes (n = 34)	Controls (n = 16)
Age (years)	60.0 ± 10.2	54 ± 6.4
BMI (kg/m^2)	22.6 ± 6.7	26.7 ± 5.8
Duration (M)	88.7 ± 48.8	
FBS (mg/dl)[a]	172.9 ± 75.7	83.1 ± 22.6
HbA1C (%)	8.3 ± 2.2	
T-chol (mg/dl)[a]	194.6 ± 47.9	149.3 ± 18.9
HDL-chol (mg/dl)	40.7 ± 9.0	38.8 ± 6.7
TG (mg/dl)[a]	157.5 ± 87.1	96.0 ± 34.5
Mn-SOD activity (U/mg protein)[a]	2.6 ± 1.8	12.9 ± 7.5

[a] $p<0.05$.

Table 2. Mn-SOD activity in diabetic retinopathy subgroups and normal controls.

	Number	Mn-SOD actibity(U/mg protein)
Nondiabetic controls	16	12.9 ± 7.5
NIDDM patients	34	10.4 ± 1.8^{a}
No retinopathy	20	12.8 ± 2.0
Background retinopathy	11	8.0 ± 1.3
Proliferative retinopathy	3	5.6 ± 0.5

$^{a}p < 0.05$.

lated that it may be a more representative enzyme of intracellular oxidative stress than cytosolic Cu/Zn-SOD. Furthermore, we used mononuclear cells because they express more stable SOD activities than other materials. In the results, the Mn-SOD activities were significantly lowered in NIDDM patients. It is unclear whether it is a result or primary cause of aggravated oxidative stress in diabetic patients. However, we believe that the decreased SOD activities might be related to the pathophysiologic mechanisms of NIDDM. A more detailed experiment to elucidate these complex findings is required. There was no correlation of Mn-SOD activities with severity of diabetic retinopathy and various clinical and biochemical parameters [9]. It may be related to the small number of patients with proliferative retinopathy and the duration of the diabetic complication.

Table 3. Simple linear regression analysis of Mn-SOD activity and clinical and biochemical variables in diabetic patients.

Independent variables	Correlation coefficients	p value
BMI (kg/m^2)	0.042	0.78
FBS (mg/dl)	0.058	0.70
HbA1C (%)	0.150	0.43
Total chol (mg/dl)	−0.081	0.61
HDL-chol (mg/dl)	0.193	0.22
TG (mg/dl)	−0.234	0.14
Diabetes duration	−0.116	0.526

References

1. Oberlyey L. Free radicals and diabetes. Free Rad Biol Med 1998;5:113–124.
2. Halliwell B, Gutteridge JMC. Free Radicals in Biology and Medicine. Oxford: Clarendon Press, 1989.
3. Packer L. The role of anti-oxidative treatment in diabetes mellitus. Diabetologia 1993;36: 1212–1213.
4. Altan N, Ongun C, Hasanoglu E et al. Effect of the sulfonylurea glyburide on superoxide dismutase activity in alloxan-induced diabetic rat hepatocytes. Diabet Res Clin Prac 1994;22(2/3): 95–98.

5. Asayama K, Nyfeler F, English D, Pilkis SJ, Burr M. Alloxan-induced free radical production in isolated cell: Selective effect on islet cells. Diabetes 1984;33:1008–1011.
6. Baynes JW. Role of oxidative stress in development of complications in diabetes. Diabetes 1991; 40:405–412.
7. Gandy SE, Buse MG, Crouch RK. Protective role of superoxide dismutase against diabetogenic drugs. J Clin Invest 1982;70:650–658.
8. Rema M, Mohan V, Bhaskar A et al. Does oxidant stress play a role in diabetic retinopathy? Indian J Opthalmol 1995;43(1):17–21.
9. Baynes JW. Role of oxidative stress in the development of complications in diabetes mellitus. Diabetes 1991;40:405–412.

Etiology

Recent Advances on the Pathogenesis and Management of Diabetes Mellitus.
S.H. Shinn, M. Shichiri and K.-W. Kim, editors.

Identification of glucokinase mutations in subjects with postrenal transplantation diabetes mellitus

H.C. Lee, J.H. Nam, Y.H. Kim, Y.J. Won, Y.D. Song, K.R. Kim and K.B. Huh
Division of Endocrinology, Department of Internal Medicine, Yonsei University College of Medicine, Seoul, Korea

Abstract. Mutations in the glucokinase (GCK) gene are considered a possible cause of maturity-onset diabetes of the young (MODY). The purpose of this study was to evaluate the contribution of this gene to the development of postrenal transplantation diabetes mellitus (PTDM). Identification of GCK mutation was attempted on 58 selected renal allograft recipients with PTDM and 45 normal controls. The exons in the GCK gene were examined by polymerase chain reaction (PCR) and single-stranded DNA conformational polymorphism (SSCP). The abnormal bands were also confirmed by DNA sequencing analysis. The exons of affected family members were also investigated for mutations of the GCK gene. Two of the 58 PTDM patients (3.4%) were found to have GCK mutations. The mutation of exon 5 was identified as a substitution of CCT (proline) for CTT (leucine) at codon 164, which has never been reported before. The abnormal band on the SSCP analysis of exon 7 was identified as the insertion of base C/T at the 39th nucleotide in intron 7. We found GCK mutations in subjects with PTDM and we speculate that GCK mutation is rare but that these mutations may be one of the contributing causes of PTDM.

Keywords: glucokinase, postrenal transplantation, diabetes mellitus.

Introduction

Glucokinase (GCK) is among the few candidate genes for diabetes mellitus (DM). Mutations in the GCK gene are considered a possible cause of maturity-onset diabetes of the young (MODY). It may be difficult to make an accurate diagnosis of MODY without obtaining thorough clinical, laboratory and family histories because DM caused by mutations in the GCK gene is usually associated with mild symptoms. Therefore, it is reasonable to speculate that a considerable proportion of patients with mutations of the GCK gene may be recognized as having the common form of NIDDM with onset late in life, gestational DM and postrenal transplantation diabetes mellitus (PTDM). The purpose of this study was to evaluate the contribution of this gene to the development of PTDM.

Subjects and Methods

The subject group consisted of 45 normal controls and 58 patients who were

Address for correspondence: Hyun Chul Lee MD, Professor of Internal Medicine, Division of Endocrinology and Metabolism, Severance Hospital Yonsei University College of Medicine, 134 Shinchon-dong Seodaemun-ku, Seoul 120-752, Korea. Tel.: +82-2-361-5425. Fax: +82-2-393-6884.

diagnosed with PTDM. All patients were being followed at the Endocrinology Department of Yonsei University College of Medicine. They were previously non-diabetic renal allograft recipients with PTDM. None were prone to ketosis. The exons in the GCK gene were examined by polymerase chain reaction (PCR) and single-stranded DNA conformational polymorphism (SSCP). The abnormal bands were also confirmed by DNA sequencing analysis. The exons of affected family members were also investigated for mutations of the GCK gene.

Results

Two of the 58 PTDM patients (3.4%) were found to have GCK mutations (Table 1). One had the mutation on exon 5 and the other on intron 7. One control subject had the mutation on intron 9. The mutation of exon 5 was identified as a substitution of CCT (proline) for CTT (leucine) at codon 164, which has never been reported before (Fig. 1). The abnormal band on the SSCP analysis of exon 7 was identified as the insertion of base C/T at the 39th nucleotide in intron 7 (Fig. 2). The one mutation of 45 normal controls was C→T located at the 8th nucleotide in intron 9, which was a common polymorphism. The patient who had the LEU (CTT)→Pro (CCT) mutation was a 35-year-old male and was an allograft recipient. He did not have DM before transplantation. His ideal body weight is 94% (weight 55 kg, height 165 cm). When he was examined, his fasting and 2-h values for glucose were 133 and 289 mg/dl, and for C-peptide were 4.03 and 5.40 ng/ml, respectively. His father and sister had mutations on exon 5 and neither were diagnosed with DM. He is now being treated with diet therapy. The subject who had the intron 7 mutation was a 49-year-old male who had not been diagnosed with DM before transplantation. His mother and son had the same mutation too. His ideal body weight is 112% (weight 67 kg, height 165 cm). When he was examined, his fasting and 2-h values for glucose were 70 and 114 mg/dl, and for C-peptide were 1.03 and 1.26 ng/ml, respectively. He is now being treated with oral agent therapy.

Discussion

To date, about 40 mutations in the GCK gene have been reported in many other countries. Although mutations in the GCK gene have been identified in nine dif-

Table 1. Summary of sequence variations of glucokinase gene in Korean subjects with PTDM and controls.

Position	Codon	Sequence
Exon 5	164	Leu (CTT) → Pro (CCT)
Intron 7	C/T insertion 39 bp dowstream from 3′-end	
Intron 9	8 bp downstream from 3′-end GCCCGCC → GCCTGCC	

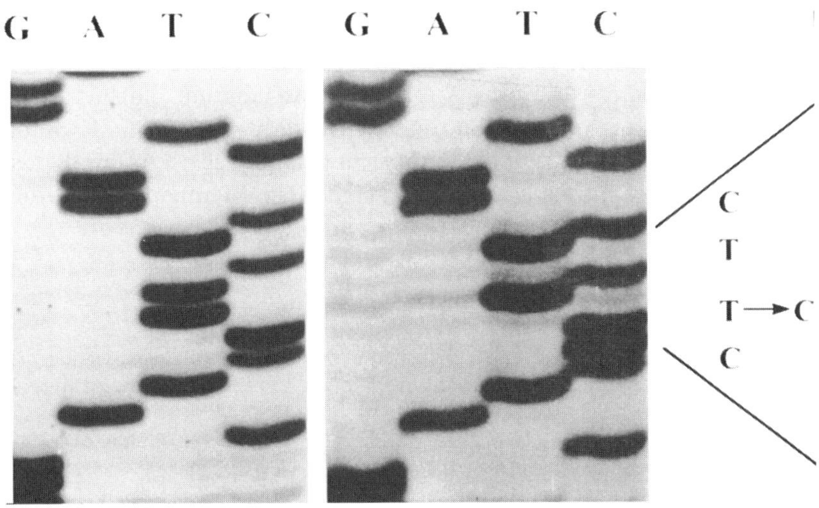

Fig. 1. The missense mutation in the exon 5.

ferent exons, the missense mutations occurring in four exons, exons 5, 6, 7, and 8 appear to be important, suggesting that these exons may encode functionally important domains of the protein [1,2]. We have identified a new missense mutation in the GCK gene in PTDM patients. This mutation was not seen in 45 controls. The effect of the $CTT^{Leu} \rightarrow CCT^{Pro}$ mutation on GCK has not been determined. However, CTT^{Leu} is located in a β-sheet surface loop that may affect conformational change and thereby alter the enzymatic properties of GCK

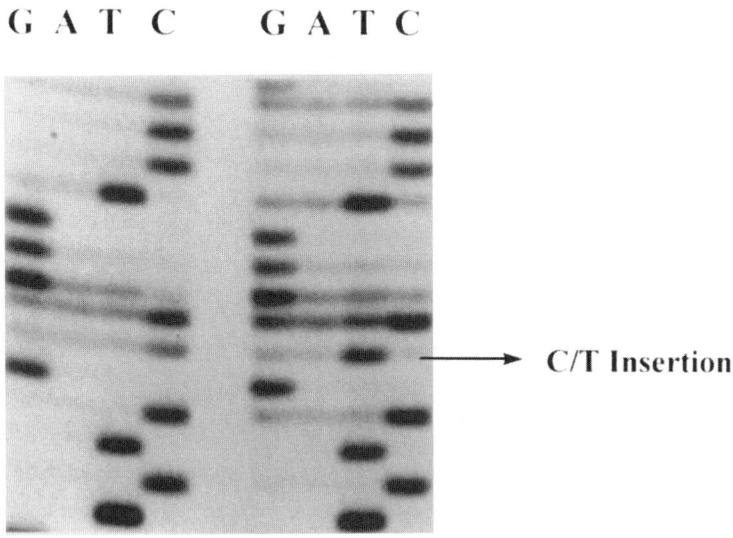

Fig. 2. The insertional mutation in the intron 7.

[3,4]. Considering the patient's insulin secretion capacity, this mutation may affect glucose disposal. The influence of the insertional mutation of intron 7 is not known because the introns have no known cellular function. Further study is required for the role of mutations of intron 7. This study suggests GCK mutations may occur in at least 3.4% of PTDM subjects without regard to family history of DM. In summary, this study indicates that PTDM might result from mutations in GCK.

References

1. Stoffel M, Froguel Ph, Takeda J et al. Human glucokinase gene: isolation, characterization, and identification of two missense mutations linked to early-onset non-insulin-dependent (type 2) diabetes mellitus. Proc Natl Acad Sci USA 1992;89:7698–7702.
2. Hughes SD, Johnson JH, Quaade C, Newgard CB. Engineering of glucose-stimulated insulin secretion and biosynthesis in nonislet cells. Proc Natl Acad Sci USA 1992;89:688–692.
3. Anderson CM, McDonald RC, Steitz TA. Sequencing a protein by X-ray crystallography. Interpretation of yeast hexokinase B 2.5 A resolution by model building. J Molec Biol 1978;123: 1–13.
4. Unger RH. Diabetic hyperglycemia: link to impaired glucose transport in pancreatic β cells. Science 1991;251:1200–1205.

Recent Advances on the Pathogenesis and Management of Diabetes Mellitus.
S.H. Shinn, M. Shichiri and K.-W. Kim, editors.

Insulin secretory defect as an early metabolic defect in offspring of NIDDM

Y.-S. Chung, K.-W. Lee and H.-M. Kim
Department of Endocrinology and Metabolism, Ajou University School of Medicine, Suwon, Korea

Abstract. *Background.* Pathogenesis of non-insulin-dependent diabetes mellitus (NIDDM) is heterogeneous; both insulin secretory defects and peripheral insulin resistance contribute to the development of NIDDM. The purpose of this study is to clarify the mechanism of early metabolic defects causing NIDDM in the offspring of Korean NIDDM patients.

Methods. Eight young control subjects and six healthy young offspring of NIDDM patients participated in this study. The 75-g oral glucose tolerance test (OGTT) with C-peptide and insulin response, euglycemic hyperinsulinemic clamp test, and hyperglycemic clamp test were performed.

Results. OGTT revealed that all of the study subjects had normal glucose tolerance levels. The offspring of NIDDM and control subjects showed similar insulin secretory capacity in OGTT. There was no significant difference in peripheral insulin sensitivity between control and offspring groups. Two out of the six offspring of NIDDM patients had decreases in the first and second phases of insulin secretion in the hyperglycemic clamp test compared to normal control subjects.

Keywords: early metabolic defect, family history, insulin secretion, offspring, pathogenesis.

Introduction

The pathogenesis of non-insulin-dependent diabetes mellitus (NIDDM) is heterogeneous, but it can be summarized as being the two major aspects of derangement in either insulin secretory defects or peripheral insulin resistance. The purpose of this study was to clarify the mechanism an of early metabolic defect causing NIDDM in the offspring of Korean NIDDM patients.

Material and Methods

Eight control subjects and six healthy offspring of NIDDM patients participated in this study. The 75-g oral glucose tolerance test (OGTT) with C-peptide and insulin responses was performed. The euglycemic hyperinsulinemic clamp test, and hyperglycemic clamp test were performed by the method described by DeFronzo et al. [1]. During the hyperglycemic clamp test, the first phase was defined as the mean of 0—10 min of insulin secretion, and the second phase as the mean of 10—120 min of insulin secretion. The serum glucose levels were measured using the glucose oxidase method. The serum C-peptide and insulin levels were measured by radioimmunoassay.

Address for correspondence: Yoon-Sok Chung MD, Department of Endocrinology and Metabolism, Ajou University School of Medicine, 5 Wonchon-Dong, Paldal-Gu, Suwon 442-749, South Korea.

Table 1. Clinical characteristics of the subjects.

	Control (n = 8)	Offspring (n = 5)
Age (years)	28.5 ± 1.6	25.4 ± 2.7
Sex (M:F)	8 : 0	3 : 2
Height (cm)	170 ± 2	169 ± 4
Weight (kg)	66.4 ± 3.3	66.4 ± 7.7
BMI (kg/m^2)	22.8 ± 0.9	22.9 ± 1.7
Body fat (%)	19.3 ± 1.4	21.0 ± 2.2

Note: BMI = body mass index.

Results

The clinical characteristics of the study subjects were similar between the two groups (Table 1). Serum glucose levels during the 75-g OGTT revealed that there was no significant difference between the two groups. Serum C-peptide areas under the curve were slightly higher in the control group compared to the offspring group. There was no significant difference in serum glucose and insulin areas under the curve during OGTT between the two groups. There was an early peak (at about 60 min) of insulin secretion in the control group. In contrast, a delayed peak (at about 90 min) of insulin secretion was observed in the offspring group (Table 2).

The peripheral glucose utilization rates in control and offspring groups were 8.71 ± 1.26 and 8.34 ± 1.01 mg/kg/min, respectively. The peripheral insulin sensitivities in control and offspring groups were 8.13 ± 1.34 and 8.87 ± 1.31 mg/kg/min/100 μU/ml insulin, respectively. There was no significant difference between control and offspring groups (Fig. 1).

In the control group, the first and second phases of insulin secretion were 37.7 ± 5.8 and 71.9 ± 19.9 μU/ml, respectively. In the offspring group, first and second phases of insulin secretion were 27.7 ± 7.1 and 46.4 ± 10.4 μU/ml, respectively. Both the first and second phases of insulin responses were slightly higher in the control group than in the offspring group (Fig. 2).

Table 2. Area under the curve during OGTT.

	Control (n = 8)	Offspring (n = 5)
Garea (mg/dl × h)	244 ± 11	242 ± 26
Carea (ng/dl × h)	13.6 ± 2.1	7.5 ± 1.1
Iarea (μU/ml × h)	75.4 ± 14.6	72.6 ± 21.1

Note: Garea = glucose area under the curve. Carea = C-peptide area under the curve. Iarea = insulin area under the curve.

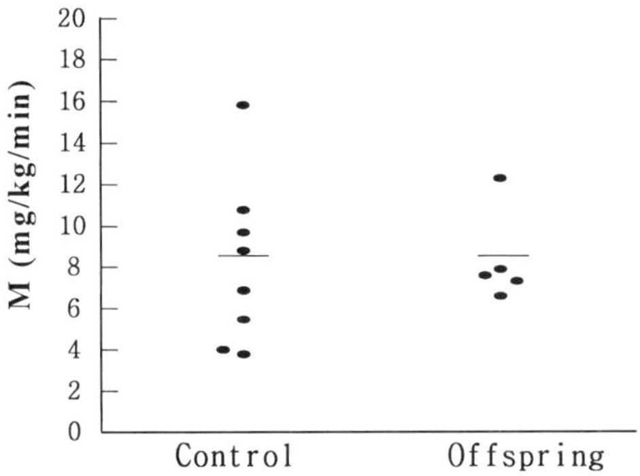

Fig. 1. Peripheral glucose utilization rate (M) during the euglycemic hyperinsulinemic clamp test.

Discussion

In this study, we tried to clarify the early metabolic defect in the development of NIDDM. We used the tools of the euglycemic hyperinsulinemic clamp test and hyperglycemic clamp test as methods of measuring peripheral insulin sensitivity and insulin secretion.

The lowest limits of peripheral insulin sensitivities were 3.8 mg/kg/min and 3.1 mg/kg/min/100 μU/ml insulin. None of the offspring of NIDDM had peripheral insulin resistance according to these criteria. The lowest limits of the first and second insulin secretory capacities in control subjects were 18 and 26 μU/ml, respectively. According to this cutoff point, two subjects from a total of six NIDDM patients' offspring revealed defects in the first and second phases of insulin secretion. The offspring of NIDDM patients had normal glucose tolerance, but they secreted less insulin in response to an intravenous glucose challenge.

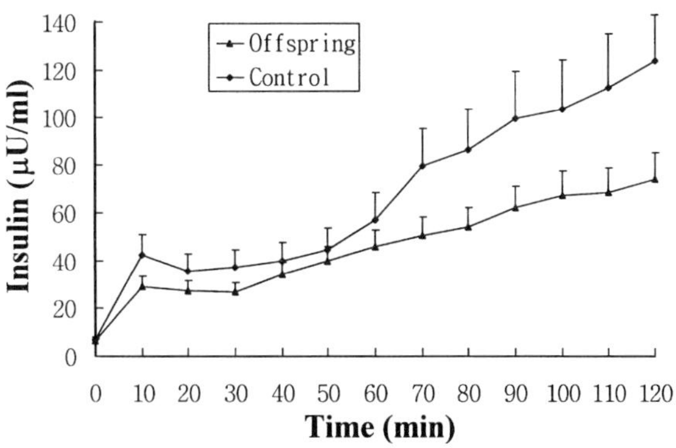

Fig. 2. Serum insulin levels during the hyperglycemic clamp test.

In Caucasians, peripheral insulin resistance with compensatory hyperinsulinemia usually precedes an insulin secretory defect [2]. But recently, Pimenta et al. [3] reported that pancreatic β cell dysfunction was the primary defect in first-degree NIDDM relatives. In this study, we also found that an insulin secretory defect was an early metabolic defect in Korean offspring of NIDDM patients. In conclusion, the early metabolic defects of Korean offspring of NIDDM patients may be related to an insulin secretory defect rather than peripheral insulin resistance.

Acknowledgements

We wish to thank H.C. Lim, B.J. Lee and Y.J. Kwak for their technical assistance, and Heather Yu for editing the research paper. This study was partly supported by a grant (#HMP-96-M-2-0018) of the 1996 Good Health R&D Project, Ministry of Health & Welfare, R.O.K.

References

1. DeFronzo RA, Tobin JD, Andres R. Glucose clamp technique: A method for quantifying insulin secretion and resistance. Am J Physiol 1979;237:E214–E223.
2. Yki-Jarvinen H. Role of insulin resistance in the pathogenesis of NIDDM. Diabetologia 1995; 38:1378–1388.
3. Pimenta W, Korytkowski M, Mitrakou A. Pancreatic beta-cell dysfunction as the primary genetic lesion in NIDDM. Evidence from studies in normal glucose-tolerant individuals with a first-degree NIDDM relative. JAMA 1995;273:1855–1861.

Recent Advances on the Pathogenesis and Management of Diabetes Mellitus.
S.H. Shinn, M. Shichiri and K.-W. Kim, editors.

Family history of diabetes and anti-GAD antibodies in nonobese NIDDM

Y. Yoshida, R. Hagura, G. Sugasawa and Y. Akanuma
The Institute for Diabetes Care and Research, Asahi Life Foundation, Tokyo, Japan

Abstract. *Background.* Genetic factors play a more important role in nonobese NIDDM than in obese NIDDM as far as the risk for development of NIDDM is concerned. On the other hand, since the frequency of nonobese patients is higher in SP-IDDM than in NIDDM, it is assumed that nonobese NIDDM patients can be expected to progress to slowly progressive IDDM (SP-IDDM) more often than obese NIDDM patients.

Methods. We compared the family history of diabetes and anti-GAD antibodies (anti-GAD Ab) in nonobese NIDDM patients (L: past maximal BMI < 23; n = 235) with those in obese NIDDM (O: past max IBM > 25; n = 729), slowly progressive IDDM (S: n = 91) and control subjects (C: n = 63).

Results. 1) The prevalence of a positive family history of diabetes in the first-degree relatives was 50%**, 49%**, 48%** and 11% in L, O, S and C, respectively (** vs. C, $p < 0.01$). 2) The prevalence of positive anti-GAD Ab in S (36.2%) was significantly higher than in L (3.0%, $p < 0.01$). Even when S cases with a past maximal BMI < 23 were examined, the prevalence of anti-GAD Ab was higher in S (33.0%) than in L. The frequency of positive anti-GAD Ab in C was 3.2%. 3) No significant difference was observed in the frequency of positive anti-GAD Ab in nonobese and obese SP-IDDM. The prevalence of positive anti-GAD Ab in S with a positive family history of diabetes (21%) was significantly lower than that in the negative family history group (50%, $p < 0.05$).

Conclusions. Our study demonstrated that there is a strong genetic factor in the etiology of nonobese NIDDM, and that autoimmunity plays an important role in the development of SP-IDDM. In SP-IDDM cases, the patients who have a positive family history of diabetes showed a significantly lower incidence of anti-GAD Ab than the patients with a negative family of diabetes. Thus, SP-IDDM is a heterogeneous disorder as far as its etiology is concerned.

Keywords: autoimmunity, etiology, slowly progressive IDDM.

introduction

Obesity is a major risk factor for NIDDM, but about 20% of all patients with NIDDM have never been obese. It is assumed that genetic factors are more strongly involved in the etiology of nonobese NIDDM than in obese NIDDM. On the other hand, we occasionally experience IDDM patients who initially had NIDDM which then showed progressive loss of β cell function, so-called slowly progressive IDDM (SP-IDDM). The frequency of obese patients is higher in NIDDM than in SP-IDDM. Thus, nonobese NIDDM patients can be expected to progress to SP-IDDM more often than obese NIDDM patients.

Therefore, we studied the family history of diabetes and the frequency of anti-

Address for correspondence: Yoko Yoshida, The Institute for Diabetes Care and Research, Asahi Life Foundation, 1-6-1 Marunouchi, Chiyoda-ku, Tokyo 100, Japan.

GAD Ab in nonobese NIDDM patients, and the results were compared with those in obese NIDDM patients, SP-IDDM patients and nonobese control subjects.

Subjects and Methods

The subjects were as follows:

1. Nonobese NIDDM patients are defined as NIDDM patients with a past maximal body mass index (BMI) of less than 23 (n = 235; M/F = 189/46; age (mean ± SD); 60 ± 9 years; duration: 14 ± 8 years).
2. Obese NIDDM patients are NIDDM patients with a maximal BMI of more than 25 (n = 729; 506/223; 58 ± 11 years; 12 ± 8 years).
3. SP-IDDM patients are defined as those initially diagnosed as NIDDM, but then progressed to insulin dependency (proneness to ketosis and dependence on exogenous insulin to sustain life) within several months or a few years. In these SP-IDDM patients, the time period until starting insulin treatment after diagnosis was more than 3 months, and the 24-h urine CPR was under 20 μg/day (n = 91; 51/40; 55 ± 14 years**; 17 ± 9 years**; (** vs. nonobese NIDDM, $p<0.01$)).
4. Nondiabetic controls: cases with a past maximal BMI of less than 23 (n = 63; 3/60; 33 ± 11 years).

A questionnaire and interviewing were used for the examination of diabetes patients and control cases. Anti-GAD Ab were assayed using an anti-GAD immunoassay kit (RIP Anti-GAD, Hoechst).

Results

1. The incidence of a positive family history of diabetes in the first-degree relatives was 50.2, 48.6, 48.4 and 11.1% in nonobese NIDDM, obese-NIDDM, SP-IDDM and the controls, respectively. The prevalence was significantly higher in each diabetic patient group than in the controls. The prevalence in nonobese NIDDM was almost the same as in obese-NIDDM and SP-IDDM.
2. The frequency of positive anti-GAD Ab in SP-IDDM (36.2%) was significantly higher than that in nonobese NIDDM (3.0%, $p<0.01$) (Table 1). Even when SP-IDDM patients with a past maximal BMI of less than 23 were studied, the frequency of anti-GAD Ab was higher in SP-IDDM (30%) than in nonobese NIDDM ($p<0.01$). Only one obese NIDDM patient among 168 cases (0.6%) was positive for these antibodies. The frequency of positive anti-GAD Ab in the controls was 3.2%, which was similar to the frequency in nonobese NIDDM.

   In the nonobese NIDDM patients positive for anti-GAD Ab the incidence of a positive family history of diabetes was 43% (3/7), while the incidence of positive islet cell antibody (ICA) was 17% (1/6). HLA-DR9 was present in 4/6. Neither DR4 nor DR2 was found.

Table 1. Comparison of frequency of positive anti-GAD antibodies.

	Nonobese NIDDM		Obese NIDDM		SP-IDDM		SP-IDDM (BMI < 23)		Control	
	%	n	%	n	%	n	%	n	%	n
Frequency of positive anti-GAD	3.0	7/235	0.6	1/168	36.2	25/69	33.3	11/33	3.2	2/63

Nonobese NIDDM vs. SP-IDDM: $p<0.01$
Nonobese NIDDM vs. SP-IDDM (BMI < 23): $p<0.01$

3. Forty-eight percent of the SP-IDDM subjects had a BMI < 23 and 52% were ⩾23. However, there was no difference in the positive rate of the anti-GAD Ab between the BMI < 23 and BMI ⩾ 223 groups. In the SP-IDDM patients, the frequency of positive anti-GAD Ab in the patients with a positive family history was significantly lower than in the patients with a negative family history (21 vs. 50%, Table 2).

Discussion

According to the WHO Study Group, NIDDM is classified into "obese" and "nonobese" subtypes. These two subtypes probably reflect underlying differences in the etiologic mechanisms [1]. Köbberling [2] showed that the siblings of nonobese diabetics have a significantly higher chance of becoming diabetic than the siblings of very obese diabetics. Genetic factors, although not clarified at present, are thought to be more strongly associated with the etiology of nonobese NIDDM. Since the prevalence of a positive family history of NIDDM in SP-IDDM was almost the same as in NIDDM, there is a possibility that not only immunogenetic but genetic factors play an important role in the development of SP-IDDM. Kobayashi et al. [3] and Cheta et al. [4] reported that the incidence of a positive family history of diabetes was higher in SP-IDDM than in acute-onset IDDM.

The incidence of anti-GAD Ab, which are thought to be a predictor of insulin dependency [5], was slightly higher in nonobese than in obese NIDDM, but the

Table 2. Family history of diabetes and frequemcy of positive anti-GAD antibodies in SP-IDDM.

	Family history of diabetes			
	Positive (%)	Negative (%)	Positive (n)	Negative (n)
Prevalence of positive anti-GAD antibodies	21.2	50.0	7/33	18/36

Note: $p<0.05$.

difference was not significant. However, more cases must be studied to draw a clear conclusion.

In this study, we found that the frequency of positive anti-GAD Ab was significantly lower in the patients with a positive family history of diabetes than in the patients with a negative family history, which indicates that SP-IDDM is etiologically heterogeneous.

Conclusion

Our study demonstrated a strong genetic factor but almost no role of autoimmunity in the etiology of nonobese NIDDM. On the other hand, autoimmunity plays an important role in the development of SP-IDDM. In SP-IDDM patients, the patients who have a positive family history of diabetes showed a significantly lower incidence of anti-GAD Ab than the patients with a negative family history of diabetes. Thus, SP-IDDM is a heterogeneous disorder as far as its etiology is concerned.

Acknowledgements

We gratefully acknowledge the skilled assistance of Miss Chika Saga.

References

1. WHO Study Group on Diabetes Mellitus. Geneva, World Health Organization, 1985 (WHO Technical Report Series, No. 727).
2. Köbberling J. Studies on the genetic heterogeneity of diabetes mellitus. Diabetologia 1971;7: 46–49.
3. Kobayashi T, Tamemoto K, Nakanishi K, Kato N, Okubo M, Kajio H, Sugimoto T, Murase T, Kosaka K. Immunogenic and clinical characterization of slowly progressive IDDM. Diabet Care 1993;16:780–788.
4. Cheta D, Dumitrescu G, Georgescu M, Cocioaba G, Lichiardopol R, Stamoran M, Ionescu-Tirgoviste G, Paunescu-Georgescu M, Mincu I. A study on the types of diabetes mellitus in first degree relatives of diabetic patients. Diabetes Metab 1990;16:11–15.
5. Zimmet PZ, Tuomi T, Mackay IR, Rowley MJ, Knowles W, Cohen M, Lang DA. Latent autoimmune diabetes mellitus in adults (LADA): The role of antibodies to glutamic acid decarboxylase in diagnosis and prediction of insulin dependency. Diabet Med 1994;11:299–303.

Recent Advances on the Pathogenesis and Management of Diabetes Mellitus.
S.H. Shinn, M. Shichiri and K.-W. Kim, editors.

Risk factor determination for pregnancy-induced impaired glucose tolerance (IGT)

N.H. Cho[1], H.M. Kim[2], K.S. Oh[3], Y.S. Chung[2], K.W. Lee[2], J.I. Yang[3], H.S. Kim[3] and H.M. Kim[4]

Departments of [1]Preventive Medicine, [2]Endocrinology, [3]Obestetrics and Gynecology, Ajou University School of Medicine, Suwon; and [4]Department of Food and Nutrition, Sookmyung Women's University, Seoul, Korea

Abstract. *Background.* A number of reports show that some genetic, demographic and maternal physical characteristics predict gestational diabetes mellitus (GDM). However, these predictive variables were influenced by ethnicity and geographic settings. Therefore, in this study, we investigated demographic and maternal physical characteristics for pregnancy-induced impaired glucose tolerance (IGT) (i.e., a single positive for screening criteria and GDM).

Methods. The study consisted of 817 subjects with normal pregnancy and 94 with IGT. The independent t test was used to compare mean differences, the χ^2 test for categorical variables, and the multiple logistic regression analysis to investigate the independent effect of putative variables for IGT.

Results. The mean maternal age (28.8 ± 3.7, 31.2 ± 4.2, $p<0.05$), BMI (20.7 ± 2.8, 22.5 ± 4 kg/m^2, $p<0.001$), diastolic blood pressure (71.1 ± 8.1, 74.5 ± 9.4, $p<0.05$), systolic blood pressure (112.9 ± 10.4, 116.5 ± 12.7, $p<0.05$), and weight at the time of examination (52.9 ± 7.5, 56.3 ± 10, $p<0.001$) were significantly higher in the IGT group. Spouse's educational level (SEL) was lower (45 vs. 68%, odds ratio (OR) = 0.58, 95% CI 0.37–0.93; $\chi^2 = 5.3$, $p<0.05$), and family history of diabetes (DM) was higher (24.2 vs. 14.3%, OR = 1.9, 95% CI 1.1–3.2; $\chi^2 = 6.1$, $p<0.05$) in the IGT group. No differences were observed in maternal educational level and parity. When these relationships were further evaluated using the multiple logistic model after controlling for potential confounders, we observed negative associations between IGT and beer imbibe status (BIS), SEL and maternal height. On the other hand, age, DBP, and DM status were positively associated with IGT. Adjusted OR for SEL was similar to unadjusted, but DM status improved (OR = 2.3, 95% CI 1.2–4.5), and BIS was magnified (OR = 0.4, 95% CI 0.19–0.88) in the adjusted model.

Conclusion. In this study, we found that maternal age, height, DBP, SEL, BIS and DM were independently associated with IGT.

Keywords: gestational diabetes mellitus, Korean women, risk factors.

Introduction

Gestational diabetes mellitus (GDM) complicates 0.5–16% of all pregnancies and it is associated with an adverse outcome of pregnancy including macrosomia, birth trauma and metabolic complications in the newborn [1–4]. Risk factors for GDM include older maternal age, obesity, family history of diabetes and previous unexplained stillbirths or babies with congenital abnormalities [5].

Address for correspondence: N.H. Cho, Department of Preventive Medicine, Ajou University School of Medicine, #5 Wonchon-Dong, Paldal-Gu, Suwon 442-749, Korea.

However, it is unclear whether these same risk factors interplay for GDM in Korean women. Therefore, the purpose of this study was to determine which pregnancy characteristics were associated with diagnosis of pregnancy-induced impaired glucose tolerance (IGT) in Korean women.

Materials and Methods

All pregnant women who visited Ajou University Hospital from 1 February 1995, to 31 March 1997, for antepartum care underwent universal screening with a 50-g glucose load at 24–28 weeks gestational age. Multiple gestations and patients with chronic medical conditions were excluded. Those with a 1-h plasma glucose $\geqslant 130$ mg/dl underwent a 3-h, 100-g oral glucose tolerance test (OGTT) after 8 h of fasting but not exceeding 14 h. Subjects were considered to have GDM if at least two values, and IGT if at least one value reached or exceeded the following: 105 mg/dl on fasting, 190 mg/dl at 1 h, 165 mg/dl at 2 h, and 145 mg/dl at 3 h [6]. Demographic, lifestyle and metabolic variables were evaluated as potential risk factors. Analysis of variance, the χ^2 test and the multiple logistic regression analysis were used to investigate the independent effect of putative variables for IGT (single positive and GDM).

Results

The study consisted of 820 subjects with normal pregnancy and 94 with IGT (48 single positives and 47 GDM). As shown in Table 1, the mean maternal age, BMI, weight, systolic blood pressure, diastolic blood pressure, beer imbibe status and family history of diabetes were significantly different among the three groups. Spouse's education level was marginally ($p = 0.07$) lower in single positive and GDM groups compared to the normal group. However, no differences were

Table 1. Demographic characteristics of the study population.

Variable	Normal	Single positive	GDM	p value
Maternal age (years)	28.8 ± 3.7	30.5 ± 4.0	31.9 ± 4.3	< 0.001
Gestational age @ exam (week)	28.1 ± 3.7	28.4 ± 4.4	28.4 ± 3.7	ns
Age at menarch (years)	14.4 ± 1.4	14.8 ± 1.9	14.3 ± 1.4	ns
BMI (kg/m^2)	20.7 ± 2.8	21.7 ± 3.1	23.4 ± 4.6	< 0.001
Weight (kg)	52.9 ± 7.5	54.0 ± 7.8	58.6 ± 11.4	< 0.001
Weight change (kg)[a]	2.4 ± 3.3	2.3 ± 2.9	2.8 ± 3.4	ns
Systolic blood pressure (mmHg)	112.9 ± 10.3	114.4 ± 12.3	118.5 ± 12.9	< 0.01
Diastolic blood pressure (mmHg)	71.0 ± 8.0	72.7 ± 8.5	76.3 ± 10.1	< 0.001
Socioeconomic status	20.7%	19.5%	13.3%	ns
Beer imbibe	29.2%	21.7%	17.8%	0.054
Family history of DM	14.3%	22.7%	25.5%	< 0.05

[a]Weight change during the past 3 months prior to the examination. Other variables evaluated: level of education, parity and level of exercise.

Table 2. Multivariate analysis: multiple logistic regression.

Variable	β	p value	Adjusted odds ratio
Beer imbibe	−0.88	<0.05	0.4 (0.2∼0.9)
Family history of DM	0.846	<0.05	2.3 (1.2∼4.5)
Spouse's education level	−0.54	<0.05	0.6 (0.4∼0.9)
Diastolic blood pressure	0.04	<0.01	
Maternal age	0.159	<0.0001	

observed in maternal educational level, age at menarch, mean weight changes during the 3 months prior to the examination, gestational age at examination, socioeconomic level and parity. When these variables were further evaluated using the multiple logistic model after controlling for potential confounders we observed negative associations between IGT and beer imbibe status, spouse educational level. Maternal age, diastolic blood pressure, and family history of diabetes were positively associated with IGT. Adjusted odds ratio (OR) for spouse's educational level was similar to unadjusted, but family history of diabetes improved (OR = 2.3, 95% CI 1.2—4.5), and beer imbibe status was magnified (OR = 0.4, 95% CI 0.19—0.88) in the adjusted model (Table 2).

Discussion

In this study we found that maternal older age, elevated diastolic blood pressure, lower spouse's educational level, beer drinking and family history of diabetes were independently associated with IGT. Similar to the previous reports, we also revealed that older maternal age and family history of diabetes were risk factors for IGT. However, we found an interesting phenomenon that drinking beer during pregnancy plays a protective role against IGT but a lower spouse's educational level and a higher diastolic blood pressure increases the risk for IGT. No association was seen with other types of alcohol. Spouse's education level was positively correlated with the women's education level, and obesity was inversely correlated with the women's education level. Thus, when we analyzed these variables with IGT using multivariate analysis, including both variables (women's educational level and obesity level), the obesity level masks an influence of the women's educational level on IGT. When the women's educational level was used alone it stayed in the model independently. A positive relationship between diastolic blood pressure and IGT was seen in other previous studies. These studies indicated that hyperinsulinemia was positively correlated with antepartum blood pressure.

References

1. Hadden DR. Geographic, ethnic, and racial variations in the incidence of gestational diabetes. Diabetes 1985;34(Suppl 2):8—12.

2. Jacobson JD, Cousins L. A population-based study of maternal and perinatal outcome in patients with gestational diabetes. Am J Obstet Gynecol 1989;161:981–986.
3. Jang HC, Cho NH, Min YK, Han IK, Jung KB, Metzger BE. Increased macrosomia and perinatal morbidity independent of maternal obesity and advanced age in Korean women with gestational diabetes mellitus. Diabet Care (In press).
4. Langer O, Levy J, Brustman L, Anyaegbunam A, Merkatz R, Divon M. Glycemic control in gestational diabetes mellitus – how tight is tight enough: small for gestational age versus large for gestational age? Am J Obstet Gynecol 1989;161:646–653.
5. Stewart M, Taylor R. Gestational diabetes mellitus. Prof Care Mother Child 1994;4(5):136–138.
6. National Diabetes Data Group. Classification and diagnosis of diabetes and other categories of glucose intolerance. Diabetes 1979;28:1039–1057.

Recent Advances on the Pathogenesis and Management of Diabetes Mellitus.
S.H. Shinn, M. Shichiri and K.-W. Kim, editors.

Peripheral blood mitochondrial DNA content can predict the development of diabetes

J.J. Koh, J.H. Song, C.S. Shin, D.J. Park, S.Y. Kim, B.Y. Cho, H.K. Lee and C.-S. Koh
Department of Internal Medicine, Seoul National University Hospital, Seoul, South Korea

Introduction

Recent studies have revealed that a mitochondrial gene mutation at 3243 is associated with insulin-dependent diabetes (IDDM), and non-insulin-dependent diabetes mellitus (NIDDM) with deafness. MtDNA abnormalities were one of the candidate diabetogenic genes, since oxidative phosphorylation in mitochondria is believed to be important for the insulin secretion. Most studies on the relationship between diabetes mellitus (DM) and mtDNA have been concerned with its qualitative changes, such as mutations and deletions but rarely on its quantitative aspects. We found that mtDNA quantity was decreased in the peripheral blood of diabetic patients in 1994, and in 1995 Antonetti et al. reported that it decreased in skeletal muscle of humans with DM [7]. This study was performed to investigate whether mtDNA contents in the peripheral blood could predict the development of diabetes.

Methods

Subjects

The peripheral blood samples were collected in the Younchon County Basal Survey in 1993, and in 1995 a second survey was carried out. Sixty-six newly developed diabetic subjects were found from stored samples of the first survey, we selected 22 samples of subjects who became diabetic converters in 1995, and 23 samples of age- and gender-matched control subjects as nonconverters.

Internal standard for quantitative PCR

DNA was extracted from a stored peripheral blood leukocyte using a QIAamp blood kit. An internal standard is needed to compare the efficacy of competitive PCR amplification in each reaction. Two independent PCR amplification using sets of mtF1 (CCTAGGGATAACAGCGCATT 2928-2947) and JS3 (GCCA-

TGGGTAGGGCTCTGCCATCTTAACAA 3317-3308 3247-3228), and (mtR1-TAGAAGAGCGATGGTGAGAG 3358-3539) and JS4 (GGCAGAGCCCTA-CCCATGGCCAACCTCCTA 3238-3247,3308-3317) produced 331 and 261 base pairs, respectively. Secondary PCR amplification using the above products and primers mtF1 and mtR1 produced 571 base pair fragments and deletion of the intervening 60 base pairs. The internal standard has the same primer templates as the target gene and can compete with the target DNA in the PCR process but was designed to generate a skipped 60 base pairs size of PCR product (Fig. 1). The reaction condition was as follows: 1 cycle of 3 min at 94°C, 1 min at 60°C, 1 min at 72°C, and 34 cycles of 40 s at 94°C, 1 min at 60°C, 1 min at 72°C, and final extension at 72°C for 10 min. Figure 1 shows a PCR product that was analyzed on agarose gel by electrophoresis. Competition equivalence points were determined by interpolation of the graph, and the calculated ratio of the signals for internal standard bands to the signals for target bands. Ligation of the 3932 bp vector and 571 bp insert makes plasmid DNA containing 4503 bp fragments. (MW of competitive template = the number of base pair × 649 daltons/base pair = 2,922,447 (2.92×10^6); 1 μg plasmid = 0.3425×10^{-12} mol = 2.055×10^{11} copy number (1 mol = 6×10^{23} molecules)).

Results

The characteristics of subjects and mean mtDNA quantities are shown in Table 1. The mean mtDNA contents of a diabetic converter's peripheral blood leukocyte (0.86 ± 0.35) was significantly decreased compared to that of a nonconverter's (1.14 ± 0.57, $p<0.05$, Fig. 2). The relationships between mtDNA and waist:hip ratios from the first and second surveys are shown in Fig. 3. The mtDNA contents as a picogram template DNA over the copy number of mtDNA was negatively correlated with the waist:hip ratio in the first and second surveys (Fig. 3). The copy number of mtDNA was negatively correlated with diastolic blood pressure and fasting glucose concentration in the second survey (Fig. 4).

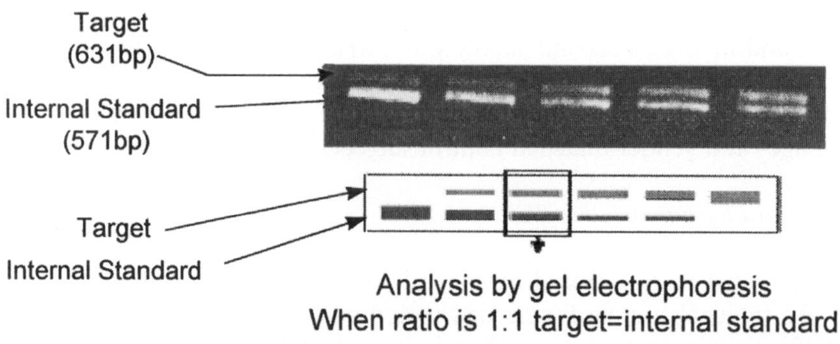

Fig. 1. Internal standard for quantitative PCR.

Table 1. Clinical characteristics of the subjects.

	Converter to diabetes (n = 23)	Nonconverter (n = 22)	p value
Age (years)	60.0 ± 11.8	57.5 ± 13.8	ns
Sex (M/F)	12/11	14/9	ns
BMI (kg/m^2)	24.8 ± 4.1	23.8 ± 3.5	ns
WHR	0.90 ± 0.05	0.89 ± 0.05	ns
Fasting glucose (mg/dl)	104.7 ± 13.4	100.5 ± 9.5	ns
PP2 (mg/dl)	118.1 ± 30.0	120.4 ± 31.4	ns
SBP (mmHg)	132.2 ± 18.8	128.4 ± 23.2	ns
DBP (mmHg)	82.5 ± 12.2	84.6 ± 17.7	ns
Cholesterol (mg/dl)	162.1 ± 37.8	156.1 ± 29.5	ns
Triglyceride (mg/dl)	155.6 ± 95.7	122.1 ± 82.1	ns
HDL-cholesterol (mg/dl)	35.4 ± 8.9	34.1 ± 9.0	ns

Conclusion and Discussion

MtDNA content of peripheral blood leukocyte was decreased in diabetic converters before the development of diabetes. The lower amounts of mtDNA were negatively correlated with weight:hip ratios in the first and second surveys, and with diastolic blood pressure and fasting glucose level in the second survey. The mtDNA contents in the peripheral blood leukocyte were able to predict the development of diabetes.

Allele-specific quantitation DNA can be very complicated and even with current technologies results are still highly variable. In our studies, single determination resulted in a 30% coefficient variation. We overcame the problem of variance with multiple measurements of single samples; at least four times. All the measurements reported in this study were done using one batch of internal standard

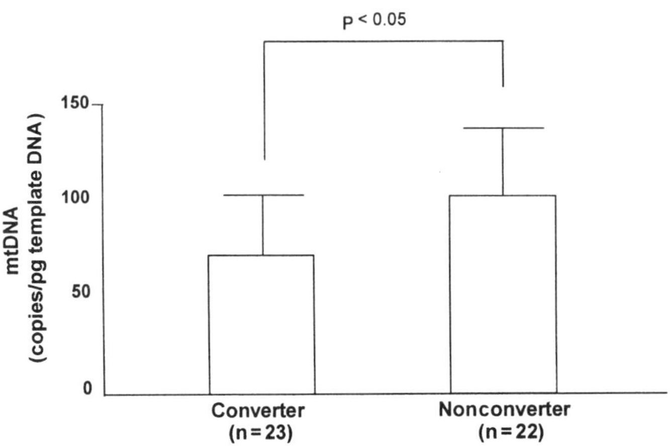

Fig. 2. Peripheral leukocyte mtDNA content.

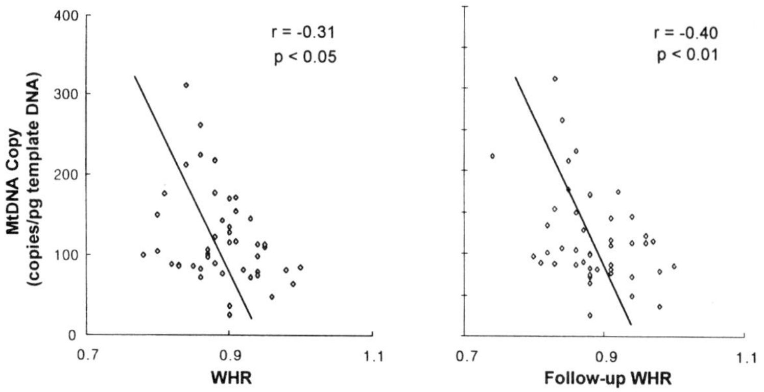

Fig. 3. Peripheral leukocyte mtDNA content and WHR.

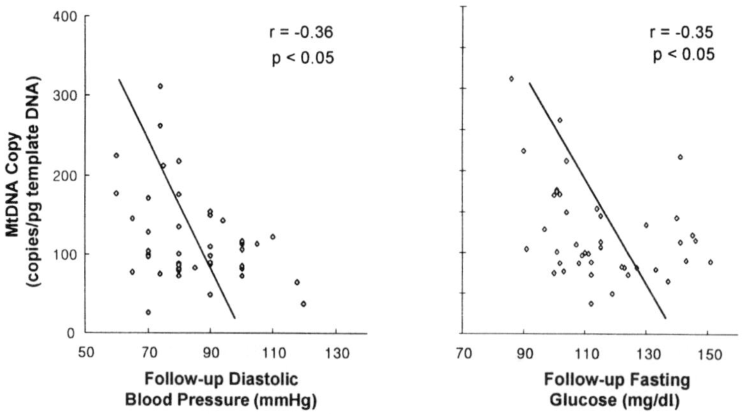

Fig. 4. Peripheral leukocyte mtDNA content and blood pressure and fasting glucose.

and reagents, a change of which sometimes resulted in a very difficult result, even for the same sample. Lower amounts of mtDNA in the peripheral blood leukocyte could not cause diabetes, hypertension or abdominal obesity. We believe that this decrease should reflect the general decrease of mtDNA in the body. The fact that heteroplasmy of mitochondric-different tissue has different mtDNA even with the same maternally inherited gene is well known. In this regard, although the question of whether the decrease in mtDNA content in the buffy coat is generalized or limited to the subpopulation of peripheral blood cells cannot be answered at this moment, the latter case does seem more likely.

Additional reading

1. Park Y, Lee H, Koh CS, Min H, Yoo K, Kim Y, Shin YP. Revalence of diabetes and IGT in Yonchon County, South Korea. Diabet Care 1995;18(4):545–548.

2. Shin CS. Quantitative abnormalities of mitochondrial DNA in non-insulin-dependent diabetes mellitus. Korean J Diabet Assos 1994;18:344–350.
3. Reaven GM. Role of insulin resistance in the pathophysiology of non-insulin dependent diabetes mellitus. Diabet Metab Rev 1993;9(Suppl 1):5S–12S.
4. Hales CN, Barker DJ. Type 2 (non-insulin-dependent) diabetes mellitus: the thrifty phenotype hypothesis [see comments]. Diabetologia 1992;35(7):595–601.
5. Gerbitz KD, van den Ouweland JM, Maassen JA, Jaksch M. Mitochondrial diabetes mellitus: a review. Biochim Biophys Acta 1995;1271(1):253–260.
6. Shigenaga MK, Ames BN. Oxidants and mitogenesis as causes of mutation and cancer: the influence of diet. Basic Life Sci 1993;61:419–436.
7. Antonetti DA, Reynet C, Kahn CR. Increased expression of mitochondrial-encoded genes in skeletal muscle of humans with diabetes mellitus. J Clin Invest 1995;95(3):1383–1388.
8. Wang H, Fliegel L, Cass CE, Penn AM, Michalak M, Weiner JH, Lemire BD. Quantification of mitochondrial DNA in heteroplasmic fibroblasts with competitive PCR. Biotechniques 1994; 17(1):76–78, 80, 82.

Recent Advances on the Pathogenesis and Management of Diabetes Mellitus.
S.H. Shinn, M. Shichiri and K.-W. Kim, editors.

Absence of a Gly40Ser mutation in the glucagon receptor genes of Japanese NIDDM and hypertension patients

N. Babaya, H. Ikegami, T. Fujisawa, E. Yamato, Y. Kawaguchi, Y. Hamada, M. Hotta, H. Ueda, M. Shintani, K. Nojima, Y. Kawabata, J. Fu, G.-Q. Shen and T. Ogihara
Department of Geriatric Medicine, Osaka University Medical School, Osaka, Japan

Abstract. A possible pathogenic mutation in the glucagon receptor gene causing a glycine to serine change at codon 40 (Gly40Ser) was reported to be associated with non-insulin-dependent diabetes mellitus (NIDDM) and essential hypertension in several Caucasian populations. Since frequencies of the mutation were much higher than that of any of the previously reported mutations in candidate genes, it is important to clarify whether this mutation contributes to the diseases universally. In this study, we investigated the association of this mutation with NIDDM and/or hypertension in a large number of Japanese patients. None of the Japanese patients with NIDDM and/or hypertension had a Gly40Ser mutation, and the frequencies of this mutation in Japanese were significantly lower than those in Caucasian populations. These results not only indicate that the Gly40Ser mutation in the glucagon receptor gene plays little, if any, role in susceptibility to NIDDM or essential hypertension in Japanese, but also indicate the genetic heterogeneity in these diseases and further emphasize the importance of studies on genetic susceptibility to complex traits in different ethnic groups.

Keywords: association, genetic susceptibility, missense mutation.

Introduction

Non-insulin-dependent diabetes mellitus (NIDDM) and essential hypertension are genetically and clinically heterogenous disorders. Although several mutations in candidate genes, such as insulin, insulin receptor and glucokinase genes [1,2], mitochondrial DNA [3] in NIDDM, and the angiotensinogen gene [4] in essential hypertension have been identified, these mutations were found only in a small number of patients with NIDDM or hypertension.

Recently, Hager et al. reported an association and linkage of a possible pathogenetic mutation in the glucagon receptor gene causing a glycine to serine change at codon 40 (Gly40ser) with NIDDM in France and Sardinia [5]. Frequencies of the mutation, about 5% in patients with familial NIDDM in France and 8% in randomly chosen diabetic patients in Sardinia, were significantly higher than those in control subjects. More recently, Chambers et al. reported that the Gly40-Ser mutation in the glucagon receptor gene was found in 5% (seven out of 130)

Address for correspondence: Hiroshi Ikegami MD, Department of Geriatric Medicine, Osaka University Medical School, 2-2 Yamadaoka, Suita, Osaka 565, Japan. Tel.: +81-6-879-3852. Fax: +81-6-879-3859.

of Caucasian patients with familial essential hypertension, whereas only 1% (one out of 90) of control subjects had the mutation. In addition, the age at onset of hypertension was significantly older in patients with the mutation than that of those without [6].

Since the frequencies of the mutation were much higher than that of any of the mutations in candidate genes reported so far, it is important to clarify whether this mutation contributes to the diseases universally or not. In this study, we investigated the frequencies of the Gly40Ser mutation in Japanese patients with NIDDM and/or hypertension.

Materials and Methods

We evaluated 383 unrelated Japanese patients with NIDDM [7], and 188 unrelated Japanese patients with hypertension [8]. NIDDM was diagnosed according to the guidelines of the National Diabetes Data group. Hypertension was diagnosed according to the criteria of WHO. A Gly40Ser mutation of the glucagon receptor gene was detected using the PCR-RFLP method, as reported previously [5]. Statistical analysis was performed using Fisher's exact test.

Results

All 383 NIDDM patients in the present study were homozygotes for the wild-type allele, and none of the patients had the Gly40Ser mutation of the glucagon receptor gene. None of the patients with hypertension had the Gly40Ser mutation in the glucagon receptor gene either. The frequencies of Gly40Ser mutation in NIDDM and hypertension were significantly lower than those reported in Caucasian populations (Figs. 1 and 2) [5,6,9].

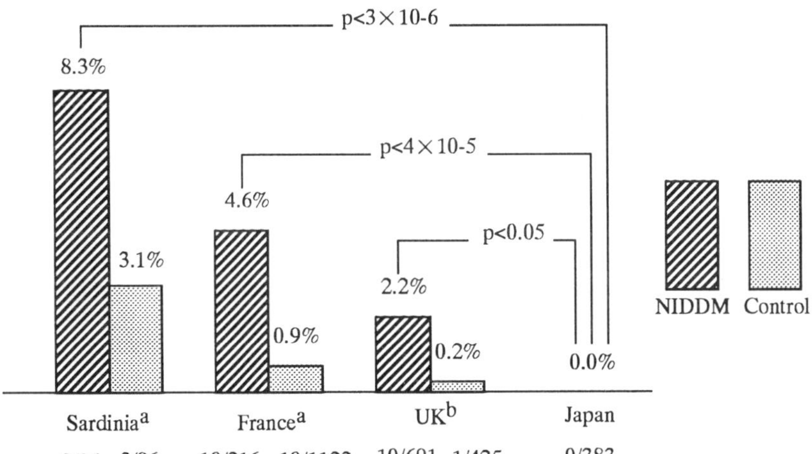

Fig. 1. Gly40Ser mutation of the glucagon receptor gene in NIDDM. [a]Data from [5]. [b]Data from [9].

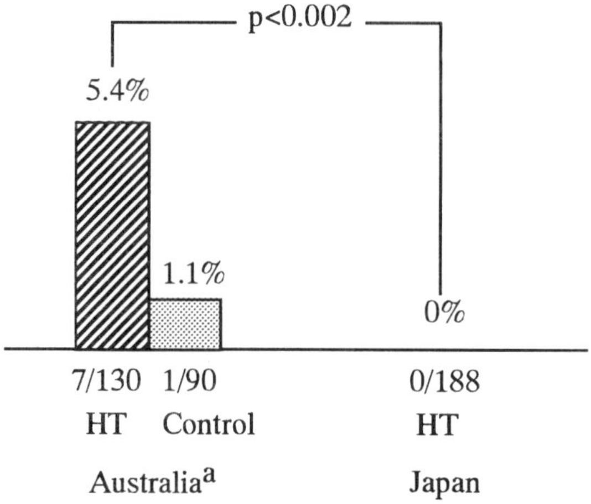

Fig. 2. Gly4OSer mutation of the glucagon receptor gene in essential hypertension. [a]Data from [6].

Discussion

In Japanese patients with NIDDM and/or hypertension, the frequencies of the mutation were significantly lower than those in other countries. The absence of the Gly40Ser mutation in the Japanese patients suggests that the contribution of this mutation to genetic susceptibility to NIDDM or essential hypertension is not universal, or that a founder effect was not observed in our isolated population. Given the likely heterogeneity of the pathogenesis of NIDDM and essential hypertension, the role of the glucagon receptor gene in the genetic predisposition to NIDDM and hypertension may vary in different ethnic groups.

Racial differences in association of candidate genes with NIDDM were previously reported. Association of the glucokinase gene polymorphism with diabetes was observed in African Americans [10] and Japanese [1,2], but not in Caucasians [11]. Similarly, the glycogen synthase gene polymorphism was associated with NIDDM in Finnish [12] and French [13], but not in Japanese [14]. Different frequencies of the 3243 mutation in mitochondrial DNA among different ethnic groups were also reported [3]. Given the likely heterogeneity of NIDDM, the importance of the glucagon receptor gene in susceptibility to NIDDM may also vary in different ethnic groups.

The frequencies of this mutation in Japanese patients with hypertension were also significantly lower than that reported in Caucasian populations [6]. The reason for the different frequencies in the two studies possibly originates from the difference in genetic background among races, i.e., the frequencies of this polymorphism exhibit a marked diversity among different ethnic groups [5,6,9]. Another possible explanation is that there is no tight relationship between the Gly40Ser mutation and essential hypertension. Evidence for this second hypothesis comes from the Caucasian data, as the observed frequency of the mutation in the hypertensive group (5%, seven out of 130) was not significantly different from that in the control group (1%, one out of 90; $p = 0.09$, by Fisher's exact test) [8]. In addition, it is unlikely that an amino acid substitution in the glucagon receptor protein directly contributes to the elevation of blood pressure, because functional alteration associated with the Gly40Ser mutation in itself may cause a low secretion of insulin [6], whereas hyperinsulinemia/insulin resistance is well-accepted to be implicated in the the pathogenesis of hypertension.

In conclusion, these results not only indicate that the Gly40Ser mutation in the glucagon receptor gene plays little, if any, role in susceptibility to NIDDM or essential hypertension in Japan, but also indicate the genetic heterogeneity in these diseases and further emphasize the importance of studies on genetic susceptibility to complex traits in different ethnic groups.

Acknowledgements

We thank Miss Yumiko Ueno for her skillful technical assistance. This work was supported in part by a Grant for Diabetes Research from the Ministry of Health and Welfare, Grants-in-Aid for Scientific Research from the Ministry of Education, Science, Sports and Culture, Japan, a Grant from the SANDOZ Foundation for Gerontological Research, and a Grant from the Kato Memorial Trust for Nambyo Research.

References

1. Takekawa K, Ikegami H, Fukuda M et al. Early-onset type 2 (non-insulin-dependent) diabetes mellitus is associated with glucokinase locus, but not with adenosine deaminase locus, in the Japanese population. Diabetes Res Clin Pract 1994;23:141–146.
2. Noda K, Matsutani A, Tanizawa Y et al. Polymorphic microsatellite repeat markers at the glucokinase gene locus are positively associated with NIDDM in Japanese. Diabetes 1993;42: 1147–1152.
3. Kadowaki T, Kadowaki H, Mori Y et al. A subtype of diabetes mellitus associated with a mutation of mitochondrial DNA. N Engl J Med 1994;330:962–968.
4. Kamitani A, Rakugi H, Higaki J et al. Association analysis of a polymorphism of the angiotensinogen gene with essential hypertension in Japanese. J Hum Hypertens 1994;8:521–524.
5. Hager J, Hansen L, Vaisse C et al. A missense mutation in the glucagon receptor gene is associated with non-insulin-dependent diabetes mellitus. Nature Genet 1995;9:299–304.
6. Chambers SM, Morris BJ et al. Glucagon receptor gene mutation in essential hypertension. Nature Genet 1996;12:122.
7. Fujisawa T, Ikegami H, Yamato E et al. A mutation in the glucagon receptor gene (Gly40Ser): heterogeneity in the association with diabetes meilitus. Diabetologia 1995;38:983–985.
8. Fujisawa T, Ikegami H, Babaya N et al. Gly40Ser mutation of glucagon receptor gene and essential hypertension in Japanese. Hypertension 1996;28:1100.
9. Gough SCL, Saker PJ, Pritchard LE et al. Mutation of the glucagon receptor gene and diabetes mellitus in the UK: association or founder effect? Hum Molec Genet 1995;4:1609–1612.
10. Chiu KC, Province MA, Permutt MA. Glucokinase gene is genetic marker for NIDDM in American Blacks. Diabetes 1992;41:843–849.
11. Permutt MA, Chiu KC, Tanizawa Y. Glucokinase and NIDDM: a candidate gene that paid off. Diabetes 1992;41:1367–1372.

12. Groop LC, Kankuri M, Schalin-Jäntti C et al. Association between polymorphism of the glycogen synthase gene and non-insulin-dependent diabetes mellitus. N Engl J Med 1993;328: 10–14.
13. Zouali H, Velho G, Froguel P. Polymorphism of the glycogen synthase gene and non-insulin-dependent diabetes mellitus. N Engl J Med 1993;328:1568.
14. Kadowaki T, Kadowaki H, Yazaki Y. Polymorphism of the glycogen synthase gene and non-insulin dependent diabetes mellitus. N Engl J Med 1993;328:1568–1569.

Recent Advances on the Pathogenesis and Management of Diabetes Mellitus.
S.H. Shinn, M. Shichiri and K.-W. Kim, editors.

The β3-adrenergic receptor gene polymorphism (Trp64Arg) in Korean NIDDM

H.R. Li, J.H. Lee, S.W. Lee, M.S. Nam, B.S. Cha, Y.J. Won, Y.D. Song, S.K. Lim, H.C. Lee and K.B. Huh

Department of Internal Medicine, Yonsei University College of Medicine, Seoul, Korea

Abstract. A possible pathogenic mutation in the β3-adrenergic receptor (β3-AR) gene (Trp64Arg) has been reported to be associated with an earlier age of onset of non-insulin-dependent diabetes mellitus (NIDDM), the insulin resistance syndrome and abnormal lipid and carbohydrate metabolism in Pima Indian, Finnish, French and Japanese subjects. To clarify the role of the mutation (Trp64Arg) of the β3-AR gene in Korean NIDDM patients, we measured the anthropometric and biochemical parameters and analyzed the β3-AR gene in 134 subjects with NIDDM and 30 nondiabetic subjects. The results showed that the allelic frequency of the Trp64Arg mutation was similar in the NIDDM and nondiabetic subjects (11 and 12%, respectively); the mean age of onset of NIDDM was not significantly different in NIDDM with the mutation and without it (45 ± 12 and 44 ± 12 years, respectively); in the clinical and biochemical characteristics there was no significant difference between NIDDM with the mutation and without it. These results suggested that the Trp64Arg allele of β3-AR may not contribute to the development of Korean NIDDM.

Keywords: β3-adrenergic receptor gene (β3-AR gene), mutation, non-insulin-dependent diabetes (NIDDM).

Introduction

Genetic factors play a major role in the development of non-insulin-dependent diabetic mellitus (NIDDM), but the candidate gene, the location of the gene locus and the mode of transmission are unclear. On the other hand, the genes responsible for the common forms of obesity, insulin resistance and NIDDM are unknown.

The β3-adrenergic receptor (β3-AR), located mainly in adipose tissue, is involved in the regulation of lipolysis and thermogenesis. There have been several reports about the association of β3-AR gene polymorphism with an earlier age of onset of NIDDM, insulin resistance syndrome and abnormal lipid and carbohydrate metabolism in Pima Indian, Finnish, French and Japanese subjects [1–4]. To clarify the role of polymorphism of the β3-AR gene in Korean NIDDM patients, we investigated the relationship between β3-AR gene polymorphism and the clinical and biochemical features of NIDDM patients.

Address for correspondence: Dr Hai- Ri Li, Department of Internal Medicine, Yonsei University College of Medicine, 134 Shinchondong, Sudaemungu, Seoul 120-752, Korea. E-mail: endohuh@yum-c.yonsei.ac.kr

Methods

We examined 134 randomly selected Korean patients with NIDDM and 30 nondiabetic controls. All patients were recruited from the Severance Hospital. All subjects fulfilled the diagnostic criteria of the WHO. All subjects gave written informed consent and the study was approved by the ethics committee of Yonsei University College of Medicine.

We studied the frequency of a cytosine-to-thymidine mutation that results in the replacement of tryptophan by arginine at position 64 (Trp64Arg) of the β3-AR by restriction-enzyme digestion with *Bst OI.* Clinical examinations and anthropomorphic measurements (height, weight, BMI, WHR, maximal weight and BMI) were made by physicians specifically trained for the study. Biochemical parameters (fasting and 2-h postprandial glucose, insulin and C-peptide, cholesterol, triglyceride, HDL-chol and LDL-chol) were also measured.

Results

The allelic frequency of the Arg 64 mutation was similar in the NIDDM subjects and in the nondiabetic controls (11 and 12%, respectively). There was no difference in the age of onset of NIDDM between NIDDM subjects with and without the mutation (45 ± 12 and 44 ± 12 years, respectively). The clinical and biochemical characteristics were not statistically different between the NIDDM subjects with and without the mutation. In nondiabetic controls, there were no differences in the clinical and biochemical characteristics between the nondiabetic subjects with and without the mutation. The frequency of high WHR, BMI and maximal BMI was not significantly different between the NIDDM subjects with and without the mutation.

Discussion

The relationship between a missense variant (Trp64Arg) in the gene encoding the β3-AR and obesity and NIDDM has been reported. Pima Indian and Japanese subjects homozygous for the Trp64Arg β3-AR mutation have an earlier onset of NIDDM and tend to have a lower resting metabolic rate (this mutation may accelerate the onset of NIDDM by altering the balance of energy metabolism in visceral adipose tissue). The Trp64Arg allele of the β3-AR is associated with abdominal obesity and resistance to insulin and may contribute to the early onset of NIDDM in Finland. People with the Trp64Arg mutation of the gene for the β3-AR may have an increased capacity to gain weight in France. β3-AR was associated with increased obesity but not with insulin resistance or dyslipidaemia in the UK.

Although there were similar tendencies towards a higher frequency of the Arg/Arg genotype of β3-AR among NIDDM patients in the Japanese, Pima Indian and Finnish populations, this mutated genotype was not significantly associated with NIDDM. A few papers reporting the opposite results have also been published. Some authors observed that the Arg64 allele was not significantly associated with lower values of total and percentage of body fat, percentage of abdominal fat, body weight, BMI, systolic and diastolic blood pressures and fasting insulin levels. Their preliminary data confirm other studies in that there is little evidence for this allele having a major role in fat distribution and, in particular, abdominal fat in normal female twins. Other authors have found that the three groups (homozygous for the Trp64Arg, heterozygous and homozygous for the normal type allele) were similar in age, percentage of body fat and waist-to-thigh ratio. There were no differences in fasting plasma nonesterified fatty acid (NEFA) concentration, NEFA rate of appearance or basal lipid oxidation rates between the three genotypes. Basal, isoproterenol-stimulated, and insulin-inhibited lipolysis in abdominal subcutaneous adipocytes were also similar in the three groups. These data indicate that the Trp64Arg variant in the β3-AR gene, even when expressed in its homozygous form, does not affect in vivo or in vitro lipid metabolism in Pima Indians. This is consistent with a recent report that the human Trp64Arg β3-AR is pharmacologically and functionally indistinguishable from the normal type form when expressed in cultured cells. Therefore, the pathophysiological mechanism by which this variant is causing a 4-year earlier onset of NIDDM in Pima Indians remains to be demonstrated. One possibility is that the Trp64Arg AR gene variant is in linkage disequilibrium with nearby genes affecting the age of onset of NIDDM.

We observed results similar to some of the afore-mentioned results, i.e., the allelic frequency of the Arg 64 mutation was similar in NIDDM subjects and in nondiabetic controls; there was no difference in age of onset of NIDDM between NIDDM subjects with and without the mutation; in diabetic and nondiabetic controls the clinical and biochemical characteristics were not statistically different between the subjects with and without the mutation; the frequency of high WHR, BMI and maximal BMI was not significantly different between the NIDDM subjects with and without the mutation.

Despite the small number of subjects studied, the consistent finding that the Arg64 allele was associated with lower risk-factor values, suggests that this mutation is not a major genetic determinant of obesity, regional fat distribution or other secondary characteristics such as NIDDM and hypertension. The reason for the different results may have been in the selection of patients, the difference in race and the use of different methods.

Conclusion

Our results suggest that the β3-AR gene mutation may not be a major determinant of the development of NIDDM in Korea.

References

1. Walston J et al. Time of onset of non-insulin-dependent diabetes mellitus and genetic variation in the β3-adrenergic-receptor gene. N Engl J Med 1995;333:343–347.
2. Widen E et al. Association of a polymorphism in the β3-adrenergic-receptor gene with features of the insulin resistance syndrome in Finns. N Engl J Med 1995;333:348–351.
3. Clement K et al. Genetic variation in the β3-adrenergic receptor and an increased capacity to gain weight in patients with morbid obesity. N Engl J Med 1995;333:352–354.
4. Fujisawa T et al. Association of Trp64Arg mutation of the β3-adrenergic-receptor with NIDDM and body weight gain. Diabetologia 1996;39:349–352.

Recent Advances on the Pathogenesis and Management of Diabetes Mellitus.
S.H. Shinn, M. Shichiri and K.-W. Kim, editors.

Non-HLA genetic markers for Korean insulin-dependent diabetic patients

Sunghee Lee[1], Yongsoo Park[1], Youhern Ahn[1], Taewha Kim[1], Mokhyun Kim[1] and Seiwon Yang[2]
[1] *Department of Internal Medicine, Hanyang University College of Medicine, Seoul; and* [2] *Department of Pediatrics, Seoul National University College of Medicine, Seoul, Korea*

Abstract. *Background.* Genes within the HLA class II region on chromosome 6 are the most important genetic factors for determining susceptibility to IDDM. However, they alone are not sufficient to account for the entire genetic contribution to this disease. Recent studies have demonstrated that LMP, TAP and other non-HLA genes such as the IDDM-2 (INS) and CTLA-4 genes are associated with susceptibility to IDDM in Caucasian subjects.

Methods. 130 Korean IDDM patients were selected from the Korean Seoul Registry and 120 non-diabetic unrelated controls were recruited from the same geographic area. A total of 49 IDDM simplex families were also studied. The INS gene typing was studied by PCR-RFLP (Pst I+1127), and LMP7 polymorphisms were also identified by the same method using the restriction enzyme Hha I. Association analysis was used to evaluate a candidate region near the CTLA-4 gene using 49 Korean IDDM families as well as unrelated cases and controls.

Results. The frequency of the INS +/+ homozygous genotype was not different between IDDM patients and controls (94.4 vs. 95.5%) and it was not polymorphic. There was no significant difference in the frequency of LMP7 A/A homozygotes between IDDM and controls (7.4 vs. 10.9%). Furthermore, when we divided and compared the subjects according to their HLA types (haplo-identical subjects), we could not detect any association of the LMP7 A/A homozygous genotype with IDDM. The transmission/disequilibrium test (TDT) revealed a highly significant deviation of transmission for alleles at the A/G polymorphism within the CTLA-4 gene ($p = 0.03$). However, case/control comparisons could not confirm the association.

Conclusions. We could assess that the polymorphism in the INS gene region or LMP7 region appeared to be of less value as a genetic marker for IDDM in Koreans. Non-HLA markers for IDDM such as the CTLA-4 gene might contribute to IDDM susceptibility in Koreans. Other candidate genes might be involved in IDDM susceptibility.

Keywords: CTLA-4 gene, genetic susceptibility marker, IDDM, IDDM2 gene, LAP gene.

Introduction

IDDM is a disease characterized by an absolute deficiency of insulin caused by destruction of the pancreatic β cells through an autoimmune mechanism. The development of the disease is influenced by the interaction of a large number of

Address for correspondence: Yongsoo Park MD, Department of Internal Medicine, Hanyang University Hospital, 249-1 Kyomun-dong, Kuri, Kyunggi-do, Seoul 471-020, Korea.

susceptibility genes and environmental factors. Recent genome-wide mapping studies have indicated that a lot of genes contribute to IDDM susceptibility and predisposing genetic loci have been precisely mapped through the entire human genome [1]. It is well-established that a major portion of genetic susceptibility and resistance to IDDM is associated with alleles of the HLA class II DQ and DR loci [2]. However, they alone are not sufficient to account for the entire genetic contribution to this disease. In addition to DR and DQ genes, recent studies have demonstrated that the large multifunctional protease (LMP) gene transporter associated with antigen processing (TAP) gene and other non-HLA genes such as IDDM2 and cytotoxic T lymphocyte associated (CTLA)-4 gene are associated with susceptibility to IDDM in Caucasian subjects [3—11]. In the Asian populations, it has been known that clinical and immunogenetic characteristics of IDDM are quite different from those in Caucasians. Therefore, we investigated the effect of the insulin gene polymorphism (IDDM2), LMP7 gene and CTLA-4 polymorphism on IDDM susceptibility in Korean patients with IDDM.

Materials and Methods

130 cases of IDDM patients were selected randomly from the Korean Seoul Registry. The criteria for classification of IDDM were determined by the National Diabetes Data Group. Sixty-seven were male, 63 were female; their mean current age was 13 years (range: 3—22 years). Their mean age at diagnosis was 7.9 ± 4.3 years with the mean duration of diabetes being 4.8 ± 3.4 years. 120 nondiabetic control subjects with no family history of diabetes were selected from the same geographical area; 58 were male and 62 were female. All the patients and control subjects gave their informed consent to the study. A total of 129 family members from the 49 simplex IDDM families also participated in this study. All the genotypes of the patients were precisely assessed by the family study.

Genomic DNA was obtained from all donors for the molecular typing of the generic typing of HLA-DRB1 and most common HLA-DQ A and B chain gene allelic forms. The gene frequencies were obtained by counting the total number of specific HLA antigens defined by oligonucleotide probe analysis.

The INS gene typing (Pst I+1127) was studied by PCR-RFLP. The LMP7 polymorphism (G/T-37360) was also identified by same method using the restriction enzyme Hha I [9]. The CTLA-4 exon 1 polymorphism was also studied by the same method using the restriction enzyme BstE II [11].

Differences in the allelic distributions of the respective gene were determined using the χ^2 test with Yates' correction (two-tailed). When the expected frequency for one of the alleles was less than 5, Fisher's exact test was used. Intrafamilial association studies were carried out using the transmission/disequilibrium test (TDT) described by Spielman et al. [12].

Results

The distribution of IDDM2 gene genotype or allele in patients with IDDM

The INS +/+ genotype was carried by 94.4% patients with IDDM and by 95.5% of the control subjects, and the gene was not actually polymorphic in Koreans, and neither the distribution of the INS +/+ homozygous genotype nor that of the INS + allele between IDDM and controls was significantly different.

The distribution of LMP7 genotype or allele in patients with IDDM

Neither the frequency of LMP7 A/A homozygotes nor that of the LMP7 A allele was significantly different between IDDM (7.4%; 42.4%) and controls (10.9%; 40.5%). To entirely eliminate possible influences from the nearby HLA class II molecules, we analysed LMP7 polymorphisms using direct extended haplotype-matched comparisons (Table 1). However, the frequencies of LMP7 genes on the same HLA haplotypes were not significantly different between IDDM and controls. Thus, this result suggests that the LMP7 gene polymorphism does not contribute to IDDM susceptibility irrespective of HLA molecules.

Association analysis to evaluate a candidate region near the CTLA-4 gene

The transmission/disequilibrium test (TDT) revealed a highly significant deviation of transmission for alleles at the A/G polymorphism within the CTLA-4 gene ($p = 0.03$) (Table 2). However, case/control comparisons could not confirm the association. There were more IDDM patients with alanine in the homozygous (58.8 vs. 50.0% of the controls) and fewer patients with threonine in the homozygous (2.1 vs. 10.7% of the controls), however, this did not reach statistical significance. These data indicate that the CTLA-4 gene polymorphism may contribute to IDDM susceptibility in Koreans.

Table 1. LMP7 association with IDDM in HLA haplo-identical subjects.

HLA haplotypes	IDDM			Control		
DRB1-DQB1	AA	AB	BB	AA	AB	BB
03 – 0201	1	9	14	0	1	5
0405 – 0302	0	5	10	0	0	1
0405 – 0401	0	16	14	1	11	17
09 – 0303	7	23	13	2	12	14
15 – 0601	0	0	1	1	3	10
15 – 0602	0	2	1	4	7	3
12 – 0301	1	0	1	3	6	6
Others	7	50	41	15	50	66
Total	16	105	95	26	90	122

Table 2. Transmission of the CTLA-4 G (Ala) allele from heterozygous parents to diabetic children.

Transmitted	Not transmitted	p value
13 (76.5%)	3 (23.5%)	0.03

Discussion

The insulin gene region on chromosome 11p15 (IDDM2 gene) has been reported to be significantly associated with IDDM in Caucasians and this association extends into its 5′ and 3′ flanking region [3,4]. The INS region contains several polymorphic loci outside the coding sequences, suggesting that IDDM susceptibility may derive from altered expression and/or regulation of the INS gene [5,6]. However, there have been some reports suggesting that it is not polymorphic in Asians and our results demonstrated that the IDDM2 gene was not polymorphic and was not associated with IDDM in Koreans in contrast to Caucasians.

Large multifunctional proteasome (LMP2) and LMP7 reside in a cluster of genes within 50 kb upstream of the HLA-DQB gene. They are speculated to play a role in the generation of endogenous peptides for the presentation by class I molecules to cytotoxic T cells [7,8]. Thus, the LMP genes may be good candidates for the additional IDDM susceptibility factors [9]. However, our results showed that the polymorphism of the LMP7 gene was not associated with Korean IDDM and did not contribute to IDDM susceptibility irrespective of HLA molecules.

These results suggest that the polymorphisms in the IDDM2 and LMP7 genes appear to be of less value than genetic markers for Korean IDDM. These differences between the Korean and Caucasian data may result from the differences in the genetic make-up of the control population or those in the patterns of linkage disequilibrium.

The cytotoxic T lymphocyte associated (CTLA)-4 gene is another strong candidate gene for a T-cell-mediated autoimmune disease because it encodes a T cell receptor that mediates T cell apoptosis and is a vital negative regulator of T cell activation. The CTLA-4 G (Ala) allele has been found to be associated with IDDM in Spanish and Italian families, providing evidence that this allele is related to the IDDM susceptibility [10,11]. Our results showed that the CTLA-4 gene polymorphism might confer susceptibility to Korean IDDM. However, case/control comparisons could not confirm this association. In our case/control studies, the increase of the GG genotype in patients compared to controls was consistent with the increase of transmission of the G allele from heterozygous parents to diabetic offspring, although statistical significance was not reached. It is important to note that family-based association studies are much more reliable and should be the preferred experimental design for association studies.

In conclusion, we could assess that neither the frequencies of the INS +/+ nor those of LMP7 A/A homozygous genotype was different between IDDM patients and controls. Furthermore, when the subjects were divided and compared according to their HLA types (haplo-identical subjects), we could not detect any association to the LMP7 A/A homozygous genotype with IDDM. However, non-HLA markers for IDDM such as the CTLA-4 gene may contribute IDDM susceptibility in Korean IDDM. Other candidate genes might be involved in the etiology of IDDM in Korea.

References

1. Davies JL, Kawaguchi Y, Bennett ST, Copeman JB, Cordell HJ, Pritchard LE, Reed PW, Gough SCL, Jenkins C, Palmer SM, Balfour KM, Rowe BR, Farrall M, Barnett AH, Bain SC, Todd JA. A genome-wide search for human type 1 diabetes susceptibility genes. Nature 1994;371: 130–136.
2. She JX. Susceptibility to type 1 diabetes: HLA-DQ and DR revisited. Immunol Today 1996;17: 323–329.
3. Bell GI, Karam JH, Rutter WJ. Polymorphic DNA region adjacent to the 5′ end of the human insulin gene. Proc Natl Acad Sci USA 1981;78:5759–5763.
4. Lucassen AM, Julier C, Beressi JP, Boitard C, Froguel P, Lathorp M, Bell JI. Susceptibility to IDDM maps to a 4.1 kb segment of DNA spanning the insulin gene and associated VNTR. Nature Genet 1993;4:305–310.
5. Julier C, Hyer RN, Davies J, Merlin F, Soularu P, Briant L, Cathelineau G, Deschamps I, Rotter JI, Froguel P, Boitard C, Bell JI, Lathorp GM. Insulin-IGF2 region on chromosome 11p encodes a gene implicated in HLA-DR4-dependent diabetes susceptibility. Nature 1991;354: 155–159.
6. Bain SC, Prins JB, Hearne CM, Rodrigues NR, Rowe BR, Pritchard LE, Ritchie RJ, Hall JRS, Undlin DE, Ronningen KS, Dunger DB, Barnett AH, Todd JA. Insulin gene region-encoded susceptibility to type 1 diabetes is not restricted to HLA-DR4-positive individuals. Nature Genet 1992;2:212–215.
7. Deverson EV, Gow IR, Coadwell WJ, Monaco JJ, Butcher GW, Howard JC. MHC class II region encoding proteins related to the multidrug resistance family of transmembrane transporters. Nature 1990;348:738–741.
8. Monaco JJ, Cho S, Attaya M. Transport protein genes in the murine MHC: possible implications for antigen processing. Science 1990;250:1723–1726.
9. Deng GY, Muir A, Maclaren NK, She JX. Association of LMP2 and LMP7 genes within the major histocompatibility complex with insulin-dependent diabetes mellitus: population and family studies. Am J Hum Genet 1995;56:528–534.
10. Nistico L, Buzzetti R, Pritchard LE, Auwera BV, Giovannini C, Bosi E, Larrad MTM, Rios MS, Chow CC, Cockram CS, Jacobs K, Mijovic C, Bain SC, Barnett AH, Vandewalle CL, Schuit F, Gorus FK, Belgian Diabetes Registry, Tosi R, Pozzilli P, Todd JA. The CTLA-4 gene region of chromosome 2q33 is linked to, and associated with, type 1 diabetes. Hum Molec Genet 1996; 5:1075–1080.
11. Donner H, Rau H, Walfish PG, Braun J, Siegmund T, Finke R, Herwig J, Usadel KH, Badenhoop K. CTLA4 alanine-17 confers genetic susceptibility to Graves' disease and to type 1 diabetes mellitus. J Clin Endocrinol Metab 1997;82:143–146.
12. Spielman RS, McGinnis RE, Ewens WJ. Transmission test for linkage disequilibrium: The insulin gene region and insulin-dependent diabetes mellitus (IDDM). Am J Hum Genet 1993;52: 506–512.

Clinical diabetes

Recent Advances on the Pathogenesis and Management of Diabetes Mellitus.
S.H. Shinn, M. Shichiri and K.-W. Kim, editors.

C-peptide and clinical presentation follow-up study in newly onset diabetes of the young

H.S. Kim, J.H. Lee, B.S. Cha, Y.D. Song, S.K. Lim, K.R. Kim, H.C. Lee and K.B. Huh

Division of Endocrinology, Department of Internal Medicine, Yonsei University College of Medicine, Seoul, Korea

Abstract. To evaluate the change of insulin secretary function of β cells by measuring the follow-up C-peptide level in newly onset diabetes of the young in Korea, we examined, retrospectively, 65 patients aged between 15 and 35 years who were admitted within 1 year after the clinical onset and who had been followed-up for more than 2 years. According to the basal C-peptide level at the initial visit, patients were divided into three groups (G1, <0.6 ng/ml; G2, 0.6–1.0 ng/ml; and G3, >1.0 ng/ml). The clinical characteristics, laboratory parameters and follow-up basal C-peptide level were measured and the results obtained showed that BMI ((in G3 compared to G1 and G2) 23.1 ± 4.7 vs. 17.6 ± 1.5, 18.8 ± 2.1, $p<0.01$) and family history ((FH) 53 vs. 0%, 29%, $p<0.05$) were significantly higher. In the follow-up measurement of basal C-peptide level, almost all patients (7/8) in G1 showed decreased basal C-peptide and these seven were classified as IDDM. In G2, 53% (9/17) of patients had a decreased follow-up basal C-peptide, and all of these nine patients except one were classified clinically as IDDM. In G3, 18% (7/40) of the patients had prominent deteriorations of the β cell function, and among these seven patients had a high ICA positivity (60%). So ICA might be a significant marker in predicting the secretary capacity of β cell function in these patients. In conclusion, the follow-up of serum C-peptide level is a useful parameter for the classification of newly onset young diabetic patients.

Keywords: C-peptide, diabetes of the young.

Introduction

Correct classification of diabetic patients at the time of diagnosis is often difficult because of the discrepancy in clinical and immunogenetic characteristics during the follow-up. But it is important in clinical practice in the decision of appropriate treatment and in the understanding of the pathogenesis and clinical course of the diabetes. Therefore, we compared the clinical classification at the initial onset and the follow-up period and evaluated the change of insulin secretory function of β cells by measuring the follow-up C-peptide level in newly onset diabetes of the young.

Address for correspondence: Hyun Soo Kim MD, Department of Internal Medicine, Severance Hospital Yonsei University College of Medicine, 134 Shinchon-Dong, Seodaemun-ku, Seoul 120-752, Korea. Tel.: +82-2-361-5410. Fax: +82-2-393-6884.

Subjects and Methods

In 65 young adult onset diabetic patients aged between 15 and 35 years who were admitted to our hospital within 1 year after the clinical onset and who were followed-up for more than 2 years, clinical and immunogenetic characteristics and basal C-peptide level were determined. According to the basal C-peptide level at the initial visit, patients were divided into three groups: the basal C-peptide level of group 1 was below 0.6 mg/ml. Group 2 was between 0.6 and 1.0 ng/ml, and group 3 was above 1.0 ng/ml. The clinical characteristics studied were age, sex, BMI, family history (FHx), and history of DKA. The laboratory parameters measured were fasting blood glucose (FBG), basal C-peptide, HbA1c, HLA typing, and ICA.

Results

Among the three groups, there were no significant differences in FBS, HBA1C level, and prevalence of HLA-DR4 and ICA. However, in group 3 compared to groups 1 and 2, BMI was significantly higher with an average of 23.1 kg/m^2 and familial tendency was significantly higher at 53%. In group 1, the plasma basal C-peptide level decreased in all the patients except one and these seven patients were classified as IDDM. In group 2, (where the initial plasma basal C-peptide level was between 0.6 and 1.0) nine patients out of 17 had a decreased follow-up C-peptide level below 0.6, and three patients had an increased follow-up C-peptide level above 1.0 ng/ml after the follow-up period. In group 3, there was no deterioration of the β cell function in 60% (24/40) of the patients. However, 18% (7/40) of the patients had prominent deteriorations of the β cell function and the islet cell antibody might be a significant marker in these patients. The initial clinical and immunogenetic characteristics of the patients whose follow-up C-peptide level dropped to group 1 (G1→1, first G; G2→1, second G; and G3→1, third G) were also reviewed. In contrast with the initial study, all three groups had no significant differences in BMI and familial history. However, age was significantly lower in the second and third group compared to the first group. The interesting fact was that ICA was shown in 60% of the third group, where the follow-up C-peptide level dropped by the largest amount. But because of the small subjects number of the measured ICA, it is difficult to compare statistically.

Conclusion

The follow-up of the serum C-peptide level is a useful parameter for the classification of newly diagnosed young adult onset diabetes. Long-term prospective studies are necessary to elucidate the pathogenetic mechanism of these young diabetic patients.

Recent Advances on the Pathogenesis and Management of Diabetes Mellitus.
S.H. Shinn, M. Shichiri and K.-W. Kim, editors.

The patterns of clinical characteristics according to body weight and weight changes in Korean NIDDM patients

Young Sun Hong, Jee Young Oh, Hee Jin Kim, Yeon-Ah Sung and Nan Ho Kyung
Department of Internal Medicine, College of Medicine, Ewha Women's University, Seoul, Korea

Abstract. *Background.* It is known that Korean NIDDM patients are mainly nonobese and have experienced weight loss frequently during the course of the disease. Our study was designed to determine the characteristics of diabetes in Korea by examining the differences in the clinical features according to the current weight and the weight changes.

Methods. From 308 Korean NIDDM patients, we obtained the data about the changes of weight and measured the current weight and height. We also evaluated the presence of diabetic retinopathy, nephropathy and neuropathy. We designated the patients with BMI 21 kg/m^2 and less as the lean group, the patients with BMI 21 to <26 kg/m^2 as the middle-range group and the patients with 26 kg/m^2 and over as the obese group.

Results. At the time of maximal weight, 61.4% of the patients were obese, however, 40.3% were obese at diagnosis and only 33.8% were obese at recruitment. In the lean group, C-peptide was low and the frequency of insulin therapy was high. Although there was no statistical significance, diabetic complications were more frequent in the lean group. The percentage of the patients who lost weight (loss of 10% from the maximal weight) was 65.9% in the lean group, 42.3% in the middle-range group and 32.7% in the obese group. The prevalence of the retinopathy and the neuropathy were higher in the group with weight loss, although not significantly.

Conclusion. Many Korean NIDDM patients experienced weight loss before and after the diagnosis. In such patients, insulin secretory capacity was low and the frequency of insulin therapy was high. Our study showed that the lean group and the patients who lost weight tended to have a higher prevalence of the complications. The mass prospective study about the clinical characteristics according to weight changes in Korean NIDDM patients will be needed.

Keywords: complications, Korea, weight loss.

Introduction

In 1995, a WHO multinational study reported the positive association of BMI with age, blood pressure, and cholesterol and the negative association with duration of diabetes, retinopathy, and use of insulin. Also, weight loss, particularly in the lean diabetic patients, was associated with an increased mortality risk [1].

In Korea, NIDDM patients are mainly nonobese and have experienced weight loss frequently during the course of the disease. But there have been few studies about the patterns of treatment and complications according to the weight changes [2–4]. So, the purpose of this study was to determine the characteristics

Address for correspondence: Young Sun Hong, Department of Internal Medicine, Ewha Women's University Tongdaemun Hospital, Chongro 6-ka, Chongro-ku, Seoul, Korea.

of diabetes in Korea by examining the difference in the clinical features according to the current weight and the weight changes.

Material and Methods

From 308 Korean NIDDM patients, we obtained the data on the weight at the time of maximal obesity and diagnosis of diabetes and measured the current weight and height.

We also evaluated the presence of diabetic retinopathy, nephropathy and neuropathy. The nonproliferative and proliferative retinopathy were diagnosed by an ophthalmologic specialist after pupil dilation. The nephropathy was diagnosed when overt proteinuria was present. The neuropathy was diagnosed by symptoms, physical examination, abnormal nerve conduction velocity and loss of R-R interval variation in EKG during the deep respiration.

We designated the patients with BMI of 21 kg/m^2 and less as the lean group, the patients with BMI of 21 to <26 kg/m^2 as the middle-range group, and the patients with 26 kg/m^2 and over as the obese group.

We defined significant weight loss as the loss of more than 10% from the maximal weight.

Results

At the maximal weight, 61.4% of the patients were obese, however, 40.3% were obese at diagnosis and only 33.8% were obese at recruitment. In the lean group, C-peptide and serum cholesterol were significantly lower and the frequency of insulin therapy was significantly higher than both that of the middle-range and the obese group. Also, serum triglyceride was significantly lower than the obese

Table 1. Clinical characteristics of subjects according to current BMI.

	$BMI \leqslant 21$	$21 < BMI < 26$	$BMI \geqslant 26$
Number	41 (13.3%)	163 (52.9%)	104 (33.8%)
Sex (M:F)	21:20 (1:0.95)	77:86 (1:1.12)	36:68 (1:1.89)
Age (years)	54.3 ± 13.7	56.6 ± 11.4	55.2 ± 11.5
Duration (years)	9.0 ± 7.1	8.8 ± 7.4	7.3 ± 6.5
FBS (mmol/l)	9.6 ± 4.2	8.8 ± 3.0	9.0 ± 3.1
HbA1c (%)	8.8 ± 2.5	8.2 ± 1.9	8.5 ± 2.1
C-peptide (n/mol)	0.63 ± 0.46^a	0.76 ± 0.70	0.96 ± 0.53
Systolic BP (mmHg)	121.0 ± 32.8	126.5 ± 18.6	126.7 ± 26.0
Diastolic BP (mmHg)	75.9 ± 18.8	78.7 ± 8.9	78.8 ± 14.9
Cholesterol (mg/dl)	179.5 ± 38.3^a	196.4 ± 39.5	204.8 ± 42.8
Triglyceride (mg/dl)	142.4 ± 67.3^b	177.6 ± 137.1	224.5 ± 162.0
Insulin therapy (%)	61.0^a	41.1	31.7

Values are the means ± SD. $^a p<0.05$ $BMI \leqslant 21$ vs. BMI 21–26, $BMI \geqslant 26$; $^b p<0.05$ $BMI \leqslant 21$ vs. $BMI \geqslant 26$.

Table 2. The prevalence of complications among the groups according to current BMI.

	Lean (n = 41)	Middle-range (n = 163)	Obese (n = 104)
Complications (%)			
retinopathy	52.6	43.2	32.3
nephropathy	35.9	25.8	26.6
neuropathy	65.0	60.4	51.0

group (Table 1).

We classified the obese patients at the time of maximal obesity into two groups. One group contained the patients who lost weight from obese group weight to middle-range or lean group weight and the other group contained the patients who have maintained their weight. In the weight-maintaining group, the proportion of female patients was significantly higher.

The prevalence of diabetic complications was not significantly different among the three groups but it tended to be more frequent in the lean group (Table 2). After the correction of the effect of the duration, there was no statistical significance in the prevalence of complications among the groups. However, the p value in the prevalence of retinopathy was 0.058 suggesting the minimal significance.

In the lean group, the percentage of the patients who lost weight significantly was 65.9%. The frequency of insulin therapy was higher in the group without weight loss (85.7 vs. 48.2%). Although there was no statistical significance, the prevalence of retinopathy and neuropathy was higher in the group with weight loss. In the middle-range group, the percentage of the patients with weight loss was 42.3%. The patients with significant weight loss were older (59.0 vs. 54.9 years). The duration of the diabetes was longer in the group without weight loss (10.6 vs. 6.4 years). The prevalence of complications was higher in the group with weight loss, although not significantly. In the obese group, the percentage of the patients with weight loss was 32.7%. The patients who lost weight tended to have a higher prevalence of the complications. (Data not shown.)

In total, the prevalence of retinopathy was significantly higher in the patients with weight loss (Table 3).

Table 3. The prevalence of complications between the groups according to the changes in BMI (in total).

	Patients with significant weight loss (n = 130)	Patients without significant weight loss (n = 178)
Complications (%)		
retinopathy	47.9[a]	35.6
nephropathy	30.3	25.2
neuropathy	62.2	54.7

[a]$p < 0.05$.

Table 4. The prevalence of complications between the groups according to the use of insulin.

	Insulin therapy (n = 125)	No insulin therapy (n = 183)
Complications (%)		
retinopathy	53.9[a]	31.5
nephropathy	42.0[a]	17.0
neuropathy	78.7[a]	43.5

[a]$p < 0.001$.

The prevalence of retinopathy, nephropathy and neuropathy was significantly higher in the patients who used insulin (Table 4).

Discussion

It is known that Korean NIDDM patients, in contrast to Caucasians, are mainly nonobese and have experienced severe weight loss during the course of disease. In our study, 42.2% of 308 NIDDM patients experienced weight loss before and after the diagnosis and only 33.8% were obese at recruitment. In the lean group, insulin secretory capacity was low and the frequency of insulin therapy was high. It was suggested that a proportion of patients with such clinical characteristics may be slowly progressive IDDM patients [5]. Our study showed that the lean group and the patients who have lost weight tended to have a higher prevalence of the complications. Some researchers suggested that leaner people with NIDDM have an increased genetic burden and therefore a more severe form of the disease and an increased likelihood of complications [6]. The severity of retinopathy was found to be associated inversely with body mass index in the Wisconsin epidemiologic study of diabetic retinopathy [7].

In our study, the proportion of female patients was significantly higher in the weight-maintaining obese group. It may be related with the difference in stress, exercise and alcohol intake. Also postpartum or postmenopausal weight gain can influence but it must be elucidated.

Considering the different characteristics of Korean NIDDM compared with Caucasians, a mass prospective study about the clinical features according to weight changes in Korean NIDDM will be needed.

References

1. Chaturvedi N, Fuller JH. Mortality risk by body weight and weight change in people with NIDDM. Diabetes Care 1995;18:766–774.
2. Park JY, Kim HK, Kim MS et al. Body weight changes of non-insulin-dependent diabetic patients in Korea. J Kor Diabetes Assoc 1993;17:51–58.
3. Cho JK, Kim HM, Lim SK et al. A study on change of body weight of non-insulin-dependent diabetes mellitus. J Kor Diabetes Assoc 1986;10:89–93.
4. Choli MS, Lee JH, Paik IK et al. Influence of duration of diabetes on nutritional status in non-insulin-dependent diabetes mellitus. J Kor Diabetes Assoc 1992;16:35–44.

5. Kim YS, Park YS, Lee MK et al. The frequency of ICSA and PCA in Koreans with diabetes mellitus. J Kor Diabetes Assoc 1990;14:45–50.
6. Kobberling J. Studies on the genetic heterogeneity of diabetes mellitus. Diabetologia 1971;7: 46–49.
7. Klein R, Klein BEK, Moss SE et al. The Wisconsin epidemiologic study of diabetic retinopathy III. Arch Ophthalmol 1984;102:527–532.

Recent Advances on the Pathogenesis and Management of Diabetes Mellitus.
S.H. Shinn, M. Shichiri and K.-W. Kim, editors.

Characteristics of NIDDM patients with fasting hyperglycemia

K. Nojima, H. Ikegami, E. Yamato, Y. Kawaguchi, T. Fujisawa, Y. Hamada, M. Hotta, H. Ueda, M. Shintani, Y. Kawabata, N. Babaya, J. Fu, G.-Q. Shen and T. Ogihara

Department of Geriatric Medicine, Osaka University Medical School, Osaka, Japan

Abstract. In NIDDM patients treated with sulfonylureas or insulin, a higher dose of agents is usually required in the morning rather than in the evening. There is, however, a subset of patients who receive more agents in the evening than in the morning, in order to suppress the fasting hyperglycemia in the morning. To clarify the mechanism underlying fasting hyperglycemia in such patients, we studied the clinical, metabolic and hormonal features of patients receiving a higher dose of agents in the evening than in the morning. The patients were characterized by higher BMI, higher serum FFA levels, and low ketone-to-body ratio with no differences in glucagon and cortisol levels. These data suggest that an increase in lipolysis and overfeeding of the substrates for the gluconeogenesis, together with the change of energy metabolism in the liver, may contribute to the fasting hyperglycemia in such patients.

Keywords: fasting hyperglycemia, FFA, hepatic glucose production, ketone body.

Background

In the case of twice a day NPH insulin injection, it is usual to inject more insulin in the morning than in the evening. Figure 1 shows daily profiles of blood glucose in an NIDDM patient treated with NPH insulin twice a day. Daily profiles, measured over four different days, are shown. The glucose levels before supper are well-controlled around 80 mg/dl by injecting 6 units of NPH insulin in the morning. In contrast, the fasting plasma glucose levels are still high at around 140 mg/dl despite the injection of 8 units of NPH insulin in the evening. As shown in this case, there is a subset of NIDDM patients who require more insulin in the evening than in the morning to suppress the fasting hyperglycemia in the morning.

Methods

Subjects were 84 NIDDM patients who attended the outpatient clinic of Osaka University Hospital. To exclude the effect of comedication, the patients who received sulfonylurea only (SU group) or insulin only (insulin group) were selected from a total of 84 patients.

Address for correspondence: K. Nojima, Department of Geriatric Medicine, Osaka University Medical School, 2-2 Yamadaoka, Suita, Osaka 565, Japan. Tel.: +81-6-879-3852. Fax: +81-6-879-3859.

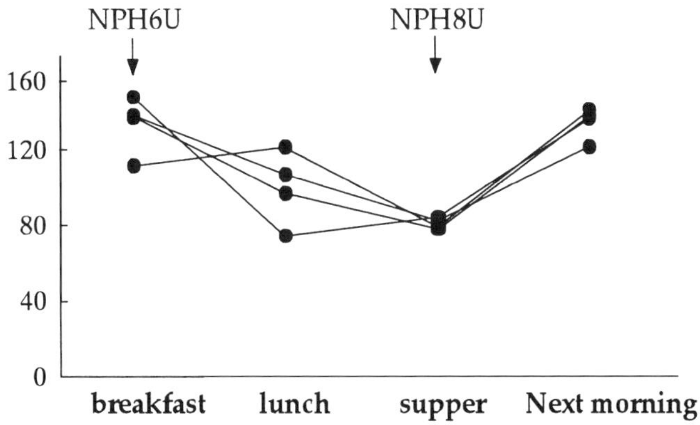

Fig. 1. Daily profiles of blood glucose in NIDDM patients treated with NPH insulin twice a day. Daily profiles measured over four different days are shown.

Patients in the SU group and the insulin group were divided into two types, the morning type and the evening type, according to the relative dose of hypoglycemic agents in the morning and in the evening.

In the SU group, the morning type was defined as the patients who received a higher dose of drugs in the morning than in the evening. The evening type was defined as the patients who received the same or a higher dose of drugs in the evening than in the morning.

In the insulin group, the morning type was defined as the patients who received less than 40% of the morning insulin in the evening. The evening type was defined as the patients who received more than 60% of the morning insulin in the evening.

Height and body weight were measured, and body mass index (BMI) was calculated. As metabolic parameters, fasting plasma glucose, HbA1c, free fatty acid, triglyceride, and ketone bodies were measured, and the ketone-to-body ratio was calculated by dividing acetoacetate by β-hydroxybutylate.

Also, the hormones regulating glucose metabolism, plasma and urinary C-peptide, plasma glucagon and cortisol levels were measured.

Since the liver is a major organ responsible for fasting plasma glucose levels, the liver function was assessed by measuring AST, ALT, γ-GTP, and cholinesterase.

Results

Table 1 shows the characteristics of the subjects. In the SU group, the morning type received the mean dosage of 0.9 tablet in the morning, and 0.1 tablet in the evening. In contrast, the evening type received 0.7 tablet in the morning, and 0.9 tablet in the evening, indicating that the evening type required a much higher dose of sulfonylurea in the evening to control fasting hyperglycemia.

Table 1. Characteristics of the patients.

	SU		Insulin	
	Morning type	Evening type	Morning type	Evening type
Dosage				
morning	0.9 ± 0.2 tab	0.7 ± 0.1 tab	13 ± 2 U	11 ± 2 U
evening	0.1 ± 0.1 tab	0.9 ± 0.1 tab	3 ± 1 U	10 ± 2 U
Sex (M/F)	6/1	7/5	1/5	4/2
Age (years)	62.0 ± 4.0	53.9 ± 5.2	61.3 ± 3.3	62.0 ± 2.5
BMI (kg/m^2)	22.9 ± 0.7	24.0 ± 0.9	20.8 ± 1.2	22.3 ± 1.2

Mean ± SEM.

In the insulin group, the morning type received the mean dosage of 13 units in the morning and 3 units in the evening. In contrast, the evening type received 11 units in the morning and 10 units in the evening, indicating that the evening type required a much higher dose of insulin in the evening to control fasting hyperglycemia. In both groups BMI was higher in the evening type than in the morning type.

Table 2 shows the metabolic characteristics. In the SU group, fasting plasma glucose was higher in the evening type than in the morning type, but HbA1c levels were similar between the two groups, indicating that overall plasma glucose level was well-controlled in the evening type at the same level as in the morning type, but the plasma glucose increased from the night to early in the morning despite receiving a higher dose of sulfonylurea in the evening. FFA level was significantly higher in the evening type than in the morning type. Ketone-to-body ratio was significantly lower in the evening type in the SU group. In the insulin group ketone body was too low to be detected.

Table 3 shows the hormones regulating glucose metabolism. The urinary C-peptide and serum C-peptide showed no remarkable differences between the two types. The glucagon:C-peptide ratio, which is known to affect the glucose

Table 2. Metabolic characteristics.

	SU		Insulin	
	Morning type	Evening type	Morning type	Evening type
FPG (mg/dl)	119 ± 11	129 ± 6.5	146 ± 18	158 ± 12
HbA1c (%)	6.5 ± 0.3	6.1 ± 0.3	7.3 ± 0.3	7.4 ± 0.3
FFA (mmol/l)	118 ± 33	239 ± 2[a]	81 ± 32	277 ± 59[a]
TG (mg/dl)	125 ± 1	110 ± 13	113 ± 24	113 ± 36
Ketone body (mmol/l)	79 ± 23	100 ± 13		
Ketone-to-body ratio	0.95 ± 0.18	0.64 ± 0.05[a]		

Mean ± SEM. [a]$p < 0.05$ vs. morning-type.

Table 3. Hormones regulating glucose metabolism.

	SU		Insulin	
	Morning type	Evening type	Morning type	Evening type
C-peptide				
Urinary (mg/gCr)	41.7 ± 12.7	33.8 ± 6.5	15.3 ± 3.3	21.6 ± 4.7
Serum (ng/ml)	2.3 ± 0.4	2.6 ± 0.4	1.2 ± 0.1	1.1 ± 0.2
Glucageon (pg/ml)	209 ± 56	139 ± 15	114 ± 18	100 ± 9
Glucagon/C-peptide	0.09 ± 0.03	0.05 ± 0.01	0.09 ± 0.01	0.09 ± 0.01
Cortisol (mg/dl)	13.0 ± 0.9	11.4 ± 0.7	13.0 ± 1.1	13.1 ± 1.1

metabolism in the liver, was similar in the two types. Glucagon and cortisol levels were also similar in the evening type and the morning type in both groups. These data suggest that endogenous insulin and counterregulatory hormones were not responsible for the fasting hyperglycemia in the evening type.

Table 4 shows the parameters related to liver function. There are no apparent differences in AST, ALT, γ-GTP and cholinesterase between the morning and the evening type.

Conclusions

NIDDM patients who received a high dose of hypoglycemic agents in the evening were characterized by high BMI, high serum FFA levels, and a low ketone-to-body ratio. These data suggest that increased lipolysis and overfeeding of the substrates for the gluconeogenesis, together with the change of energy metabolism in the liver, may contribute to the fasting hyperglycemia in the morning.

Recently, FFA has been proposed to be responsible for fasting hyperglycemia by studying the relationship between FFA and hepatic glucose production (HGP). First, FFA is the signal to control the HGP in the fasting state. Second, FFA is a substrate for gluconeogenesis. In animal models, the elevation of glycerol, lactate and alanine increase HGP in the fasting state. Overfeeding of substrates for gluconeogenesis, however, only partially explains HGP. Moreover, glucose fatty acid cycle is known to increase the peripheral insulin resistance. Both increased HGP and decreased glucose utilization in peripheral tissue seem to be

Table 4. Parameters related to liver function.

	SU		Insulin	
	Morning type	Evening type	Morning type	Evening type
AST (U/l)	16.4 ± 3.0	15.8 ± 1.7	22.0 ± 6.8	13.5 ± 1.5
ALT (U/l)	17.7 ± 5.5	22.5 ± 5.0	29.2 ± 14.4	11.8 ± 1.0
γ-GTP (U/l)	31.1 ± 7.0	31.3 ± 5.5	24.2 ± 5.8	20.0 ± 5.1
Cholinesterase (U/l)	4232 ± 311	4460 ± 193	3619 ± 330	3704 ± 278

responsible for fasting hyperglycemia.

In our study, the ketone-to-body ratio was very low in the insulin group, indicating that peripheral hyperinsulinemia in the insulin group suppressed the lipolysis much more than portal hyperinsulinemia in the SU group. In the evening type in the SU group, FFA was significantly higher and ketone-to-body ratio was significantly lower than that in the morning type, indicating that the evening type failed to suppress the lipolysis to the same level as the evening type because of the higher BMI or other factors. According to the Redox theory, there is a strong relationship between ketone-to-body ratio and energy charge in the mitochondria in the liver. Although it is not clear whether the low ketone-to-body ratio is only the result of high FFA or low ketone-to-body ratio is the cause of increased HGP, the data in the present study suggest that the energy metabolism in the liver in patients with fasting hyperglycemia is different to those without.

Additional reading

1. Sindelar DK, Chu CA, Rohlie M, Neal DW, Swift LL, Cherrington D. The role of fatty acid in mediating the effects of periferal insulin on hepatic glucose production in the concious dog. Diabetes 1997;46:187–196.
2. Rebrin K, Steil GM, Getty L, Bergman RN. Free fatty acid as a link in the regulation of hepatic glucose output by periferal insulin. Diabetes 1995;44:1038–1045.
3. Lewis GF, Zinman B, Groenewoud Y, Vranic M, Giacca A. Hepatic glucose production is regulated both by direct hepatic and extrahepatic effects of insulin in human. Diabetes 1996; 45:454–462.
4. Williamson DH, Lund P, Krebs HA. The Redox state of free nicotinamide-adenine dinucleotide in the cytoplasm and mitochondria of rat liver. Biochem J 1966;103:514–527.

Recent Advances on the Pathogenesis and Management of Diabetes Mellitus.
S.H. Shinn, M. Shichiri and K.-W. Kim, editors.

Clinical and immunogenetic characteristics of the patients occurring diabetic ketoacidosis in Korea

Hong Seung Kim, Han Hyo Lee, Mee Duk Lee, Young Goo Shin and Choon Hee Chung

Department of Internal Medicine, Wonju College of Medicine, Yonsei University, Wonju, Korea

Abstract. *Background.* Diabetic ketoacidosis (DKA) usually occurs in insulin-dependent diabetes mellitus (IDDM) patients. However, in some non-insulin-dependent diabetes mellitus (NIDDM) patients DKA also occurs. We call these patients atypical diabetes mellitus (ADM) patients. We studied DKA patients and classified them as either IDDM or ADM patients. The immunogenetic and clinical characteristics were compared in these patients for the clarification of the pathogenesis of ADM.

Methods. We studied 29 diabetic patients admitted to the Wonju Christian Hospital due to DKA from February 1994 to February 1996. We classified these patients into two groups and studied the basic clinical data, 75-g oral glucose tolerance test (OGTT), glucagon stimulation test, HLA DR typing, islet cell antibody (ICA), insulin autoantibody (IAA), antiglutamic acid decarboxylase (anti-GAD) antibody and anti-mumps IgM type antibody.

Results. Between ADM and IDDM patients, there were no significant differences in age, duration of DM, BMI and HgA1c. However, the C-peptide response area under the curve on the 75-g OGTT was significantly higer in ADM patients than IDDM patients. Autoantibodies such as ICA, IAA, anti-GAD Ab and anti-mumps IgM Ab were detected in some ADM patients but not in IDDM patients. The positivity of HLA DR3/DR4 was the same between the two groups.

Conclusions. In concordance with the above results, we suggest that ADM with DKA might be developed using another mechanism rather than autoimmunity.

Keywords: atypical diabetes mellitus, autoantibodies, IDDM.

Introduction

Diabetic ketoacidosis (DKA) generally occurs in insulin-dependent diabetes mellitus (IDDM) patients. However, in some non-insulin-dependent diabetes mellitus (NIDDM) patients DKA may occur. Recently Winter et al. [1] reported that 12 of 129 black patients with youth-onset diabetes were identified as having an unusual clinical course, with apparent insulin dependence at the time of presentation followed by absence of dependence months to years later. They called these patients atypical diabetes mellitus (ADM) patients. The HLA DR3 and DR4 were not associated with these patients and C-peptide response on the oral glucose tolerance test (OGTT) was at an intermediate level between nondiabetic controls and classic IDDM patients. Also, Banerji et al. [2] reported that long-

Address for correspondence: Choon Hee Chung, Department of Internal Medicine, Wonju College of Medicine, Yonsei University, 162 Ilsan-Dong, Wonju-Si, Kangwon-Do, Wonju 220-701, Korea.

term near-normoglycemic remission had occurred in some patients' groups following intensive treatment of insulin or oral sulfonylurea drugs. These patients were islet cell antibody (ICA) and antiglutamic acid decarboxylase antibody negative (anti-GAD). Their insulin secretions were below the normal range and in some patients DKA occurred. We studied the clinical and immunologenetic characteristics of the DKA patients in Korea for the evaluation of differences between Korean diabetic patients and classic IDDM patients.

Materials

We studied diabetic patients admitted to the Wonju Christian Hospital due to DKA between February 1994 and February 1996. We divided these patients into two groups, ADM and classic IDDM. The inclusion criteria of ADM were: 1) basal serum peptide level > 0.6 ng/ml on the 75-g OGTT; 2) serum C-peptide level > 1.8 ng/ml at 6 min on the glucagon stimulation test; and 3) daily insulin requirement < 20 U for glycemic control. The inclusion criteria of IDDM were: 1) basal serum C-peptide level < 0.6 ng/ml on the 75-g OGTT; 2) serum C-peptide level < 1.8 ng/ml at 6 min on the glucagon stimulation test; and 3) daily insulin requirement for glycemic control > 20 U.

Methods

We checked height, weight, body mass index (BMI), HgA1c, urine ketone body and serum pH in all patients. After intensive treatment of diabetic ketoacidosis and clinical status was stabilized, we performed a 75-g OGTT with measurement of C-peptide and insulin. Also, we measured C-peptide after 6 min following a 1-mg glucagon i.v. bolus injection. We performed HLA-DR typing by mixed leukocyte reaction. We checked ICA using a commercial ELISA kit (Biomerica, USA), IAA using a commercial EIA kit (Biomerica, USA), anti-GAD antibody using a commercial EIA kit (Elias USA, Inc., USA), and also that its cutoff value was calculated as the mean $\pm$ 3SD of 530 mGAD-U/ml, and anti-mumps IgM type antibody by IFA method (Bion, USA).

Table 1. Clinical characteristics of the patients.

	IDDM (n = 18)	ADM (n = 11)
Sex (M:F)	13:5	6:5
Mean age (years)	36.8 ± 16.4	44.8 ± 13.7
DM duration (years)	5.6 ± 4.5	5.1 ± 4.7
BMI (kg/m^2)	19.6 ± 3.9	19.6 ± 2.2
CRA (ng/ml/min)	3.2 ± 4.6	4.2 ± 2.3[a]
HbA1c (%)	11.6 ± 3.9	13.0 ± 2.8

Note: CRA = C-peptide response area under the curve. [a]$p < 0.05$ by Mann-Whitney U test.

Table 2. Immunogenetic characteristics of the patients.

	IDDM	ADM
IAA	33%	–
ICA	22%	–
anti-GAD Ab	11%	–
anti-mumps IgM Ab	27%	–
HLA DR3/DR4	55%	50%

Results

Between the two groups, age, duration of DM, BMI and HbA1c were not significantly different, but the C-peptide response area under the curve on the 75-g OGGT was significantly higher in ADM patients than IDDM patients (Table 1).

The islet cell antibody, insulin autoantibody (IAA), anti-GAD antibody and anti-mumps IgM type antibody showed positivity of 22, 33, 11 and 27% in IDDM patients, respectively. However these autoantibodies and anti-mumps IgM type antibody were not detected in ADM patients. The HLA DR3 or DR4 showed a positivity of 50 and 55% in ADM patients and IDDM patients, respectively (Table 2).

Discussion

We suggest that ADM-occurring DKA might be developed by another mechanism such as genetic predisposition, environmental and nutritional status rather than autoimmunity. We need a long-term follow-up of these patients.

References

1. Winter WE. Maclaren N, Reley W, Clarke DW, Kappy MS, Spillar RP. Maturity-onset diabetes of youth in black Americans. N Engl J Med 1987;316:287–291.
2. Banerji MA, Chaiken RL, Harold E. Lebovitz HE. Long-term normoglycemic remission in black newly diagnosed NIDDM subjects. Diabetes 1996;45:337–341.

Recent Advances on the Pathogenesis and Management of Diabetes Mellitus.
S.H. Shinn, M. Shichiri and K.-W. Kim, editors.

Anemia in nonuremic diabetic patients

Y.S. Yun, B.S. Cha, Y.D. Song, S.K. Lim, H.C. Lee, J.S. Hahn and K.B. Huh
Division of Endocrinology, Department of Internal Medicine, Yonsei University College of Medicine, Seoul, Korea

Abstract. We evaluated the causes and characteristics of anemia in diabetic patients without uremia (creatinine clearance $\geqslant 30$ ml/min/m^2) and investigated whether inappropriate erythropoietin response was involved in the unexplained anemia of diabetics. As evaluative causes of anemia, iron deficiency (21.7%) and chronic disorders (18.8%) were frequent intercurrent illnesses. However, the causes of anemia could not clearly be explained in 35 (50.7%) out of 69 patients. In this group, serum EPO levels (17.1 ± 8.0 mU/ml) were significantly lower than those of nondiabetic anemic patients (144.9 ± 108.0 mU/ml, $p < 0.01$). It is suggested that a blunted EPO response to anemia may play some role in the maintenance of unexplained anemia of long-term diabetes.

Keywords: anemia, erythropoietin.

Introduction

Anemia is a frequently noted disorder in long-term diabetes [1]. Causes of anemia in diabetic patients are thought to be intercurrent illnesses such as iron deficiency, chronic disorder or uremia due to diabetic nephropathy [2]. However, in some groups, causes of anemia cannot be explained clearly. This suggests that there may be a specific type of anemia associated with long-term diabetes [3]. Erythropoietin (EPO) is synthesized by the kidney in response to anemic or hypoxic stimulation and bears a negative relationship to hemoglobin concentration and hematocrit percentage [4]. Therefore, we investigated the characteristics and possible causes of anemia in nonuremic diabetic patients and evaluated whether blunted renal EPO production is involved in the pathogenesis of anemia of these patients.

Material and Methods

Among the 779 nonuremic diabetic patients followed up by the diabetic clinic at Yonsei University College of Medicine from January 1991 to December 1995, 192 anemic patients (14 IDDM and 178 NIDDM) were recruited for this study. All patients were nonuremic with a creatinine clearance rate $\geqslant 30$ ml/min/m^2. Studies for the causes of anemia could be completed in 69 subjects. Routine

Address for correspondence: Yong Seok Yun MD, Department of Internal Medicine, Severance Hospital Yonsei University College of Medicine, 134 Shinchon-Dong Seodaemun-Gu, Seoul 120-752, Korea. Tel.: +82-2-361-5422. Fax: +82-2-393-6884. E-mail: endosong@yumc.yonsei.ac.kr

laboratory tests were performed: blood count, serum iron, total iron-binding capacity, vitamin B_{12} and folate level, reticulocyte, Coombs' test, serum haptoglobulin, peripheral blood smear or bone marrow study. Serum erythropoietin levels were measured by radioimmunoassay with an EPO-Tranc^{TM} RIA kit (23200, INCSTAR Corporation Stillwater, Minnesota, USA). The amount of EPO was expressed in mU/ml and the average EPO value was 17.7 ± 7.5 mU/ml with a normal range of 9.1–30.8 mU/ml. As a control, serum EPO levels were measured in 20 nondiabetic anemic patients with other hematologic diseases.

Results

The mean hemoglobin value was 11.6 ± 1.1 g/dl in 180 patients and red cell indices were normocytic in 134 (69.8%) out of 192 patients. The hemoglobin values were inversely correlated with diabetic duration ($p = 0.03$) and the amount of albuminuria ($p = 0.01$). In 69 anemic patients who underwent the baseline study for anemia, iron deficiency and chronic disorder were frequent causes of anemia. However, causes of anemia cannot be explained exactly in spite of a baseline study of anemia in 35 (50.7%) patients. Mean serum EPO levels of unexplained anemic patients were 17.6 ± 8.1 mU/ml. Each value was almost within the normal range and did not show an appropriate increased response when considering the anemic condition. These values were significantly lower than those of nondiabetic patients with anemia (144.9 ± 108.0 mU/ml, $p < 0.01$).

Discussion

In this study, the prevalence of anemia was 24.6% (192 out of 772 patients) in non-uremic diabetic patients. In most patients, the severity of anemia was mild and the erythrocyte indices were normocytic normochromic patterns. As definable causes of anemia, iron deficiency and chronic disorders such as tuberculosis were noted frequently. These may be associated with the dietary pattern and nutritional status of diabetic patients. However, in many patients, the causes of anemia could not be explained exactly despite the baseline studies of anemia. Such findings suggest that there may be a specific type of anemia associated with long-term diabetes. Our finding of inadequate erythropoietin responses in these patients was consistent with the finding of anemia of chronic disease or chronic renal failure. There were at least three possible mechanisms for reduction of EPO response in diabetic patients: damage to the renal parenchyme, which includes the EPO-producing site [5], defect of the autonomic nervous system, such as β-2 adrenergic antagonist, and protein malnutrition can reduce EPO response.

It must be carefully considered that a long-term diabetic condition should be included in the category of chronic disorders associated with anemia. Inappropriate EPO response may be involved in maintenance of anemia in some diabetic patients and further studies will be warranted to evaluate the certain processes which blunt the feedback mechanisms regulating the serum EPO production.

References

1. Kojina K, Totsuka Y. Anemia due to reduced serum erythropoietin concentration in non-uremic diabetic patients. Diabet Res Clin Pract 1995;27:229–233.
2. Erslew AJ, Wilson J, Caro J. Erythropoietin titers in anemic, non-uremic patients. J Lab Clin Med 1987;429–433.
3. Robert LJ, Charles MP. Hematologic alterations in diabetes mellitus. Am J Med 1981;70: 339–352.
4. Schwster SJ, Wilson JH, Ersler AJ, Coro J. Physiologic regulation and tissue localization of renal erythropoietin messenger RNA. Blood 1987;70(1):316–318.
5. Lacombe C, Dasilra JL, Bruneval P, Fourdier JG, Wendling F, Casaderall N, Camiller JP, Bariety J, Varet B, Tambourin P. Peritubular cells are the site of erythropoietin synthesis in the murine kidney. J Clin Invest 1988;81:620–623.

Recent Advances on the Pathogenesis and Management of Diabetes Mellitus.
S.H. Shinn, M. Shichiri and K.-W. Kim, editors.

Comparison of World Health Organization and National Diabetes Data Group criteria to detect abnormal glucose tolerance in Korean pregnant women

M.H. Kang, H.Y. Park and S.K. Lee
Department of Internal Medicine, Chung Ang Gil Hospital, Inchon, Korea

Abstract. *Background.* Currently the one-step WHO test and the two-step procedure proposed by National Diabetes Data Group (NDDG) are recommended for the diagnosis of gestational diabetes mellitus (GDM). WHO criteria, though simpler, are seldom used in Korea. This study is to compare the WHO and NDDG criteria in the effectiveness of detecting abnormal glucose tolerance and its related complications in Korean pregnant women.

Methods. Pregnant women in the latter half of the gestational period had both a 1-h and a 2-h glucose concentration measurement after an oral 75-g load, and those who had a 1-h glucose concentration $\geqslant$140 mg/dl, underwent a 100-g, 3-h glucose tolerance test. In order to determine the effectiveness of the two tests, we compared the frequency of abnormal pregnancy outcomes such as macrosomia, cesarian section, neonatal hypoglycemia and premature labor.

Results. Out of 64 women who had post-75-g, 1-h plasma glucose $\geqslant$140 mg/dl and a 100-g test, nine had DM and 38 had IGT by WHO criteria, and 17 had GDM by NDDG criteria. Thirty women with a normal test by NDDG criteria had an abnormal glucose tolerance according to WHO criteria, mostly IGT (28). From the 15 women delivering macrosomic infants, 13 (87%) were abnormal on the WHO test and nine (60%) were abnormal on the NDDG test. Of the 24 women who delivered by cesarean section, 16 (67%) had an abnormal WHO test, and eight (33%) had an abnormal NDDG test. Of the six cases of neonatal hypoglycemia, five were associated with an abnormal WHO test and all six were associated with an abnormal NDDG test.

Conclusion. The simpler one-step WHO test was at least as good as the NDDG test in predicting adverse outcomes related to abnormal glucose tolerance in Korean pregnant women.

Keywords: abnormal pregnancy outcomes, cesarian section, gestational diabetes mellitus, macrosomia, NDDG test, WHO test.

Introduction

Gestational diabetes mellitus (GDM) is associated with complications for both the mother and the infant in the perinatal period [1]. Two sets of criteria are currently being used for the diagnosis of abnormal glucose tolerance during pregnancy. One is the one-step WHO test which defines both diabetes and impaired glucose tolerance, based on a 75-g oral glucose tolerance test (OGTT) used in nonpregnant adults [2]. The other is the two-step procedure proposed by the National Diabetes Data Group (NDDG) [3]. In almost all of Korea the NDDG criteria are being used. But the NDDG criteria require two tests, four blood samples over 3 h and a high glucose load, making the procedure more cumbersome than the one-step WHO procedure. Thus there has been strong argument for adopting the WHO test as a standard diagnostic criterion for the diagnosis of

Table 1. Results of 100-g, 3-h OGTT according to 2-h glucose concentration after 75-g glucose load in the 84 subjects with 1-h glucose ⩾140 mg/dl.

75g 2-h glucose		100 g test		
mg/dl	n	No test done	Normal	Abnormal
<140	37	16	17	4
140–199	38	4	28	6
⩾200	9	0	2	7
Total	84	20	47	17

glucose intolerance during pregnancy [4–6]. This study followed methods modified from the study performed on Pima Indians by Pettit et al. [6], with the intention of comparing the WHO and NDDG criteria in the effectiveness of detecting abnormal glucose tolerance and its related complications in Korean pregnant women.

Materials and Methods

384 pregnant women in the latter half of their gestation period had both a 1-h and a 2-h glucose concentration measurement after an oral 75-g load, and those who had a 1-h glucose concentration ⩾140 mg/dl were referred for a 100-g, 3-h glucose tolerance test. Diagnosis was made as DM or IGT according to 2-h plasma glucose levels after 75-g load under WHO criteria and as GDM based on 100-g OGTT under NDDG criteria. The effectiveness of the two tests was evaluated by comparing the frequency of adverse outcomes known associated with maternal hyperglycemia including macrosomia (⩾4,000 g), delivery by cesarian section, prematurity (delivery before 37 weeks' gestation) and neonatal hypoglycemia (plasma glucose <40 mg/dl). Comparison of frequency of adverse pregnancy outcomes between the two tests was done on the 64 of 84 women with a 1-h plasma glucose ⩾140 mg/dl after a 75-g glucose load who completed a 100-g, 3-h test and delivery.

Results

Table 2. Neonatal complications by abnormal WHO or NDDG glucose tolerance tests in 64 women.

	Number	Abnormal WHO test n (%)	Abnormal NDDG test n (%)
Macrosomia (>4.0 kg)	15	13 (87%)	9 (60%)
Hypoglycemia	6	5 (83%)	6 (100%)
Prematurity (<37 weeks)	5	3 (60%)	2 (40%)
Congenital anomaly	1	1 (100%)	0 (0%)

Table 3. Maternal complications by abnormal WHO or NDDG glucose tolerance tests in 64 women.

	Number	Abnormal WHO test n (%)	Abnormal NDDG test n (%)
Cesarean section	24	16 (67%)[a]	8 (33%)[a]
Polyhydraminosis	5	5 (100%)	4 (80%)
Pre-eclampsia	2	1 (50%)	1 (50%)

[a]$p < 0.05$.

Of the 384 women who received a 75-g glucose load, 84 had a 1-h plasma glucose ⩾140 mg/dl (22%). All those with a 1-h plasma glucose < 140 mg/dl also had a 2-h plasma glucose < 140 mg/dl, and nine (2.3%) had DM and 38 (8.8%) IGT according to the WHO criteria. Out of 84 women with a 1-h plasma glucose ⩾140 mg/dl, 20 had no 100-g test and 17 (4.7%) had GDM by NDDG criteria. Thirty women with a normal glucose tolerance by NDDG criteria had an abnormal glucose tolerance according to WHO criteria, mostly IGT (28) and four with a normal test by WHO criteria had an abnormal glucose tolerance according to NDDG criteria (Table 1).

Fifteen of the 64 women delivered macrosomic infants. Thirteen of these women tested abnormal on the WHO test and nine tested abnormal on the NDDG test (Table 2). Of the 24 women who delivered by cesarean section, 16 had abnormal WHO tests, while only eight had abnormal NDDG tests (Table 3). Out of six cases of neonatal hypoglycemia, five were associated with an abnormal WHO test and all six were associated with an abnormal NDDG test. Of the five women with premature labor, three were abnormal by WHO criteria and two were abnormal by NDDG criteria. Of the five women with polyhydroamniosis, all five had abnormal WHO tests and four had abnormal NDDG tests. A higher percentage of women delivering by cesarian section was identified as abnormal by WHO criteria than NDDG criteria. Also, the two tests were not significantly different in predicting the other abnormal pregnancy outcomes.

Discussion

Both NDDG and WHO criteria are used for the diagnosis of glucose intolerance during pregnancy and international agreement still remains to be reached as to commonly acceptable diagnostic criteria. In almost all of Korea the two-step procedure proposed by NDDG is used. But the two-step NDDG procedure is more cumbersome to perform than the one-step WHO procedure, because it needs greater glucose load and more sampling time points. Thus it would be necessary to attempt comparing the two methods in the diagnosis of gestational diabetes in Korean women. Several other studies showed that the nonfasting 2-h glucose concentration after a 75-g glucose load strongly identifies adverse maternal and fetal outcomes [6—8]. This study also suggests that the simpler WHO criteria are at least as good as NDDG criteria in predicting abnormal outcomes in pregnant Korean women.

The 75-g load used in this study might produce a higher 1-h plasma glucose concentration than the 50-g screening load recommended by NDDG, particularly in subjects with abnormal glucose tolerance [9]. Though it is unlikely that any woman who would have had a plasma glucose concentration $\geqslant$140 mg/dl 1 h after a 50-g load might have not been so identified using a 75-g load. The rate of positive screening test in this study was 22%, a little higher than 14–16% in another study using a 50-g load [10], but similar to those of the studies in which the threshold values were lowered to 130 or 135 mg/dl [11,12].

There is debate over on the requirement of fasting before an oral glucose tolerance test. Fasting or nonfasting adds little to the glucose tolerance test because the glucose concentrations during the test are affected little by the time since the last meal [13]. Also, nonfasting helps improve compliance since pregnant women often have difficulty with fasting until the test.

Apart from maternal glucose intolerance, other factors such as maternal age, adiposity, ethnic origin, past obstetric experience and family history of diabetes also affect the risk for abnormal pregnancy outcomes [1]. In this study there was no difference in maternal BMI, age, frequency of family history of diabetes and gestational age at the time of the test between the abnormal WHO test group and the NDDG test group, and predictability of abnormal pregnancy outcomes was as good as or better using WHO criteria than it is using NDDG criteria. Most discrepancies in the diagnosis of glucose intolerance during pregnancy lie between IGT by WHO criteria and normal glucose tolerance by NDDG criteria, suggesting the need for improvement of sensitivity in the NDDG criteria. In fact there have been attempts to improve their sensitivity by lowering the cutoff point on the screen [11,14–16] or modifying the definition of abnormality [12,15,16]. Although the relationship between the degree of glucose intolerance and the risk of adverse maternal, fetal and neonatal outcomes remains to be elucidated, the WHO test was at least as good as the NDDG test in identifying abnormal pregnancy outcomes. It is also simpler to perform and has the advantage of comparability with a 75-g test at postpartum follow-up.

References

1. Metzger BE. Summary and recommendations of the third international workshop-conference on Gestational Diabetes Mellitus. Diabetes 1991;40(Suppl 2):197–201.
2. World Health Organization. Diabetes mellitus: report of a WHO study group. Geneva, WHO, 1985 (Tech Rep. Ser, no. 727).
3. National Diabetes Data Group. Classification and diagnosis of diabetes mellitus and other categories of glucose intolerance. Diabetes 1979;28:1039–1057.
4. Lind T, Phillips PR. Influence of pregnancy on the 75-g OGTT. A prospective multicenter study. Diabetes 1991;40(Suppl 2):8–13.
5. Martin FI. The diagnosis of gestational diabetes. Med J Aust 1991;155(2):112.
6. Pettitt DJ, Bennett PH, Narayan KMV, Knowler WC, Hanson RL. Comparison of WHO and

NDDG procedures to detect abnormalities of glucose tolerance during pregnancy. Diabet Care 1994;17:1264–1268.
7. Pettitt DJ, Bennett PH, Knowler WC, Baird R, Alerck KA. Gestational diabetes mellitus and impaired glucose tolerance during pregnancy: long-term effects on obesity and glucose tolerance in the offspring. Diabetes 1985;34(Suppl 2):119–122.
8. Pettitt DJ, Bennett PH, Saad MF, Charles MA, Nelson RG, Knowler WC. Abnormal glucose tolerance during pregnancy in Pima Indian women: long-term effects on offspring. Diabetes 1991;40(Suppl 2):126–130.
9. Castro A, Scott JP, Grettie DP, Macfarlane D, Bailey R. Plasma insulin and glucose response of healthy subjects to varing glucose loads during three-hour oral glucose tolerance tests. Diabetes 1970;19:842–851.
10. Dooley SL, Metzger BE, Cho NH. Gestational diabetes mellitus: the influence of race on disease prevalence and perinatal outcome in a U.S. population. Diabetes 1991;40(Suppl 2):25–29.
11. Jang HC, Cho N, Jung KB et al. Screening for gestational diabetes mellitus in Korea. Int J Gynecol Obstet 1995;51:115.
12. Sacks DA, Abu-Fadil S, Greenspoon JS, Fotheringham N. Do the current standards for glucose tolerance testing in pregnancy represent a valid conversion of O'Sullivans's original criteria? Am J Obstet Gynecol 1989;161:638–641.
13. Gough WW, Shack MJ, Bennett PH, Burch TA, Miller M. Evaluation of glucose in the Pima Indians by longitudinal studies. Diabetes 1970;19(Suppl 1):388 (Abstract).
14. Jang HC, Cho NH, Min YK et al. Gestational diabetes mellitus in Seoul, Korea and Chicago IL: Similarities and differences in racial/ethnic groups. Diabetes 1994;43(Suppl 1):136A (Abstract).
15. Carpenter MW, Coustan DR. Criteria for screening tests for gestational diabetes. Am J Obstet Gynecol 1982;144:768–773.
16. Tallarigo L, Giampietro O, Penno G, Miccoli R, Gregori G, Navalesi R. Relation of glucose tolerance to complications of pregnancy in nondiabetic women. N Engl J Med 1986;315:989–992.

Immunology

Recent Advances on the Pathogenesis and Management of Diabetes Mellitus.
S.H. Shinn, M. Shichiri and K.-W. Kim, editors.

HLA-DRB1/DQB1 genes and susceptibility to IDDM in Koreans

Yongsoo Park[1], Youhern Ahn[1], Taewha Kim[1], Mokhyun Kim[1], Kwangwook Ko[1] and Seiwon Yang[2]
[1]*Department of Internal Medicine and Pediatrics, Hanyang University College of Medicine, Seoul; and* [2]*Department of Pediatrics, Seoul National University College of Medicine, Seoul, Korea*

Abstract. *Background.* The HLA class II region is known to encode the most important genetic factors in IDDM and both DQ and DR are presumed to influence IDDM susceptibility. Although the nature of association for a particular allele in the HLA class II region may be very different in various ethnic groups, we can assume that the effect of a given allele on IDDM susceptibility is probably consistent in all populations.

Methods. Susceptibility of HLA-DRB1 and DQB1 genes to IDDM in Koreans was assessed by association analyses using 151 IDDM patients and 140 nondiabetic controls.

Results. DQB1*0201 was the only DQB1 allele that is positively associated while DQB1*0602, *0601 and *0301 were negatively associated with IDDM. Three DRB1 alleles (DR3, DRB1*0407 and DR9) were positively associated while four DR alleles (DR15, DR12, DR10 and DR14) were negatively associated with IDDM. However, haplotype analyses confirmed that the susceptibility effects of all DRB1 and DQB1 alleles were consistent in Koreans and all other populations.

Conclusions. The ethnic differences in allelic associations are due to different linkage disequilibrium of DRB1 and DQB1 alleles. Our analyses also indicate that the counterbalancing effect between susceptible DRB1 and protective DQB1, and vice versa, is the major factor responsible for the low incidence of diabetes in Koreans.

Keywords: HLA DQ, HLA DR, insulin-dependent diabetes mellitus.

Introduction

Recent genome-wide mapping studies have indicated that a large number of genes contribute to the genetic susceptibility to IDDM and the HLA class II region encodes the most important genetic factors in IDDM [1,2]. Several studies have clearly demonstrated that both DQ and DR influence IDDM susceptibility [3,4]. It has now become evident that there are both susceptible and protective alleles at DRB1, DQA1 and DQB1 loci. Although the nature of association (positive, neutral or negative) for a particular allele may be very different in various ethnic groups, the effect of a given allele on IDDM susceptibility is probably consistent in all populations. The ethnic discrepancies of allelic associations are explained by different linkage disequilibrium of DR and DQ genes, which results in a different counterbalancing effect between DR/DQ molecules [5].

Address for correspondence: Yongsoo Park MD, Department of Internal Medicine, Hanyang University Hospital, 249-1 Kyomun-dong, Kuri, Kyunggi-do, Seoul 471-020, Korea.

The frequencies of IDDM-associated HLA antigens correlate with the worldwide diabetes incidences [6], which differ by ethnicity as well as geographic regions. However, DR-DQ linkage disequilibrium is probably a more important factor explaining the interracial differences in diabetes incidences [5]. According to the Seoul Registry [7], the incidence of diabetes among children under the age of 15 years in Korea was 0.6/100,000/year. This low incidence rate in the Korean population may also be explained by the distribution of HLA genes. However, little is known regarding HLA allele polymorphism in the IDDM and the general population in Korea. To assess the effect of HLA-DR and DQ genes on IDDM, we performed HLA-DR and HLA-DQ molecular typing in 151 randomly selected cases of IDDM and compared those with the data of 140 healthy nondiabetic controls.

Materials and Methods

151 cases of IDDM patients were selected randomly from the Korean Seoul Registry [7]. The criteria for classification of IDDM were determined by the National Diabetes Data Group. Seventy-eight were male, 73 were female; their mean current age was 13 years (range: 3—22 years). Their mean age at diagnosis was 8.0 ± 4.3 years with the mean duration of diabetes being 4.7 ± 3.4 years.

Peripheral blood lymphocytes from all donors were used for the molecular typing of the high resolution typing of HLA-DRB1 and most common HLA-DQA and B chain gene allelic forms [8]. Amplification of HLA-DRB1 genes, HLA-DQA1 and B1 chain genes was performed according to the 11th IHW protocols using oligonucleotide primers distributed by the 11th IHW [8]. HLA DRB1/DQA1/DQB1 was genotyped using PCR-SSO techniques.

The gene frequencies were obtained by counting the total number of specific HLA antigens defined by oligonucleotide probe analysis. Differences in the HLA allele distributions were determined using the χ^2 test with Yates' correction (two-tailed). When the expected frequency for one of the alleles was less than 5, Fisher's exact test was used. Estimates of the relative risk (RR) in the different individuals were calculated using Woolf's method, as modified by Haldane for small sample sizes when appropriate [8].

Results

DR3 and DR9 had increased frequencies in diabetic patients compared to controls (RR = 6.1 and 1.6, respectively). DR4 as a group was not significantly increased in diabetic patients compared to controls. Among the DR4 subtypes, DRB1*0401 and DRB1*0405 had increased frequencies in patients compared to controls albeit the differences were not statistically significant. Surprisingly, DRB1*0407 was significantly increased (RR = 14.1). Two DR4 subtypes (0403 and 0406) had lower frequencies in patients than controls but statistical significance was not reached. As expected, DR15 confers strong protection. DR12 was also strongly protective. DR10 and DR14 were also weakly protective. Only DQB1*0201 had significantly higher frequencies in patients than controls (RR = 2.4), while three DQB1 alleles (0301, 0601, 0602) had significantly lower frequencies in patients compared to controls. It is noteworthy that DQB1*0302 (RR = 1.6) was not significantly increased in the patients.

Five haplotypes (DRB1*03-DQB1*0201, DRB1*0401-DQB1*0302, DRB1*-0405-DQB1*0302, DRB1*0407-DQB1*0302 and DRB1*0901-DQB1*0303) had increased frequencies in diabetic patients than controls. Five other haplotypes (DRB1*15-DQB1*0601, DRB1*15-DQB1*0602, DRB1*08-DQB1*0601 and DRB1*10-DQB1*05) had lower frequencies in patients than controls. All other haplotypes did not show significant differences between the two.

Nine genotypes (DR1/4, DR1/9,...) showed higher frequencies in patients than controls (RR = 7.3—12.8). These nine genotypes involve combinations of six haplotypes (DR1, DR3, DR4, DR7, DR8, DR9 and DR13). A total of 53 out of 115 (46%) patients had one of these nine genotypes, whereas only three out of 140 (2.1%) normal controls had these genotypes. As a group, the risk to IDDM for subjects with these genotypes is very high (RR = 39). It is worth noting that DR3/3 homozygotes did not confer strong susceptibility and DR4/4 homozygotes as a group may even confer some weak protection.

Discussion

We have analyzed the associations of IDDM with individual DR and DQ alleles; however, analyses of haplotypes are more informative than analyses of individual genes to understand the complex association of HLA and IDDM. As expected, the associations between IDDM and DRB1, DQB1 and their haplotypes in Koreans are very similar to those reported in Japanese [9] and Chinese [10], with some differences. In Koreans, DR3 and DR9 were positively associated with IDDM while the DR4 group was neutral. The Korean population also differs from the Japanese by the relatively higher frequency of DR3 which is almost nonexistent in Japanese.

A review of most available data indicates that DR4 subtypes have consistent effects on IDDM in all ethnic groups [5,9,10]. The DRB1*0405, 0402, 0401 confer strong susceptibility, while 0403, 0406 and 0408 confer strong protection. The distribution and susceptibility effects of various DR4 subtypes in Koreans are very similar to the observations in Chinese and Japanese. Notably, DRB1*0403 and 0406 confer protection while 0405 confers strong susceptibility. The susceptibility effect of the most common DR4 subtype in Koreans, DRB1*0405 (55% of DR4 alleles) was not revealed by association analyses of individual DRB1 alleles in the overall data set or in the DR4+ subset. However, it became more evident when the risk conferred by DRB1*0405-DQB1*0302 was examined (RR = 4.4). The susceptibility effect of DRB1*0405 could not be revealed by allelic association analyses because of strong linkage disequilibrium between the highly susceptible DRB1*0405 and protective DQB1*0401. Around

90% (37 out of 41) of the DRB1*0405 haplotypes are found with DQB1*0401, which confers protection. The counterbalance between susceptible DRB1 and protective DQB1 allele rendered the DRB1*0405-DQB1*0401 haplotype neutral (RR = 1.3).

DRB1*0403 is found in Asians and Caucasians. It confers dominant protection against IDDM in all populations studied. In Koreans its protective effect is evident even though it is associated with the highly susceptible DQB1*0302 allele. DRB1*0406, which is only found at high frequency in Asian populations, also confers strong protection. This Korean data set revealed a strong susceptibility effect of DRB1*0407, which is rare in the two other Asian populations as well as most other populations. DRB1*0404 is negatively associated with IDDM in this Korean data set, as revealed by analyses in the entire data set as well as by analyses with DR4+ subjects. The effect of DRB1*0404 is difficult to determine because inconsistent associations were reported in the literature. The increased risk of the DRB1*0404-DQB1*0302 haplotype in Koreans (RR = 3.3) is consistent with a neutral to weakly susceptibility effect for DRB1*0404. Finally, DRB1*0401 and 0402 are rare in all Asian populations; however, our observations are consistent with the susceptibility effect in Koreans.

The associations between IDDM and DQB1 alleles in the Koreans are exactly identical to those observed in the Chinese [10] and Japanese populations [9]. However, major differences were seen between the Asian populations and other groups. The most significant difference is the neutral associations of DQB1*0302 and DQB1*0401 in all three Asian populations (RR = 1.6 and 1.3, respectively in Koreans), whereas DQB1*0302 is highly susceptible and DQB1*0401 is protective in Caucasians. These transracial differences can be explained by linkage disequilibrium in these racial groups [5]. The majority of the DQB1*0302 haplotypes (70%) are associated with protective DR4 subtypes (DRB1*0403 or DRB1*0406) in the general population in Korea. This linkage disequilibrium between DQB1*0302 and protective DR4 subtypes has also been observed in Chinese and Japanese, and is believed to be responsible for the neutral association between DQB1*0302 and IDDM observed in Asian populations, even if DQB1*0302 is a strong IDDM susceptibility allele in Asians as well as in Caucasians.

While haplotype analyses are very informative in revealing the effect of DR and DQ alleles; genotypes of DR/DQ are most useful in predicting the risk to IDDM for each individual. We have calculated the relative risk associated with each genotype and some groups of genotypes. Only nine groups of genotypes confer a significantly higher risk to IDDM in Koreans. These nine genotypes involve seven haplotypes (DR1, 3, 4, 7, 8, 9 and 13). Three of the nine genotypes are found in IDDM patients in all ethnic groups (i.e., DR3/4, DR1/4, DR4/13). Two are found in Japanese IDDM patients (DR4/8 and DR9/13) and one in Chinese (DR3/9). The three other genotypes are only found in Koreans (DR1/9, DR9/9 and DR4/7). The increased risk associated with these genotypes are due to the synergistic effect, which can be explained by the heterodimers formed between DQB1 and DQA1 alleles on two different haplotypes. However, the effect of DR1/9 and DR9/9 cannot be explained by DQ heterodimers. It is important to note that since the frequencies of the high-risk genotypes such as DR3/4 are very low in the Korean population, the "iceberg" phenomenon may be very relevant in explaining the appearance of so many genotypes associated with risk to IDDM in Koreans.

Genotype analyses also revealed that DR4/4 and DR3/3 homozygotes are not associated with high risk to IDDM in Koreans. In all DR4/4 homozygous control subjects, at least one protective DR4 subtype (such as 0403 or 0406) or one protective DQB1 allele (0301 or 0401) is found. The counterbalance effect between DR and DQ molecules may explain why DR4/4 homozygous genotypes are not at high risk to IDDM in Koreans. However, it is unclear why DR3/3 confers high risk in Chinese but not in Koreans. This may be due to random variation in our samples or, if confirmed, it would indicate that other susceptibility genes on the DR3 haplotype are different between Chinese and Koreans.

The frequencies of HLA alleles and linkage disequilibrium observed in Koreans are consistent with the low frequency of diabetes in this population. As in Japanese and Chinese, linkage disequilibrium between susceptible DQB1 (DQB1*0302) and protective DRB1 (0403 and 0406), as well as between susceptible DRB1 (0405, 0401) and protective DQB1 (0401) is the major factor responsible for the low incidence of IDDM in Koreans. It is remarkable to note that the slightly higher incidence of IDDM in Chinese compared to Japanese and Koreans can be attributed, at least partly, to the low frequency of DR3/3 in Japanese and low susceptibility of DR3/3 in Koreans.

References

1. Nepom GT, Erlich H. MHC class-II molecules and autoimmunity. Ann Rev Immunol 1991;9: 493–525.
2. Thomson G. HLA disease associations: models for insulin dependent diabetes mellitus and the study of complex human genetic disorders. Ann Rev Genet 1988;22:31–39.
3. Noble JA, Valdes AM, Cook M, Klitz W, Thomson G, Erlich HA. The role of HLA class II genes in insulin-dependent diabetes mellitus: Molecular analysis of 180 Caucasian, multiplex families. Am J Hum Genet 1996;59:1134–1148.
4. Erlich HA, Zeidler A, Chang J, Shaw S, Raffel LJ, Klitz W, Beshkov Y, Cosin G, Pressman S, Bugawan T, Rotter JI. HLA classes II alleles and susceptibility and resistance to insulin dependent diabetes mellitus in Mexican-American families. Nature Genet 1993;3:358–364.
5. She J-X. Susceptibility to type I diabetes: HLA-DQ and DR revisited. Immunol Today 1996;17: 323–329.
6. Todd JA, Bell JI, McDevitt HO. HLA DQ gene contributes to susceptibility and resistance to insulin-dependent diabetes mellitus. Nature 1985;329:559–694.
7. Karvonen M, Tuomilehto J, Libman I, LaPorte R, for the World Health Organization DIAMOND Project Group. A review of the recent epidemiological data on the worldwide incidence of type 1 (insulin-dependent) diabetes mellitus. Diabetologia 1993;36:883–892.
8. Tsuji K, Aizawa M, Sasazuki T. HLA 1991: The 11th International Histocompatibility Workshop DNA component, vol 2. Oxford: Oxford University Press, 1992.

9. Awata T, Kanazawa Y. Genetic markers for insulin-dependent diabetes mellitus in Japanese. Diabet Res Clin Pract 1994;24(Suppl):S83–S87.
10. Huang HS, Peng JT, She JY, Zhang LP, Chao CC, Liu KH, She JX. HLA-encoded susceptibility to insulin-dependent diabetes mellitus is determined by DR and DQ genes as well as their linkage disequilibrium in a Chinese population. 1995;44:210–219.

Recent Advances on the Pathogenesis and Management of Diabetes Mellitus.
S.H. Shinn, M. Shichiri and K.-W. Kim, editors.

Molecular cloning of new autoantigens reactive with prediabetic NOD sera

Yup Kang, Kyeong Sook Choi, Ki-Hwan Kim, Hyeon-Man Kim, Kwan-Woo Lee, Yoon-Sok Chung, In-Young Ko and Ji-Won Yoon
Laboratory of Endocrinology, Institute for Medical Science, Ajou University, Suwon, Kyunggi-Do, Korea

Abstract. *Background.* Insulin-dependent diabetes mellitus (IDDM) is believed to be an autoimmune disease and is characterized by the activation of immunity against insulin-producing pancreatic β cell. The NOD (nonobese diabetic) diabetic mice are the best models for studying the pathogenesis of human IDDM. The identification of new autoantigens reactive with the activated immune system of diabetic patients would open the study of pathogenesis, diagnosis and prevention of this disease.

Methods. A λ gt11 expression library containing MIN6N8a cDNAs was constructed using the directional cDNA cloning method. The positive clones were selected by immunoscreening of the expressed MIN6N8a proteins with prediabetic NOD sera. The N-terminal nucleotide sequence of new autoantigen genes was determined by cyclic sequencing of cloned λ gt11 DNAs.

Results. The nine positive clones were selected from 2×10^5 phage plaque. As a result of N-terminal sequencing and database searching, it was shown that the clones 2-1, 3-1, 3-2, 3-3, 8-1 and 10-1 contained a part of the retrovirus envelope protein gene and the clones 3-5, 9-1 and 9-2 had the unreported new gene.

Conclusions. The four new autoantigen genes reactive with prediabetic NOD sera were screened from λ gt11-MIM cDNA library. One new autoantigen was confirmed to be the retroviral envelope protein and the remaining three autoantigens had the unreported new peptide.

Keywords: cDNA library, λ gt 11, IDDM (insulin-dependent diabetes mellitus), immunoscreening, MIN (mouse insulinoma), retrovirus.

Introduction

Insulin-dependent diabetes mellitus (IDDM) results from the progressive destruction of insulin-producing pancreatic β cells by an activated immune system [1]. Although the destruction of β cells is mediated by T lymphocyte [2], the pathogenic induction of IDDM is associated with the presence of autoantibodies to islet cell components including insulin, GAD 65 (glutamic acid decarboxylase), 38 kDa, ICA69 (islet cell antibody), ICA512, etc. [3]. Therefore, the identification of more autoantigens reactive with diabetic sera would widen the knowledge of the pathogenic mechanism of IDDM. Despite the acute clinical onset of the disease, there is a subclinical latency period. Autoantibodies directed against islet antigen are detectable in the serum of individuals with or at risk of IDDM,

Address for correspondence: Yup Kang, Laboratory of Endocrinology, Institute for Medical Science, Ajou University, Woncheon-Dong San 5, Paldal-Gu, Suwon, Kyunggi-Do 442-749, Korea.

thus representing important markers for the detection of anti-islet autoimmunity before the appearance of clinical symptom. Theoretically, the tolerance induction against β-cell-specific immunity involved in pathogenesis of IDDM during preclinical stage can be applied as the new therapeutic approach to prevent IDDM. The identification of more new antigens involved in pathogenesis of IDDM would be applicable to a diagnostic or preventive study of IDDM. Therefore, we have tried to find novel β-cell-specific autoantigens reactive with activated humoral immune system using NOD mice.

Materials and Methods

Cell line and sera

Mouse insulinoma cell line, MIN6N8a, was used for construction of β cell line cDNA library. This cell line was kindly provided by Dr Myazaki (University of Tokyo, Japan). This cell was cultured in 10% FBS (fetal bovine serum) of DMEM with 1 g/l glucose. The pool of 12 prediabetic NOD (nonobese diabetic) mice (8, 12 and 16 weeks old) sera was used for screening autoantigens.

Construction of MIN6N8a cDNA library

The mRNA was isolated from cultured MIN cell by using polyA-tract mRNA isolation system (Promega Biotech, Madison, WI, USA). The first strand cDNA was synthesized with Not I-dT primer (5′-AATTCGGGCCGC$(T)_{15}$). The second strand was synthesized with RNase H and DNA polymerase I. After trimming each end of cDNA with T4 DNA polymerase, EcoRI adaptor (5′-AATTCCGTTGCTGTCG, 5′-CGACAGCAACGG) was attached to each end of cDNA. After cutting with Not I, cDNAs were inserted into the corresponding site of λ gt 11 vector. Phage λ gt 11 MIN library was constructed through in vitro packaging and infection to *Escherichia coli* Y1090.

Immunoscreening

Phage lawn was made by infection of recombinant phages to *E. coli* Y1090 and pouring on LB (Luria broth) plate. MIN cDNA proteins were expressed and transferred by overlaying IPTG (isopropyl thio galactopyranoside)-saturated nitrocellulose (NT) paper onto phage lawn. The positive clones were screened by binding with 100-fold diluted NOD serum and alkaline phosphate-conjugated antimouse IgG antibody, respectively, and developing with BCIP (bromo chloro indoryl phosphate)/NBT (nitroblue tetrazolium).

Determination of N-terminal nucleotide sequence

The pure positive phage clones were selected through second and third immunoscreening. The cloned DNAs were isolated through phage amplification, PEG (polyethylene glycol) concentration, and phenol/chloroform extraction. The cyclic reaction of phage DNA with ^{32}P-labeled λ gt 11 forward primer (5′-GGTGGCGACGACTCCTGGAGCCCG) by using OmniBase sequencing polymerase (Promega Biotech) was carried out. After fractionation of the synthesized DNAs on urea gel, the nucleotide sequences were read on autoradiographic film.

Results

In order to find out new autoantigens reactive with prediabetic NOD sera, MIN6N8a cDNA library was constructed and positive clones were screened. Figure 1 shows the third screening of purified phage clones. The nine positive clones were selected from 200,000 phage library clone. The clone 3-5 has the strongest and largest signal intensity. The clones 3-1, 3-2, 3-3 and 8-1 showed fairly strong signals. In contrast, the signal intensities of clones 2-1, 9-1, 9-2 and 10-1 were pretty weak but stronger than the uncloned phage negative clone (−).

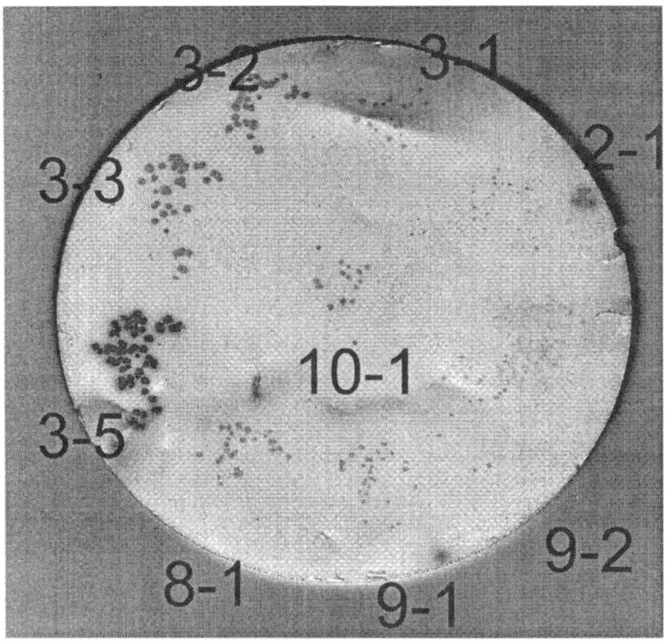

Fig. 1. Third screening of λ gt 11 MIN6N8a cDNA library with diluted prediabetic NOD sera. Phage lawn was made by infection of recombinant phage to *E. coli* Y1090 and pouring onto LB agar. Cloned proteins were expressed and transferred by overlaying IPTG saturated NT membrane on phage lawn. The positive signal was detected by binding with NOD sera and alkaline phosphate conjugated anti-mouse IgG antibody and developing with BCIP/NBT. The positive phage plaques were picked and purified by second screening. This picture depicts the third screening of positive phage clones. Around 20—30 positive phages were infected to grown *E. coli*. After induction and transfer of cloned proteins, the positive signals on NT membrane were developed by BCIP/NBT staining.

To establish which gene the positive clones were, we determined the nucleotide sequence of the N-terminal end of positive clones and compared them with the nucleotide sequence of already reported genes from Genbank database. Interestingly, the six clones 2-1, 3-1, 3-2, 3-3, 8-1 and 10-1 have a partial sequence of retrovirus envelope gene. In contrast, the clones 3-5, 9-1, and 9-2 contained the new nucleotide sequences. Table 1 lists the size of insert and the matched gene of positive clones.

Discussion

We cloned four new autoantigen genes from MIN6N8a cell reactive with prediabetic NOD sera. None of our clones were matched with the published autoantigens reactive with activated immune system in IDDM. In fact, most of the reported autoantigens were selected with activated human immune system [3]. Although it was reported that the NOD immune system also activated an immune system against GAD and HSP [4], the humoral reactivity against NOD antigens seemed to be different from that against human antigens. Although our autoantigens were selected with activated NOD immune system, more studies will be required to clarify whether our autoantigens are specific for the NOD immune system. At this moment we are producing the autoantigen proteins using the *E. coli* expression system and investigating the humoral reactivity with ICR sera. We will also investigate the generation and production period of autoantibody from individual NOD mice. Retrovirus envelope protein as an autoantigen was very interesting. It was reported that the pathogenesis of IDDM in NOD mice was associated with the expression of retrovirus. Several groups, including our group, have already reported specific expression of retrovirus in NOD pancreatic islet [5]. More studies, such as selective expression of our cloned retroviral gene in pancreatic islet, the T cell reactivity against our retroviral envelope protein, and the tolerance induction with retroviral envelope (ecotropic retroviral envelope gene) protein in NOD mice, are necessary to identify the role of retro-

Table 1. Homology matching of cloned new autoantigens.

Clone	Size of insert (kb)	Matched gene	Homology (%/size)
2-1	1.1	Env[a]	97/181
3-1	1.0	Env	97/169
3-2	1.2	Env	97/188
3-3	0.9	Env	99/226
3-5	1.8	New[b]	
8-1	1.0	Env	98/224
9-1	1.2	New	
9-2	1.0	New	
10-1	1.1	Env	99/255

[a]Env: ecotropic retroviral envelope gene; [b]New: unreported new gene in Genbank database until March 1997.

virus in the pathogenesis of IDDM. Clone 3-5 had the strongest and largest signal of our all clones. The gene of clone 3-5 was completely new. We subcloned clone 3-5 gene to *E. coli* expression vector pET 30b and expressed in *E. coli* BL21. The size of expressed protein was around 15 kDa. The small size of clone 3-5 protein on phage lawn seemed to help it to diffuse easily. NOD sera appears to contain the autoantibody recognizing conformational epitope of clone 3-5 protein, since the treatment with DTT (dithiothreitol) and SDS (sodium dodecyl sulfate) completely abolishes the immunoreactivity of NOD sera.

Acknowledgements

This study was supported by a grant (HMP-96-M-2-0018) of the 1996 Good Health R & D Project, Ministry of Health and Welfare, ROK.

References

1. Atkinson MA, Maclaren NK. The pathogenesis of insulin-dependent diabetes mellitus. N Engl J Med 1994;331:1428–1436.
2. Bach J-F. Insulin-dependent diabetes mellitus as an autoimmune disease. Endocrine Rev 1994;15:516–542.
3. Yoon JW, Park YH, Santamaria P. Autoimmunity of insulin-dependent diabetes. In: Flatt PR, Ionnides C (eds) Drugs, Diet and Disease Mechanistic Approaches to Diabetes 2. London: Ellis Howard of Simon and Schuster International Group, 1995;57–97.
4. Roep BO. T-cell response to autoantigens in IDDM. Diabetes 1996;45:1147–1156.
5. Yoon JW, Jun HS. Role of viruses and autoimmunity in the pathogenesis of type I diabetes. J Biomed Res 1995;4:18–28.

Recent Advances on the Pathogenesis and Management of Diabetes Mellitus.
S.H. Shinn, M. Shichiri and K.-W. Kim, editors.

Increased prevalence of autoimmune diseases in IDDM patients

Yoonju Cho[1], Yongsoo Park[1], Youhern Ahn[1], Taewha Kim[1], Mokhyun Kim[1] and Sinkyu Kim[2]
Departments of [1]Internal Medicine and [2]Clinical Pathology, Hanyang University College of Medicine, Seoul, Korea

Abstract. *Background.* IDDM is frequently associated with other autoimmune diseases including autoimmune thyroid diseases (ATD). The broad concept of polyendocrinopathies takes into consideration that patients affected by at least one endocrine disease may also possess a positive serological reactivity against other organs.

Methods. Because particular HLA alleles are the major predisposing factors for IDDM, we investigated whether they are shared by other autoimmune diseases. In addition, to investigate potential clustering of autoimmune diseases among IDDM family members, antithyroid autoantibody (ATA) by RIA, antinuclear antibody (ANA) and antineutrophile cytoplasmic antibody (ANCA) by indirect IF, rheumatoid factor (RF) by latex agglutination were studied in 128 cases of IDDM patients and their 96 first-degree family members.

Results. Twenty-five percent of IDDM patients were ATA(+), whereas 8% of age-matched controls were ATA(+). Twenty-six percent of IDDM family members had ATA. In contrast, 16% of IDDM patients were ANA(+), while no patients were ANCA(+) or RF(+). Seven percent of IDDM family members had ANA. IDDM patients with ATA had longer duration of disease, whereas those with ANA did not. There were no differences in the distribution of HLA alleles between those with and without respective autoantibodies.

Conclusions. From this, we could assess that individuals with IDDM and their relatives frequently develop polyclonal autoantibodies, perhaps due to common susceptibility genes that are shared among first-degree relatives.

Keywords: HLA DQ, HLA DR, IDDM, polyendocrinopathy.

Introduction

IDDM is a disease characterized by an absolute deficiency of insulin caused by destruction of the pancreatic β cells through an autoimmune mechanism. Genetic backgrounds are important in the pathogenesis of IDDM, and like many autoimmune diseases, IDDM is associated with particular HLA alleles [1]. During the long prodromal period, a lot of autoantibodies to pancreatic β cell antigens may arise and persist even after the disease has become clinically overt. IDDM patients and their relatives with or without clinical manifestations of other autoimmune disease also have a high prevalence of thyroid microsomal, gastric parietal, and adrenal antibodies [2,3]. In addition, the broad concept of polyendocrinopathies takes into consideration that patients affected by at least one

Address for correspondence: Yongsoo Park MD, Department of Internal Medicine, Hanyang University Hospital, 249-1 Kyomun-dong, Kuri, Kyunggi-do, Seoul 471-020, Korea.

endocrine disease may also possess a positive serological reactivity against other endocrine cell targets [4]. However, there has been no plausible explanation for the phenomenon. In this study, we measured antithyroid autoantibodies, antinuclear antibodies, antineutrophile cytoplasmic antibodies, rheumatoid factor, ICA, anti-GAD, and IA-2/ICA512 autoanbodies in IDDM patients with an onset age below 15 years in order to investigate potential clustering of other autoimmune diseases in IDDM patients and their family members. We also wanted to investigate whether IDDM-susceptible HLA DR/DQ alleles are shared by the IDDM patients with other autoimmune diseases to explain their coassociation.

Materials and Methods

128 cases of IDDM patients were selected randomly from the Korean Seoul Registry [5]. The criteria for classification of IDDM were determined by the National Diabetes Data Group. Sixty-six were male, 62 were female; their mean current age was 13 years (range: 3—22 years). Their mean age at diagnosis was 7.9 ± 4.3 years with the mean duration of diabetes being 4.8 ± 3.4 years. Thirty-six nondiabetic control subjects, with no family history of diabetes, matched by sex and age, were selected from the same geographical area. Eighteen were male and 18 were female. Their mean current age was 13.4 years (range: 1.4—20 years). All the patients and control subjects gave their informed consent to the study. A total of 96 family members from the 42 simplex IDDM families also participated in this study. Forty-two were male and 54 were female. Their mean current age was 34 years (range: 12—64 years).

Thyroid peroxidase antibodies and thyroglobulin antibodies were measured by radioimmunoassay using commercial kits developed by RSR Ltd. (UK). The titer was expressed in "Uml^{-1}". A value of more than 0.3 Uml^{-1} was considered positive, which was 3SD above the mean of the 50 healthy individuals. Rheumatoid factor (RF) was measured by latex agglutination. Antinuclear antibodies (ANA) and antineutrophile cytoplasmic antibodies (ANCA) were measured by indirect IF using the cultured cell line of IT-1. Islet cell antibody (ICA) was measured by indirect IF on the cryostat sections of fresh frozen pancreas from a blood group O donor obtained during a surgical operation.

Human IA-2/ICA512 (amino acids 256—979) cDNA subcloned into PCRII vector (Invitrogen, San Diego, CA) was transcribed and translated in vitro in the presence of ^{35}S-methionine using the TNT-coupled rabbit reticulocyte system. The IA-2/ICA512 radioassay was performed using a 96-well plate format as described previously [6]. The antibody levels were expressed as an index defined as: (cpm in the unknown sample – negative control)/(positive control – negative control). "Positive" was based on the 100th percentile of sera from 208 healthy control subjects, being an index of 0.071.

Soluble porcine GAD was purified from fresh pig brain and prepared for the radioimmunoprecipitation assay as previously described [7]. For immunoprecipitation, 40 μl of ^{125}I-GAD (50,000 cpm) was added to 25 μl of test plasma diluted

1:2 in cold wash buffer (20 mmol/l Tris pH 7.4, 150 mmol/l NaCl, Triton X-100 0.5% weight/volume). Samples were held overnight at 4°C, then with 50 μl of 50% protein A-Sepharose (1 h, 4°C), and then centrifuged. The radioactivity of the precipitate was then counted. The activity of test sera was expressed as a percentage of the counts precipitated by the reference serum. The upper limit for a normal result, as determined using sera from blood donors is 18 μ, which exceeds the mean ± 3SD.

Genomic DNAs from all donors were used for the molecular typing of the generic typing of HLA-DRB1 and most common HLA-DQ A and B chain gene allelic forms [7]. The gene frequencies were obtained by counting the total number of specific HLA antigens defined by oligonucleotide probe analysis. Differences in the HLA allele distributions and in the proportions of patients positive and negative for various autoantibodies were determined using the χ^2 test with Yates' correction (two-tailed).

Results

Twenty-nine of 115 (25.2%) IDDM patients had either antiperoxidase positive or antithyroglobulin positive, whereas three out of 36 (8.3%) age- and sex-matched controls had antithyroid autoantibodies (RR = 3.7, $p<0.05$). Twenty-six out of 96 (26.9%) IDDM family members had antithyroid autoantibodies (ATA). The IDDM patients with ATA had a longer duration of IDDM and were mainly composed of females (Table 1). In contrast, 16% of IDDM patients were ANA(+), while no patients were ANCA(+) or RF(+). Seven percent of IDDM family members had ANA. IDDM patients with ANA did not have a longer duration of IDDM. There were no differences in the distribution of sex between those with and without ANA.

Table 1. Clinical characteristics of IDDM patients with and without ATA.

Characteristics	IDDM patients	
	With ATA	Without ATA
n	29	86
Age of onset (years)	7.7 ± 3.6	8.1 ± 4.3
Mean duration of disease (years)	5.9 ± 3.8	4.2 ± 3.3[a]
Present age (years)	13.4 ± 4.2	12.3 ± 5.3
Sex ratio (male/female)	6/23	51/35[b]
Diabetic ketoacidosis at onset (n(%))	10 (34.5)	23 (26.7)
Family history of diabetes (n(%))	9 (31.0)	25 (29.1)
Current BMI (kg/m^2)	16.0 ± 2.5	16.1 ± 2.3
Current insulin dose (U/kg)	0.85 ± 0.42	0.82 ± 0.34
Fasting plasma c-peptide (nmol/l)	0.08 ± 0.09	0.09 ± 0.08

Note: Values are numbers or mean ± SD. [a]$p<0.05$ vs. IDDM patients with ATA. [b]$p<0.001$ vs. IDDM patients with ATA.

There was no difference in either the titer or the prevalence of ICA and anti-GAD between the patients with and without ATA. In contrast, IDDM patients with ATA had decreased levels of IA-2/ICA512 autoantibody (0.11 ± 0.24 vs. 0.26 ± 0.45, $p<0.05$). However, when we compared the IA-2/ICA512 antibody prevalence controlling for the duration, we could not find any significant difference. When we analyzed the anti-GAD titer according to duration of diabetes, we were able to find a significant difference. In long-standing IDDM patients with ATA ($\geqslant$3.6 years), the prevalence of anti-GAD was higher than in those without ATA (68.4 vs. 40.5%, $p<0.05$), but the titer was not significantly different. In contrast, in patients with short-duration diabetes with ATA (<3.6 years), the prevalence and levels of anti-GAD were not different from those in patients without ATA.

When we compared the distribution patterns of HLA-DR/DQ polymorphisms between the IDDM patients with and without ATA, no differences of the distribution of HLA alleles (or IDDM susceptibility alleles) and genotypes between the two were found. We could not find any significant differences in HLA-DR/DQ polymorphisms between the IDDM patients with and without other autoantibodies. We also measured HLA-DR/DQ polymorphisms in the first-degree family members of IDDM probands. To date, 42 IDDM probands, 40 siblings and 56 parents have participated. Six parent-offspring ATA(+) families have been identified; three with ATA(+) mothers, two with ATA(+) fathers and one with both parents affected. Three parental HLA DRB1/DQA1/DQB1 haplotypes have been defined in six of these families; four with DR4/DQA1*0301/DQB1*0302, one with DR3/DQA1*0501/DQB1*0201 and one with DR9/DQA1*0301/DQB1*0303.

Discussion

In Korean IDDM patients as well as in Caucasians, autoimmune thyroid diseases (ATD) is the most common coexisting organ-specific autoimmune disease. Individuals with IDDM even without clinical manifestations of ATD are reported to have a high frequency of thyroid autoantibodies [2,3,8]. However, these studies showed a wide range of the prevalence of ATD. From our study, we found a 25% prevalence of ATD by antithyroid antibody positivity in IDDM patients even at a young age, compared with 8% in age- and sex-matched controls. It may be feasible that more frequent screening of TFT ± antithyroid antibody may facilitate the identification of the individuals who are at risk for development of ATD.

As shown in Table 1, the duration of IDDM since onset in patients with ATA was significantly longer than that in IDDM patients without ATA, with no difference of age at onset. This finding was not consistent with that of Kawasaki et al. [8], in that they found a difference of age at onset rather than duration. Furthermore, they insisted that the prevalence of coma or ketoacidosis at the onset of IDDM in patients with ATD was significantly lower than that in patients without

ATD and that IDDM patients with ATD were clinically characterized by a late and slow onset of diabetes. But having no difference of basal insulin (c-peptide) secretory capacity might be an unlikely finding to explain IDDM patients with ATD as such. Neither could we confirm these findings. These differences might result from the numbers, the patient's age at onset, and the way of defining ATD.

There have been some reports indicating that high levels of anti-GAD were present in IDDM patients with ATD, compared with those without ATD [8,9]. In those studies, autoantibodies to GAD were determined by radioimmunoassay using the purified pig brain GAD. Using a similar assay, when we analyzed other IDDM patients with variable IDDM duration and age onset, we found a higher frequency of anti-GAD positivity in IDDM patients with older onset of age than in those with younger onset [7]. In the study by Kawasaki et al. [8], it was suggested that this may lead to a spurious increase in anti-GAD prevalence and titer in IDDM patients with ATD, who were older than those without ATD.

The broad concept of polyendocrinopathies takes into consideration that patients affected by at least one endocrine disease may also possess a positive serological reactivity against other endocrine cell targets [4]. To date, we speculate that the reasons for their coassociation are the following:

1. It might be caused by a high response by nonspecific B lymphocyte activation.
2. Other autoantibodies in IDDM patients might recognize the antigen itself or common epitopes in different antigens of both the pancreas and other tissues.

Several others have until now aimed to study the clustering of ATD [10] or other autoimmune endocrine diseases in IDDM patients and their family members [11]. However, none of the studies examined the degree of their coassociation precisely, nor did they investigate the possible cause. The present study was undertaken not only to determine the frequency of autoimmune diseases amongst IDDM patients but also to study the possible cause for their clustering in patients with IDDM and their family members. It was attempted to investigate whether IDDM-susceptible HLA DR/DQ alleles were shared between the IDDM patients with and without other autoimmune diseases to explain their coassociation. We could not find any differences in the distribution of HLA-DR and HLA-DQ alleles and genotypes between the patients with and without various autoantibodies. Furthermore, when we measured HLA-DR/DQ polymorphisms in the first-degree family members of IDDM probands, three parental HLA DRB1/DQA1/DQB1 haplotypes were defined in the affected parent-offspring ATD families: DR4/DQA1*0301/DQB1*0302, DR3/DQA1*0501/DQB1*0201 and DR9/DQA1*0301/DQB1*0303. All are the IDDM-susceptible haplotypes in the Korean population. It has been hypothesized that the autoimmune endocrine diseases are due to antigen-specific defects in suppressor T lymphocyte function [4]. There is an organ-specific suppressor T lymphocyte defect in IDDM that is separate from that of ATD, and the reduced activation of IDDM suppressor T lymphocytes by GAD is specific for IDDM. The observation that IDDM is associated with ATD or other autoimmune diseases very closely and associated with similar HLA genes suggests a very similar pathogenesis for these entities and this might be the reason why they often coassociate. It may well be that each disease has separate genes and a separate organ-specific defect in immunoregulation. The fact that some patients develop both of the diseases might be related to the inheritance of each closely related genes.

References

1. Thomson G. HLA disease associations: models for insulin dependent diabetes mellitus and the study of complex human genetic disorders. Ann Rev Genet 1988;22:31–50.
2. Christie MR, Genovese S, Cassidy D, Bosi E, Brown TJ, Lai M, Bonifacio E, Bottazzo GF. Antibodies to islet 37k antigen, but not to glutamate decarboxylase, discriminate rapid progression to IDDM in endocrine autoimmunity. Diabetes 1994;43:1254–1259.
3. Bottazzo GF, Doniach D. Polyendocrine autoimmunity: an extended concept. In: Volpe R (ed) Autoimmunity and Endocrine Disease. New York: Marcel Dekker, 1985;375–404.
4. Volpe R. Autoimmune endocrinopathies: Aspects of pathogenesis and the role of immune assays in investigation and management. Clin Chem 1994;40:2132–2145.
5. Ko KW, Yang SW, Cho NH. The incidence of IDDM in Seoul from 1985 to 1988. Diabet Care 1994;17:1473–1475.
6. Verge CF, Gianani R, Kawasaki E, Yu L, Pietropaolo M, Jackson RA, Chase HP, Eisenbarth GS. Prediction of type 1 diabetes in first-degree relatives using a combination of insulin, GAD, and ICA512bdc/IA-2 autoantibodies. Diabetes 1996;45:926–933.
7. Park Y, Lee H, Koh C-S, Min H, Rowley M, Mackay IR, Zimmet P, McCarthy B, McCanlies E, Dorman J, Trucco M. The low prevalence of immunogenetic markers in Korean adult-onset IDDM patients. Diabet Care 1996;19:241–245.
8. Kawasaki E, Takino H, Yano M, Uotani S, Matsumoto K, Takao Y, Yamaguchi Y, Akazawa S, Nagataki S. Autoantibodies to glutamic acid decarboxylase in patients with IDDM and autoimmune thyroid disease. Diabetes 1994;43:80–86.
9. Kontiainen S, Schlenzka A, Koskimies S, Rilva A, Maenpaa J. Autoantibodies and autoimmune diseases in young diabetics. Diabet Res 1990;13:151–156.
10. Dorman J, Burke J, McCanlies E, Swan J, Foley T. IDDM and Hashimoto's thyroiditis: Do they cluster in families? Diabetes 1994;43(Suppl 1):27A.
11. Badenhoop K, Walfish PG, Rau H, Fischer S, Nicolay A, Bogner U, Schleusener H, Usadel KH. Susceptibility and resistance alleles of human leukocyte antigen (HLA) DQA1 and HLA DQB1 are shared in endocrine autoimmune diseases. J Clin Endocrinol Metab 1995;80: 2112–2117.

Recent Advances on the Pathogenesis and Management of Diabetes Mellitus.
S.H. Shinn, M. Shichiri and K.-W. Kim, editors.

Expression of Fas in murine pancreatic β cells and its significance

Myung-Shik Lee[1], Sunshin Kim[2], Jae Hoon Chung[1], Moon-Kyu Lee[1] and Kwang-Won Kim[1]

[1]Department of Medicine, Samsung Medical Center; and [2]Clinical Research Center, Samsung Biomedical Research Institute, Seoul, Korea

Keywords: apoptosis, insulinoma, NOD.

Introduction

CD4+ lymphocytes are the most important effector cells in autoimmune diabetes of NOD mice which cause pancreatic β-islet cell destruction [1,2]. However, it is not known how CD4+ lymphocytes are able to destroy β-islet cells that most likely do not express MHC class II molecules. Apoptotic cell death mediated by an interaction of Fas-Fas ligand may be a mechanism by which MHC class II negative pancreatic β cells are destroyed by CD4+ T lymphocytes. We have examined the expression of Fas molecules in pancreatic islet cells as well as a NOD-derived mouse insulinoma cell line (MIN6N8) [3]. In addition, the role of Fas-mediated apoptosis in MIN6N8 cell death was explored in vitro.

Materials and Methods

We used flow cytometry, RT-PCR, in vitro CTL assays, RNase protection assays, and MTT assays.

Results

Although Fas expression was not detected by flow cytometric analysis of MIN6N8 cells using anti-Fas antibody, Fas transcripts were demonstrated in MIN6N8 cells and pancreatic islet cells by sequencing analysis of the cloned RT-PCR products using Fas-specific primers. IFN-γ, TNF-α, IL-1 and their combinations failed to enhance Fas expression. Unsorted activated splenocytes from diabetic NOD mice had CTL activity of a small degree against IFN-γ-treated MIN6N8 cells with FasL upregulation. However, agonistic anti-Fas antibody with or without cycloheximide did not exert cytotoxicity against MIN6N8 cells or pancreatic islets.

Address for correspondence: Myung-Shik Lee, Division of Endocrinology and Metabolism, Department of Medicine, Samsung Medical Center, 50 Ilwon-dong, Kangnam-ku, Seoul 135-230, Korea.

Discussion

Our data indicate that pancreatic β-islet cells express a small amount of Fas molecules, however, the role of Fas expression in the pathogenesis of autoimmune diabetes remains to be clarified further using other model systems enabling direct in vivo approaches to the significance of Fas expression on pancreatic β cells.

References

1. Wang Y et al. Autoimmune diabetes in NOD mice is L3T4 T-lymphocyte dependent. Diabetes 1987;36:535.
2. Wicker L et al. Transfer of autoimmune diabetes with splenocytes from nonobese diabetic (NOD) mice. Diabetes 1986;35:855.
3. Yagi N et al. Expression of intercellular adhesion molecules 1 on pancreatic b-cells accelerates b-cell destruction by cytotoxic T-cells in murine autoimmune diabetes. Diabetes 1995;44:744.

Recent Advances on the Pathogenesis and Management of Diabetes Mellitus.
S.H. Shinn, M. Shichiri and K.-W. Kim, editors.

Islet-specific autoantibodies and HLA DRB/DQA/DQB polymorphism in Korean IDDM

Jinho Shin[1], Yongsoo Park[1], Youhern Ahn[1], Taewha Kim[1], Mokhyun Kim[1] and Seiwon Yang[2]

[1]Department of Internal Medicine, Hanyang University College of Medicine, Seoul; and [2]Department of Pediatrics, Seoul National University College of Medicine, Seoul, Korea

Abstract. *Background.* Korea has the lowest incidence of IDDM in the world and prevalences of islet-specific autoantibodies are reported to be low compared with Caucasians. A different genetic susceptibility marker or a low frequency of high-risk HLA alleles could explain the lower prevalence of islet-specific autoantibodies and the low incidence of IDDM.

Methods. This was investigated by determining the frequencies of anti-GAD, ICA512/IA-2 autoantibodies, ICA, HLA-DRB1/DQA1/DQB1 alleles, in 150 cases of IDDM in Korea, selected for an age at diagnosis of IDDM of less than 15 years.

Results. Fifty-six percent were positive for anti-GAD, 36% for ICA512/IA-2 and 38% for ICA. The highest prevalence of anti-GAD was observed in those homozygous for DR4 (87.5%), exceeding that (47.8%) in those without this allele, and those with one DR4 (63.5%), whereas the highest prevalence of ICA was found in those homozygous for DR3 (100%), exceeding that in those with one DR3 (64.3%) or in those without this allele (36.7%). There was a significant difference in numbers of HLA DQ susceptibility heterodimers in anti-GAD positive or negative patients. No association of HLA alleles and ICA512/IA2 antibody positivity was found.

Conclusions. The prevalence of islet-specific autoantibodies in Koreans with IDDM is comparable to that in Caucasians and the immunogenetic markers for IDDM among Caucasians confer disease susceptibility among Koreans. Seropositivity to islet antigens was also associated with the HLA genotypes common to Caucasians. Low frequency of high-risk HLA alleles might explain the low incidence of IDDM in Korea.

Keywords: anti-GAD, HLA DQ, HLA DR, ICA, ICA512/IA-2, IDDM.

Introduction

During the prodromal period of IDDM, multiple autoantibodies to pancreatic β-cell antigens, including glutamic acid decarboxylase (GAD) ICA512/IA-2 and other unspecified antigens of islet cells (ICA), may arise and persist after the disease has become clinically overt [1–3]. However, a few patients with IDDM show no evidence of autoimmunity to these autoantigens [4]. There have been some data on differences in the prevalence of anti-GAD and ICA between Caucasians and Koreans with IDDM [5]. Genetic differences between ethnic groups might contribute to heterogeneity in the autoimmune response to the autoantigens. A different genetic susceptibility marker could explain the lower prevalence

Address for correspondence: Yongsoo Park MD, Department of Internal Medicine, Hanyang University Hospital, 249-1 Kyomun-dong, Kuri, Kyunggi-do, Seoul 471-020, Korea.

of islet-specific autoantibodies. In fact, IDDM is much less frequent in Korea than in countries with a predominantly Caucasian population [6]. However, what is common to the two populations is that the presence of high-risk HLA alleles increases the prevalence of autoantibodies specific for islet cells, as well as the incidence of IDDM, and the presence of low-risk alleles decreases these. Therefore, to estimate the degree to which genetic determinants influence the low incidence of IDDM in Korea, and to determine whether genetic factors contribute to differential autoimmune responses to islet-specific autoantigens, we examined the HLA-DR and -DQ associations with seropositivity to GAD, ICA512/IA-2 and ICA in Korean patients with IDDM.

Materials and Methods

150 IDDM cases were selected randomly from the Korean Seoul Registry [6]. The criteria for classification of IDDM were determined by the National Diabetes Data Group. Seventy-eight were male, 72 were female; their mean current age was 13 years (range: 3—22 years). Their mean age at diagnosis was 8.0 ± 4.3 years with the mean duration of diabetes being 4.7 ± 3.4 years.

Human ICA512 (amino acids 256—979) cDNA subcloned into PCRII vector (Invitrogen, San Diego, CA) was transcribed and translated in vitro in the presence of ^{35}S-methionine using the TNT-coupled rabbit reticulocyte system. The ICA512 radioassay was performed using a 96-well plate format as described previously [7]. The antibody levels were expressed as an index calculated from the cpm for the test sample and the positive and negative samples. “Positive” was based on the 100th percentile of sera from 208 healthy control subjects, being an index of 0.071.

The full-length GAD65 cDNA subcloned into pcDNA II vector (pEx9) was transcribed and translated in vitro using the same TNT-coupled reticulocyte lysate systems in the presence of ^{35}S-methionine as that in ICA512/IA-2 autoantibody assay. The anti-GAD65 assay was performed using a 96-well plate format as described previously [8]. The results of the anti-GAD65 assays were expressed as an index and the upper limits of the normal ranges for anti-GAD65 (index of 0.032) were established as the 99th percentile of the levels in 205 healthy control subjects.

ICAs were assessed using the immunoenzymatic method. End-point titers of ICA after serial dilution were expressed in Juvenile Diabetes Foundation (JDF) units by comparison with a standard curve constructed using a JDF standard reference serum and a value of more than 2.5 JDF units was considered positive.

Peripheral blood lymphocytes were used for the molecular typing of the generic typing of HLA-DRB1 and most common HLA-DQ A and B chain gene allelic forms [9]. Generic amplification of HLA-DRB1 genes were performed according to the 11th IHW protocols using oligonucleotide primers distributed by the 11th IHW [9]. HLA DQA1/DQB1 was genotyped using PCR-SSO techniques according to previous reports [10].

Differences in the HLA allele distributions and in the proportions of patients positive for islet-specific autoantibodies were determined using the χ^2 test with Yates' correction (two-tailed). When the expected frequency for one of the alleles was less than 5, Fisher's exact test was used.

Results

Antibodies to GAD were present in 84 (56%), and to ICA512/IA-2 were in 54 (36%) of the 150 cases of IDDM. ICA were found in 57 (38%) patients. In the IDDM cases, HLA DR3 (RR = 7.5, $p<0.00001$) and DR4 (RR = 2.3, $p<0.001$) were increased, while DR2 (RR = 0.2, $p<0.0001$), DR5 (RR = 0.3, $p<0.001$) and DR10 (RR = 0.1, $p<0.05$) were decreased. Among the DR genotypes, DR3/9 (RR = 24.3, $p<0.0001$), DR9/9 (RR = 12.2, $p<0.05$), DR3/4 (RR = 5.8, $p<0.001$) and DR3/X (X: other than 3, 4; RR = 7.6, $p<0.01$) were susceptible genotypes for IDDM. The HLA DQA1*0301 allele (RR = 2.0, $p<0.0001$) and the DQB1*0201 allele (RR = 2.6, $p<0.01$) were increased, and the DQB1*0301 allele (RR = 0.2, $p<0.001$), and the DQB1*0602 allele (RR = 0.2, $p<0.01$) were decreased.

When the frequencies of HLA-DR alleles, according to the presence or absence of each of the islet-specific autoantibodies were compared, we could not find any significant difference. When we compared HLA DQA1/DQB1 allele frequencies between patients positive or negative for anti-GAD, there was a significantly higher frequency of HLA-DQB1*0605 and a lower frequency of HLA-DQB1*0602. The relative prevalence of autoantibodies according to HLA-DR genotypes (Table 1) showed a decrease in prevalence of anti-GAD according to

Table 1. Prevalence of glutamic acid decarboxylase (GAD) antibodies and islet cell antibodies (ICA) according to HLA-DR genotype in Korean IDDM patients.

HLA-DR genotype	Anti-GAD present n (%)	Anti-GAD absent n (%)	Relative risk	p value
DR 4/4	7 (87.5)	1 (12.5)	7.3	<0.05[c]
DR 4/3 or DR 4/X[a]	41 (58.6)	29 (41.4)		
DR Y/Y[b]	26 (49.0)	27 (51.0)		
Total	74	57		
HLA-DR genotype	**ICA present n (%)**	**ICA absent n (%)**	**Relative risk**	**p value**
DR 3/3	1 (100)	0 (0)	6.1	
DR 3/4 or DR 3/X[a]	17 (53.1)	15 (46.9)	2.3	<0.05[d]
DR Z/Z[e]	32 (32.7)	66 (67.3)		
Total	50	81		

[a]X is an HLA-DR antigen other than DR3 or DR4. [b]Y is an HLA-DR antigen other than DR4. [c]One-side p value, when compared with the prevalence (49%) in patients without DR4 allele. [d]One-side p value, when compared with the prevalence (32.7%) in patients without DR3 allele. [e]Z is an HLA-DR antigen other than DR3.

homozygosity for DR4 (87%), heterozygosity for DR4 (59%) and those lacking this allele (49%), and a decreasing prevalence of ICA according to homozygosity for DR3 (100%), heterozygosity for DR3 (53%) and absence of this allele (33%). Finally, we ascertained a significant difference in numbers of HLA-susceptible heterodimers according to positivity or negativity for anti-GAD (Table 2). However, we could not find any association of HLA genotypes and ICA512/IA2 antibody positivity.

Discussion

From this study, we can conclude that IDDM in Korea is caused by an autoimmune mechanism on a similar type of genetic background as found in Caucasians, since the overall prevalence of islet-specific autoantibodies was comparable to Caucasians. We could assess that islet-specific autoantibodies may be good predictive markers for IDDM.

We found an association between IDDM and HLA DQ alleles, but the ORs given by HLA DQ genes were relatively small. Not only the presence of sequences coding for arginine in position 52 of the DQA1 gene (RR = 1.6, $p < 0.05$), but also that coding for an amino acid other than aspartate in the 57th position of the DQ B1 molecule (RR = 1.7, $p < 0.05$) were found to be independent markers for IDDM, but their strength of association was rather weak. The higher observed prevalence of 24% of nil heterodimers that confer susceptibility among IDDM cases in our low-risk Korean population corresponded to the distribution in nondiabetic controls, among whom the frequency of these genotypes was likewise higher. The genotype distribution among IDDM cases in a given area will reflect the proportions in the general population. The frequen-

Table 2. Frequency distribution of diabetic heterodimers composed of susceptible HLA DQ A1 (position 52) and HLA DQ B1 (position 57) alleles in 131 IDDM patients according to antibody status.

Susceptible heterodimers	Anti-GAD present n (%)	Anti-GAD absent n (%)	Relative risk	p value
4	16 (76.2)	5 (23.8)	3.6	$<0.05^a$
2	17 (50.0)	17 (50.0)	1.1	
1	26 (59.1)	18 (40.9)	1.6	
0	15 (46.9)	17 (53.1)		
Total	74 (100)	57 (100)		
Susceptible heterodimers	**ICA present n (%)**	**ICA absent n (%)**	**Relative risk**	**p value**
4	9 (42.9)	12 (57.1)	2.3	
2	14 (41.1)	20 (58.9)	2.1	
1	19 (43.2)	25 (56.8)	2.3	
0	8 (25.0)	24 (75.0)		
Total	50 (100)	81 (100)		

Note: Data are n (%) of 131 IDDM patients. [a]$p < 0.05$ vs. 0 heterodimer.

cies of IDDM-associated HLA antigens in the general population are correlated with the worldwide diabetes incidence [11]. Low frequency of high-risk susceptible heterodimers might explain the low incidence of IDDM in Korea.

It is interesting to note that the three susceptible DR genotypes found in our IDDM patients were all DR3-containing, suggesting that DR3 is important on IDDM susceptibility in Koreans. However, when we consider that only 25.2% of our IDDM patients have DR3 and therefore nearly three-quarters of our patients develop IDDM in the absence of DR3, individuals with DR3 are at a higher risk for IDDM, but DR3 is neither necessary nor sufficient for the development of the disease. Our findings in Koreans are similar to those reported in Mexican-Americans [12] and Chinese [13]. In both populations, a recessive effect of DR3 requiring another susceptible haplotype was observed. The heterozygote effect of DR3/DR4 is well-documented [11] and that of DR3/DR9 may be explained by transcomplementation of DQ molecules [13].

Autoantibodies to islet-cell antigens, including ICA512/IA-2 and GAD in addition to ICA have been described in patients with IDDM [1–4]. Anti-GAD is present in most but not all newly diagnosed IDDM patients [1,5]. The levels and prevalence of ICA and ICA512/IA-2 antibodies fall rapidly with increasing duration of IDDM, but this is not seen with anti-GAD [4,5,7]. Thus even though our cases were not recent-onset cases and the incidence of IDDM was low in our population, it was possible to ascertain an adequate number of IDDM subjects positive for anti-GAD to demonstrate an association between HLA-DR4 and anti-GAD, noting that statistical significance can be attained in a small sample if the differences are marked. However, the relatively long duration of IDDM might be seen as a limitation to our study, which could give a spurious lack of association between ICA, ICA512/IA-2 antibodies and HLA. Although we found a significant relation between HLA-DR3 and ICA, we should consider the possibility of an association between other alleles and ICA. Recognition of the significant associations between anti-GAD and HLA-DR4 genotype, as well as between ICA and HLA-DR3, merits a further investigation. Furthermore, we found a significantly increased prevalence of anti-GAD in patients with four susceptible HLA-DQ heterodimers compared with all other groups, as well as 0 heterodimer group. In our IDDM patients, 10 out of 13 patients with the DQ0302/0201 genotype had anti-GAD (RR = 3.8, $p < 0.05$), whereas 13 out of 19 patients with the DR3/4 genotype had anti-GAD. In Japanese subjects with IDDM, HLA DR9 has been found at a higher frequency in those with autoantibodies other than ICA [14]. According to Serjeantson et al. [5], it appeared that it was the persistence of anti-GAD that correlated with high-risk HLA-DR, DQ genotypes, at least in patients with a relatively late age of onset. Although HLA class II genes are important in IDDM, their influence on the expression of IDDM-associated antoantibodies is still unclear. Different genetic/environmental interactions might be involved in the etiology of IDDM among ethnic groups, or there may be a difference in persistence of autoantibodies in those with different genetic backgrounds.

References

1. Kaufman DL, Erlander MG, Clare-Salzler M, Atkinson MA, Maclaren NK, Tobin AJ. Autoimmunity to two forms of glutamate decarboxylase in insulin-dependent diabetes mellitus. J Clin Invest 1992;89:283–292.
2. Rabin DU, Pleasic SM, Shapiro JA, Yoo-Warren H, Oles J, Hicks JM, Goldstein DE, Rae PMM. Islet cell antigen 512 is a diabetes-specific islet autoantigen related to protein tyrosine phosphatases. J Immunol 1994;152:3183–3188.
3. Greenbaum CJ, Palmer JP, Nagataki S, Yamaguchi Y, Molenaar JL, Van Beers WAM, Maclaren NK, Lernmark A and Participating Laboratories. Improved specificity of ICA assays in the fourth international immunology of diabetes exchange workshop. Diabetes 1992;41:1570–1574.
4. Myers MA, Rabin DU, Rowley MJ. Pancreatic islet cell cytoplasmic antibody in diabetes is represented by antibodies to islet cell antigen 512 and glutamic acid decarboxylase. Diabetes 1995;44:1290–1295.
5. Serjeantson SW, Kohnen-Corish MJ, Rowley MJ, Mackay IR, Knowles W, Zimmet P. Antibodies to glutamic acid decarboxylase are associated with HLA-DR genotypes in both Australians and Asians with type 1 (insulin-dependent) diabetes mellitus. Diabetologia 1992;35: 996–1001.
6. Karvonen M, Tuomilehto J, Libman I, LaPorte R, for the World Health Organization DIAMOND Project Group. A review of the recent epidemiological data on the worldwide incidence of type 1 (insulin-dependent) diabetes mellitus. Diabetologia 1993;36:883–892.
7. Verge CF, Gianani R, Kawasaki E, Yu L, Pietropaolo M, Jackson RA, Chase HP, Eisenbarth GS. Prediction of type 1 diabetes in first-degree relatives using a combination of insulin, GAD, and ICA512bdc/IA-2 autoantibodies. Diabetes 1996;45:926–933.
8. Grubin CE, Daniels T, Toivola B, Landin-Olsson M, Hagopian WA, Li L, Karlsen AE, Boel E, Michelesen B, Lernmark A. A novel radiobinding assay to determine diagnostic accuracy of isoform-specific glutamic acid decarboxylase antibodies in childhood IDDM. Diabetologia 1994;37:344–350.
9. Tsuji K, Aizawa M, Sasazuki T. HLA 1991: The 11th International Histocompatibility Workshop DNA component, vol 2. Oxford: Oxford University Press, 1992.
10. Park Y, Lee H, Koh C-S, Min H, Rowley M, Mackay IR, Zimmet P, McCarthy B, McCanlies E, Dorman J, Trucco M. The low prevalence of immunogenetic markers in Korean adult-onset IDDM patients. Diabet Care 1996;19:241–245.
11. Todd JA, Bell JI, McDevitt HO. HLA DQ gene contributes to susceptibility and resistance to insulin-dependent diabetes mellitus. Nature 1985;329:559–694.
12. Erlich HA, Zeidler A, Chang J, Shaw S, Raffel LJ, Klitz W, Beshkov Y, Cosin G, Pressman S, Bugawan T, Rotter JI. HLA classes II alleles and susceptibility and resistance to insulin-dependent diabetes mellitus in Mexican-American families. Nature Genet 1993;3:358–364.
13. Chuang L-M, Lin BJ, Wu H-P, Tai T-Y, Tsai W-Y. Transcomplementation of HLA DQA1-DQB1 in DR3/DR4 and DR3/DR9 heterozygotes and IDDM in Taiwanese families. Diabet Care 1995;18:1483–1486.
14. Mimura G, Kida K, Matsuura N, Toyota T, Kitagawa T, Kobayashi T et al. Immunogenetics of early-onset insulin-dependent diabetes mellitus among the Japanese: HLA, Gm, BF, GLO, and organ-specific autoantibodies – the JDS study. Diabet Res Clin Pract 1990;8:253–262.

Recent Advances on the Pathogenesis and Management of Diabetes Mellitus.
S.H. Shinn, M. Shichiri and K.-W. Kim, editors.

Measurements of anti-GAD Ab by EIA and RIA methods in Korean diabetic patients

C.H. Chung, H.H. Lee, Y.G. Shin, M.D. Lee and H.S. Kim
Department of Internal Medicine, Wonju College of Medicine, Yonsei University, Wonju, Korea

Abstract. *Background.* Sometimes it is difficult to discriminate between IDDM and NIDDM among adult DM patients. Some NIDDM patients have autoantibodies. We labeled this as latent autoimmune diabetes of adults (LADA) or slowly progressive IDDM (SPIDDM). Anti-GAD (glutamic acid decarboxylase) Ab could be detected before the diagnosis of DM, and after the diagnosis it would be detected during the long-term follow-up period, thus it is helpful for the diagnosis of autoimmune diabetes.

Methods. Seventy-one diabetic patients who were admitted to Wonju Christian Hospital between May 1994 and February 1996 were studied. We classified them into IDDM, NIDDM and SPIDDM groups. We carried out a basic clinical study, oral glucose tolerance test, HLA DR typing, and a study of IgM antiviral Abs, ICA, IAA and anti-GAD Ab.

Results. The measurement of anti-GAD Ab by RIA had a higher sensitivity than EIA. With the RIA-IRMA method, IDDM patients showed a significantly higher positivity than NIDDM patients. Between ELA, RIA-HEXT, RIA-IRMA and RIA-RSR methods, anti-GAD titers showed a significant correlation ($p < 0.001$). Diabetic patients who had diabetes for a duration of less than 5 years showed higher positivity than the patients with diabetes of a longer duration.

Conclusions. From the above results, we concluded that in Korean diabetic patients the positivity of anti-GAD Ab by ELA and RIA method was lower than Caucasians. We suggest that other mechanisms rather than autoimmunity may be involved in the pathogenesis of diabetes mellitus in Korean patients. We need follow-up studies on the clinical and immunogenetic characteristics of these patients.

Keywords: autoantibodies, IDDM, immunogenetic, NIDDM, SPIDDM.

Introduction

Sometimes it is difficult to discriminate between IDDM and NIDDM among adult DM patients. Among these conditions is slowly progressive IDDM (SPIDDM) which has an insidious onset but eventual insulin dependency [1]. Anti-GAD (glutamic acid decarboxylase) Ab could be detected before the diagnosis of DM, and after the diagnosis it would be detected during the long-term follow-up period, therefore it is helpful for the diagnosis of autoimmune diabetes [2]. Anti-GAD Ab was positive in 78% of Caucasians with IDDM and 5% of those with NIDDM. Recently, however, Zimmet et al. reported low positivity of anti-GAD Ab in Asian IDDM patients [3]. We studied the role of autoimmunity

Address for correspondence: Choon Hee Chung, Department of Internal Medicine, Wonju College of Medicine, Yonsei University, 162 Ilsan-Dong, Wonju-Si, Kangwon-Do, Wonju 220-701, Korea.

in the pathogenesis of Korean adult DM patients using the measurements of anti-GAD Ab by several methods.

Materials

Sixty-eight diabetic patients who were admitted to Wonju Christian Hospital between May 1994 and February 1996 were studied. We classified them into IDDM, NIDDM and SPIDDM groups.

Inclusion criteria of SPIDDM (Tables 1 and 2)

1) Onset of DM after 40 years of age;
2) duration of diabetes less than 10 years;
3) maximal weight less than 110% of ideal body weight;
4) NIDDM period over 1 year;
5) basal C-peptide level less than 1.0 ng/ml;
6) C-peptide level less than 1.8 ng/ml at 6 min after 1 mg glucagon IV injection; and
7) fasting blood sugar more than 200 mg/dl.

Methods

We studied basic clinical characteristics such as duration of diabetes, percent of IBW, previous chronic alcohol drinking history (alcohol ingestion more than 44 g daily, 5 days per week, over the previous 2 years), urine ketone, HbA1C, total cholesterol, and triglyceride and 75 g oral glucose tolerance test (blood sugar, C-peptide and insulin). ICA was performed by immunohistochemical stain, IAA by ELISA kit (Biomerica, USA), anti-IgM varicella-zoster Ab by ELISA

Table 1. Clinical characteristics in IDDM, NIDDM and SPIDDM patients.

	IDDM	NIDDM	SPIDDM
Sex (m/f)	15/5 (22)	19/14 (33)	10/3 (13)
Age (years)	30.4 ± 14.8^a	52.2 ± 13.4^a	51.9 ± 8.5^a
Duration (years)	4.4 ± 4.3^a	7.4 ± 6.1^a	5.5 ± 3.7
PIBW (%)	89.6 ± 13.3^a	110.4 ± 14.8^a	95.1 ± 16.9^a
HbA1C (%)	12.1 ± 2.7^a	9.2 ± 2.7^a	10.0 ± 1.8^a
AUCC (ng/ml/h)	2.5 ± 3.9^a	9.0 ± 5.9^a	1.8 ± 0.8^a
AUIC (μU/ml/h)	8.5 ± 18.7^a	32.9 ± 26.9^a	6.4 ± 6.0^a
Triglyceride (mg/dl)	247.6 ± 373.3	248.9 ± 230.3	146.4 ± 86.3
Cholesterol (mg/dl)	167.8 ± 79.4	209.0 ± 101.8	195.1 ± 39.8
DKA history (%)	40.9^a	0^a	7.7^a
Alcohol history (%)	52.2	22.7	84.6

Notes: AUC(I)C = area under C-peptide (insulin) curve; PIBW = percent of ideal body weight. $^a p<0.05$.

Table 2. Immunogenetic characteristics in IDDM, NIDDM and SPIDDM patients.

	IDDM	NIDDM	SPIDDM
HLA DR4 (%)	27.3	12.1	38.5
VZV IgM Ab (%)	4.5	6.0	0
Mumps IgM Ab (%)	22.7	6.0	15.4
ICA (%)	9.1	3.0	0
IAA (%)	4.5	0	15.4
GADVELISA (%)	9.1	3.0	7.7
GADHEXT (%)	18.2	9.1	15.4
GADIRMA (%)	16.7[a]	0[a]	10.0
GADRSR (%)	17.6	3.0	10.0

VZV = varicella zoster virus. [a]$p < 0.05$.

kit (Radin, Italy) and anti-IgM mumps Ab by the IF method. We also performed HLA DR typing.

Anti-GAD Ab

1. ELISA (VELISA, elias, USA), cutoff value = mean ± 3SD (530 mGAD-U/ml).
2. Radioimmunoprecipitation method:
   a) anti-GAD HEXT (Japan), cutoff value = 5.4 IU/ml;
   b) IRMA, elias (Germany), cutoff value = 44.4 mGAD-U/m; and
   c) RSR Ltd. (England), cutoff value = 0.5 U/ml.

Results

The measurement of anti-GAD Ab by RIA had a higher sensitivity than ELA. Using the RIA-IRMA method, IDDM patients showed significantly higher positivity than NIDDM patients. Between ELA, RIA-HEXT, RIA-IRMA and RIA-RSR methods, anti-GAD titers showed significant correlation ($p < 0.001$). Diabetic patients who had suffered diabetes for a duration of less than 5 years showed higher positivity than the patients with diabetes of a longer duration.

Discussion

The measurement of anti-GAD Ab by RIA had higher sensitivity than ELA. Using the IRMA method, IDDM patients showed significantly higher positivity than NIDDM patients ($p < 0.05$). Between the VELISA, HEXT, IRMA and RSR methods, anti-GAD Ab titers showed significant correlation ($p < 0.001$) [4,5] (Table 3).

From the above results it can be concluded that in Korean IDDM and SPIDDM patients the positivity of anti-GAD Ab using the ELA and RIA methods was lower than in Caucasians. We suggest that other mechanisms rather

Table 3. Correlations between the anti-GAD Ab tests.

	VELISA	HEXT	IRMA	RSR
VELISA	1	0.695 ($p<0.0001$)	0.391 ($p = 0.0001$)	0.67 ($p<0.0001$)
HEXT	0.695 ($p<0.0001$)	1	0.631 ($p<0.0001$)	0.71 ($p<0.0001$)
IRMA	0.391 ($p = 0.0001$)	0.631 ($p<0.0001$)	1	0.47 ($p<0.0001$)
RSR	0.67 ($p<0.0001$)	0.71 ($p<0.0001$)	0.47 ($p<0.0001$)	1

than autoimmunity be involved in the pathogenesis of Korean IDDM and SPIDDM patients. We need further studies on the clarification of the pathogenesis of Korean adult diabetes mellitus patients.

References

1. Kobayashi T, Nakanishi K, Murase T, Kosaka K. Immunological and clinical characterization of slowly progressive IDDM. Diabet Res Clin Prac 1991;14(Suppl 1):S69.
2. Atkinson MA, Maclaren NK, Scharp DW, Lacy PE, Tiley W. 64,000 Mr autoantibodies as predictors of IDDM. Lancet 1990;1:1357–1359.
3. Zimmet P, King H et al. Classification and diagnosis of diabetes mellitus. In: Alberti KGMM, Krall LP (eds) The Diabetes Annual/3. Amsterdam: Elsevier, 1987;14.
4. Tuomi T, Groop LC, Zimmet P, Rowley MJ, Knowles W, Mackay IR. Antibodies to glutamic acid decarboxylase reveal latent autoimmune diabetes mellitus in adults with a non-insulin-dependent onset of disease. Diabetes 1993;42:359–362.
5. Rowley MJ, Mackay IR, Chen Q, Knowles W, Zimmet P. Antibodies to glutamic acid decarboxylase discriminate major types of diabetes mellitus. Diabetes 1992;41:548–551.

Recent Advances on the Pathogenesis and Management of Diabetes Mellitus.
S.H. Shinn, M. Shichiri and K.-W. Kim, editors.

The combination of multiple autoantibodies to islet-specific antigens in Korean insulin-dependent diabetic patients

Yongsoo Park[1], Youhern Ahn[1], Taewha Kim[1], Mokhyun Kim[1] and Seiwon Yang[2]

[1]Department of Internal Medicine, Hanyang University College of Medicine, Seoul; and [2]Department of Pediatrics, Seoul National University College of Medicine, Seoul, Korea

Abstract. *Background.* With the recent cloning and recombinant expression of novel islet autoantigens (ICA512 and GAD65), it is possible to investigate whether the quantitative expression of autoantibodies to these molecules is correlated with the semiquantitative titration of ICA.

Methods. To estimate the regional difference in the degree of association between these autoantibodies, autoantibodies reacting with ICA512 and GAD65 in addition to ICA were analyzed in 131 IDDM patients.

Results. Thirty-six percent of IDDM patients were ICA512 autoantibody positive and 56% of them were anti-GAD65 positive. Forty-three percent of IDDM were ICA-positive. Autoantibodies to ICA512 and anti-GAD65 were observed in 40 and 41 of 56 ICA positive subjects, respectively. The titer of ICA correlated with those of ICA512 autoantibodies ($r = 0.41$, $p < 0.0001$) and anti-GAD65 ($r = 0.49$, $p < 0.0001$). Among 131 patients with IDDM, 69% (90/131) had one or more ICA512 autoantibody, anti-GAD65, or ICA. Forty-three percent (57/131) had two or more of these autoantibodies.

Conclusions. From this, both the prevalences and the titers of ICA512 or anti-GAD65 were strongly correlated with those of ICA in Korean IDDM patients. ICA512 and anti-GAD65 in combination may be considered as an alternative to the ICA assay and they may be suitable for population screening in Korea.

Keywords: glutamic acid decarboxylase, ICA512, insulin-dependent diabetes mellitus, islet cell antibody.

Introduction

In IDDM patients, multiple autoantibodies to pancreatic β-cell antigens may arise before and persist even after the disease becomes clinically overt. Antibodies to glutamic acid decarboxylase (GAD), known as the 64KD islet cell antigen has been proved to be a sensitive and predictive antibody for IDDM [1,2]. ICA512 is another autoantigen of IDDM which was recently identified as the precursor of 40 kDa autoantigen, and has homology with the protein tyrosine phosphatase family [3]. Islet cell antibodies (ICA) are the most widely used serological markers of antiislet autoimmunity [4], but this indirect immunofluorescence assay on sections of normal human pancreas is semiquantitative and remains difficult to standardize. GAD and ICA512 have been shown to be two

Address for correspondence: Yongsoo Park MD, Department of Internal Medicine, Hanyang University Hospital, 249-1 Kyomun-dong, Kuri, Kyunggi-do, Seoul 471-020, Korea.

of the antigens that may be recognized by antibodies in the ICA test [5]. IDDM is much less frequent in Korea than in other countries with predominantly Caucasian populations [6]. There have also been some suggestions noting the marked differences in the prevalences of islet-specific autoantibodies between Caucasians and Koreans [7]. To estimate the regional difference in the degree of association between these autoantibodies of IDDM, autoantibodies reacting with ICA512 and GAD65 in addition to ICA were analyzed in Korean IDDM patients. Using these radioassays in combination, we would like to know whether these radioassays might be considered as an alternative to the ICA.

Materials and Methods

131 IDDM cases were selected randomly from the Korean Seoul Registry [8]. The criteria for classification of IDDM were determined by the National Diabetes Data Group. Sixty-eight were male, 63 were female; their mean current age was 12 years (range: 3—22 years). Their mean age at diagnosis was 7.9 ± 4.3 years with the mean duration of diabetes being 4.5 ± 3.4 years.

Human ICA512 (amino acids 256—979) cDNA subcloned into PCRII vector (Invitrogen, San Diego, CA) was transcribed and translated in vitro in the presence of ^{35}S-methionine using the TNT-coupled rabbit reticulocyte system. The ICA512 radioassay was performed using a 96-well plate format as described previously [9]. The antibody levels were expressed as an index defined as: (cpm in the unknown sample − negative control)/(positive control − negative control). "Positive" was based on the 100th percentile of sera from 208 healthy control subjects, being an index of 0.071.

The full-length GAD65 cDNA subcloned into pcDNA II vector (pEx9) was transcribed and translated in vitro using the same TNT-coupled reticulocyte lysate systems in the presence of ^{35}S-methionine as that in ICA512 autoantibody assay. The anti-GAD65 assay was performed using a 96-well plate format as described previously [10]. The results of the anti-GAD65 assays were expressed as an index calculated from the counts per minute for the test sample and the positive and negative samples. The upper limits of the normal ranges for anti-GAD65 (index of 0.032) were established as the 99th percentile of the levels in 205 healthy control subjects.

ICA were assessed using the immunoenzymatic method on cryostat sections of pancreas from a blood group O donor obtained during a surgical operation. Endpoint titers of ICA after serial dilution were expressed in Juvenile Diabetes Foundation (JDF) units by comparison with a standard curve constructed using a JDF standard reference serum, and a value of more than 2.5 JDF units was considered positive.

Results

The frequency of ICA512 autoantibodies was 36% (47/131). Fifty-six percent of

IDDM patients (73/131) had anti-GAD65, whereas 43% (56/131) had ICA. Prevalences of ICA512 autoantibodies, anti-GAD65 and ICA in recent-onset patients (duration < 1 year) were 75% (12/16), 75% (12/16) and 87% (14/16), respectively. In contrast, in a subset of these patients with long-standing diabetes (duration > 3 years), the prevalence of ICA512 autoantibodies, anti-GAD65, and ICA were decreased to 22% (17/77), 49% (38/77), and 25% (19/77), respectively (Table 1).

ICA512 autoantibodies as well as anti-GAD65 were significantly associated with the presence of ICA. Among IDDM patients, 68.7% (90/131) had one or more of anti-GAD65, ICA512 autoantibodies, or ICA; 43.5% (57/131) had two or more of these autoantibodies. ICA512 antibodies and anti-GAD65 were observed in 40 (71.4%) and in 41 (73.2%) of 56 ICA(+) subjects, respectively (Fig. 1). Only seven out of 34 (20.6%) ICA(−) patients had ICA512 antibodies. In five of these seven cases, anti-GAD65 were also detected. In the four patients who had ICA alone, the levels of ICA and ICA512 autoantibodies (8.7 ± 8.5 JDF-u; 0.02 ± 0.04) were significantly lower than those in sera with one or two additional markers (30.0 ± 51.2 JDF-u, $p<0.1$; 0.33 ± 0.46, $p<0.05$).

ICA512 autoantibodies or anti-GAD65 were found in 97% (34/35) and 100% (22/22) of subjects with ICA levels $\geqslant 20$ JDF-u and $\geqslant 40$ JDF-u, respectively. The 35 patients who had ICA levels $\geqslant 20$ JDF-u had increased indices of anti-GAD65 (0.41 ± 0.47) and ICA512 autoantibodies (0.58 ± 0.52) compared with 21 ICA(+) patients with the titer less than 20 JDF-u (0.09 ± 0.17, $p<0.01$; 0.23 ± 0.37, $p<0.01$, respectively). Analysis of autoantibody levels in individual sera revealed a significant correlation between ICA512 autoantibodies and ICA ($r = 0.41$, $p<0.0001$) or anti-GAD65 and ICA ($r = 0.49$, $p<0.0001$).

Table 1. Prevalence and levels of ICA512, anti-GAD65 and ICA in Korean IDDM patients according to the duration of disease

Characteristics	n	ICA512		Anti-GAD65		ICA	
		n (%)	Units	n (%)	Units	n (%)	Units
Newly diagnosed IDDM (< 1.0 year)	16	12 (75.0)	0.66 ± 0.59	12 (75.0)	0.33 ± 0.43	14 (87.5)	49.3 ± 52.4
Intermediate duration IDDM (1–3 years)	38	18 (47.4)	0.27 ± 0.41[b]	23 (60.5)	0.14 ± 0.27[b]	23 (60.5)	22.9 ± 35.7[a]
Longstanding IDDM (> 3.0 years)	77	17 (22.1)[c,d]	0.09 ± 0.25[c,e]	38 (49.4)	0.13 ± 0.29[b]	19 (24.7)[c,e]	14.4 ± 43.5

Note: Data are n (%) of 131 IDDM patients. Values are numbers or mean ± SD. [a]$p<0.05$ vs. newly diagnosed IDDM patients. [b]$p<0.01$ vs. newly diagnosed IDDM patients. [c]$p<0.001$ vs. newly diagnosed IDDM patients. [d]$p<0.05$ vs. intermediate duration IDDM patients. [e]$p<0.001$ vs. intermediate duration IDDM patients.

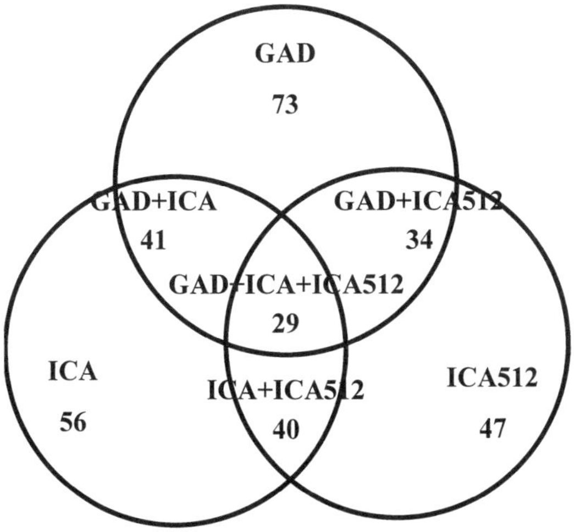

Fig. 1. The numbers of patients positive for each combination of islet-specific autoantibodies.

Discussion

In the Asian populations, it has been known that clinical and immunologic characteristics of IDDM are quite different from those of Caucasians. Countries in Asia, including Korea, have extremely low IDDM incidence rates with the rate less than one case/year/100,000 individuals [6]. The prevalences of ICA in Korean IDDM patients had been reported to be low compared with those of the Caucasians [7]. To date, not only is the detection of the islet-specific autoantibodies in a conventional way rather complicated and time-consuming, but incorrect patient definition might lead to false conclusions on the immunologic characteristics of IDDM in Korea. In this current study, we applied a new radioligand binding assay using recombinant ICA512 and GAD65 and measured the prevalence of ICA512 autoantibody, anti-GAD65 and ICA in 131 cases of IDDM, whose ages at diagnosis were less than 15 years. The overall prevalence of islet-specific autoantibodies was comparable to Caucasians, especially among those in recent-onset cases.

We found a significant association between the titers of anti-GAD65 as well as those of ICA512 autoantibodies with the levels of ICA. This suggests that not only ICA512 autoantibodies, but that GAD65 is likely to be one of the major antigens of ICA and there was a strong concordance among ICA, anti-GAD65, and ICA512 autoantibodies. Only 41 out of 73 (56.1%) anti-GAD65 positive sera from our IDDM patients were found to be ICA-positive. However, nearly all anti-GAD65-positive/ICA-negative sera were those from long-standing patients. As much as 40 out of 47 (85.1%) ICA512 autoantibody positive sera from our IDDM patients were found to be ICA-positive. Only seven out of 34 (20.6%) ICA(−) patients had ICA512 autoantibodies. This finding may reflect the greater sensitivity of radioassay compared with the immunohistochemical method used to detect ICA, because it is generally accepted that both GAD and ICA512 are ICA antigens [5].

Only 15 of 56 (26.8%) sera positive for ICA were anti-GAD65 negative. Sixteen of 56 (28.6%) sera positive for ICA were ICA512 autoantibody negative. However, four of 56 (7.1%) patients were still ICA-positive but anti-GAD65-negative/ICA512 autoantibody-negative. These ICA-positive/anti-GAD65-negative/ICA512 autoantibody-negative sera might represent the antibodies directed against a new component present in islet cells. When we admit the heterogeneity of islet-specific autoantibodies which were found in the sera of IDDM patients, and if we combine ICA512 autoantibodies and anti-GAD65 in addition to ICA, we may be able to achieve better prediction of IDDM development. Our interpretation of our data is, however, that IDDM in Korean populations has an autoimmune basis as in Caucasoids, and that there is a comparable expression of the marker autoantibodies, when we use the appropriate methodology and patient selection.

References

1. Baekkeskov S, Nielsen JH, Marner B, Bilde T, Ludvigsson J, Lernmark A. Autoantibodies in newly diagnosed diabetic children immunoprecipitate human pancreatic islet cell proteins. Nature 1982;298:167–169.
2. Baekkeskov S, Aanstoot HJ, Christgau S, Reetz A, Solimena MS, Cascalho M, Folli F, Richter-Olsen H, DeCamilli P. Identification of the 64K autoantigen in insulin-dependent diabetes as the GABA-synthesizing enzyme glutamic acid decarboxylase. Nature 1990;347:151–156.
3. Rabin DU, Pleasic SM, Shapiro JA, Yoo-Warren H, Oles J, Hicks JM, Goldstein DE, Rae PMM. Islet cell antigen 512 is a diabetes-specific islet autoantigen related to protein tyrosine phosphatases. J Immunol 1994;152:3183–3188.
4. Greenbaum CJ, Palmer JP, Nagataki S, Yamaguchi Y, Molenaar JL, Van Beers WAM, Maclaren NK, Lernmark A, and Participating Laboratories. Improved specificity of ICA assays in the fourth international immunology of diabetes exchange workshop. Diabetes 1992;41:1570–1574.
5. Myers MA, Rabin DU, Rowley MJ. Pancreatic islet cell cytoplasmic antibody in diabetes is represented by antibodies to islet cell antigen 512 and glutamic acid decarboxylase. Diabetes 1995;44:1290–1295.
6. Karvonen M, Tuomilehto J, Libman I, LaPorte R, for the World Health Organization DIAMOND Project Group. A review of the recent epidemiological data on the worldwide incidence of type 1 (insulin-dependent) diabetes mellitus. Diabetologia 1993;36:883–892.
7. Tuomi T, Zimmet P, Rowley M, Min HK, Vichayanrat A, Lee HK, Rhee BD, Vannasaeng S, Humphrey A, Mackay IR. Differing frequency of autoantibodies to glutamic acid decarboxylase among Koreans, Thais, and Australians with diabetes mellitus. Clin Immunol Immunopathol 1995;74:202–206.
8. Ko KW, Yang SW, Cho NH. The incidence of IDDM in Seoul from 1985 to 1988. Diabet Care 1994;17:1473–1475.
9. Verge CF, Gianani R, Kawasaki E, Yu L, Pietropaolo M, Jackson RA, Chase HP, Eisenbarth GS. Prediction of type 1 diabetes in first-degree relatives using a combination of insulin, GAD, and ICA512bdc/IA-2 autoantibodies. Diabetes 1996;45:926–933.
10. Grubin CE, Daniels T, Toivola B, Landin-Olsson M, Hagopian WA, Li L, Karlsen AE, Boel E, Michelesen B, Lernmark A. A novel radiobinding assay to determine diagnostic accuracy of isoform-specific glutamic acid decarboxylase antibodies in childhood IDDM. Diabetologia 1994;37:344–350.

Recent Advances on the Pathogenesis and Management of Diabetes Mellitus.
S.H. Shinn, M. Shichiri and K.-W. Kim, editors.

Antibody to GAD and islet cell autoantibody in Korean diabetic patients

Jonghyeon Yoo, Kwon Choi, Yoonsang Choi and Sangjong Lee
Department of Internal Medicine, Kangbuk Samsung Hospital, Sungkyunkwan University College of Medicine, Seoul, Korea

Abstract. *Background.* Measurement of antibodies to glutamic acid decarboxylase (anti-GAD) and islet cell autoantibody (ICA), one of the most important autoimmune markers of insulin-dependent diabetes mellitus (IDDM), could give clues regarding the possible immunological mechanism in β cell destruction. Some non-insulin-dependent diabetes mellitus (NIDDM) patients who become insulin deficient have autoantibodies. The frequency of anti-GAD and ICA in nonobese NIDDM patients tend to be higher than in the obese.

Methods. We determined the prevalence of anti-GAD and ICA in 158 Korean individuals (28 control, seven IDDM patients, 121 NIDDM patients) by radioimmunoassay (RIA) and enzyme-linked immunosorbent assay (ELISA).

Results. The prevalence of anti-GAD and ICA in the subjects of this study was 57.1% (4/7) in patients with IDDM, 3.30% (4/121) and 6.61% (8/121) in patients with NIDDM, and 3.57% (1/28) and 3.57% (1/28) in controls. NIDDM patients with short disease duration (<3 years) had ICA more frequently than those with longer disease duration (≥3 years) (6/54, 11.11% vs. 2/67, 2.90%, $p<0.05$). Nonobese patients (BMI<24) with NIDDM had ICA more frequently than obese patients (BMI ≥ 24) (5/43, 11.62% vs. 3/78, 3.64%, $p<0.04$). NIDDM patients with positive ICA had insulin treatment more frequently than those with negative ICA (4/8, 50% vs. 21/113, 18.58%, $p<0.05$).

Conclusions. These results suggest that immunological mechanisms might play a role in a certain portion of NIDDM patients with nonobese and short duration relating to insulin deficiency.

Keywords: ICA, IDDM, NIDDM.

Introduction

Insulin-dependent diabetes mellitus (IDDM) is strongly associated with the appearance of islet-specific autoantibodies, reflecting the autoimmune-mediated destruction of pancreatic β cells [1–3]. It is known that antibodies to glutamic acid decarboxylase (anti-GAD) and islet cell autoantibody (ICA) are detected in IDDM patients [4–6]. However, sometimes it is difficult to discriminate between IDDM and NIDDM among adult diabetes mellitus (DM) patients. Some NIDDM patients have autoantibodies and the course of IDDM [7–9]. In Korea, there is a higher proportion of NIDDM in DM patients, and these patients tend to be slender and have a lower insulin secretion activity when compared with

Address for correspondence: Jonghyeon Yoo, Department of Internal Medicine, Kangbuk Samsung Hospital, Sungkyunkwan University College of Medicine, 108 Pyungdong, Jongrogue, Seoul 100-752, Korea.

Western NIDDM patients. The purpose of this study was to examine the prevalence of antibodies to GAD and ICA in Korean diabetic patients and investigate the usefulness of antibodies to GAD and ICA in Korean NIDDM patients according to clinical features.

Material and Methods

The population for this prospective study was selected randomly from Korean diabetic patients who were followed and treated at Kangbuk Samsung Hospital between March 1996 and April 1997. Diagnosis of DM was made according to the National Diabetes Group Classification or WHO criteria. We examined seven patients with IDDM, 121 patients with NIDDM and 28 normal individuals for ICA and anti-GAD. The measurement of ICA was done by ELISA (Isletest-ICA, BIOMERICA, USA) and for antibodies to GAD the RIA (GAD_{65}, IRMA, Germany) was used. We also examined the prevalence of anti-GAD and ICA according to their clinical characteristics: age of onset, duration of disease, body mass index (BMI) and insulin treatment. We used Student's t test and the χ^2 test to analyze data.

Results

A total of 158 individuals (control = 28, diabetic patients = 128) were included in this study. Details of clinical characteristics of the subjects in this study are shown in Table 1. Concerning age, age at onset and BMI, IDDM patients presented significantly lower values than those of NIDDM patients. Concerning anti-GAD and ICA, patients with IDDM presented significantly higher values than those of NIDDM patients (Table 1). There was no significant difference in clinical characteristics of IDDM patients according to their GAD status (Table 2).

NIDDM patients with positive ICA had anti-GAD more frequently than those with negative ICA (37.5 vs. 0.88%) but a significant difference was not observed.

Table 1. Clinical characteristics of Korean diabetic groups and control group.

	Control (n = 28)	IDDM (n = 7)	NIDDM (n = 121)	p value[a]
Age (years)	25.48 ± 7.22	22.00 ± 6.93	47.64 ± 4.85	<0.05
Male (%)	54.22	71.4	52.1	ns
Age of onset (years)		19.57 ± 5.65	44.14 ± 3.38	<0.05
Duration (years)		1.26 ± 0.76	3.81 ± 1.95	ns
BMI (kg/m^2)	23.12 ± 4.72	20.32 ± 5.03	21.13 ± 2.42	<0.002
Fasting c-peptide (ng/ml)		0.42 ± 0.28	3.06 ± 1.29	<0.05
Anti-GAD (%)	3.57	57.1	3.30	<0.05
ICA (%)	3.57	57.1	6.61	<0.05

Note: Values represent the mean ± 2SD. ns = not significant. [a]p value – compare IDDM group with NIDDM group.

Table 2. Clinical characteristics of patients with IDDM classified according to their anti-GAD status.

	Anti-GAD(+) (n = 4)	Anti-GAD(−) (n = 3)	p value
Age (years)	18.51 ± 5.24	26.66 ± 6.89	ns
Male (%)	50	100	ns
Age of onset (years)	16.72 ± 3.14	23.31 ± 6.62	ns
Duration (years)	1.20 ± 0.31	1.34 ± 0.32	ns
BMI (kg/m^2)	18.82 ± 0.65	23.00 ± 7.52	ns
Fasting c-peptide (ng/ml)	0.34 ± 0.26	0.51 ± 0.27	ns
ICA (%)	75	66.66	ns

Note: Values represent the mean ± 2SD. ns = not significant.

NIDDM patients with positive ICA had insulin treatment more frequently than those with negative ICA (50 vs. 18.58%, $p<0.05$) (Table 3). The prevalence of ICA was higher in NIDDM patients with short duration (< 3 years) than those with long duration (⩾ 3 years) and in nonobese patients with NIDDM (BMI < 24) than obese patients with NIDDM (BMI ⩾ 24) (Table 4).

Discussion

It has been reported that the prevalence of anti-GAD is much lower in Asian patients with IDDM than in Europeans [10]. However, the prevalence in Korean patients with IDDM in our study was higher than that which has previously been documented. But the number of patients was small and any ethnic difference in prevalence remains unresolved. Due to limited reports, further studies are required. Anti-GAD have also been reported to be positive in some Caucasian NIDDM patients who become insulin deficient [7,8]. The prevalence of anti-GAD in nonobese NIDDM patients (5.3%) tends to be higher than in the obese (1.4%) [9]. In some non-Europeans, the classification into IDDM or NIDDM categories may be difficult. The WHO technical report [11] uses the term "questionable insulin dependency" for these cases. The prevalence of ICA in our NIDDM patients was higher than has previously been reported. This

Table 3. Clinical characteristics of patients with NIDDM classified according to their ICA status.

	ICA(+) (n = 8)	ICA(−) (n = 113)	p value
Age (years)	44.20 ± 10.67	48.75 ± 11.48	ns
Male (%)	51.7	48.3	ns
Duration (years)	2.20 ± 1.72	3.93 ± 3.01	ns
Age of onset (years)	41.00 ± 5.74	42.80 ± 2.04	ns
BMI (kg/m^2)	23.21 ± 5.30	28.13 ± 3.26	ns
Fasting c-peptide (ng/ml)	2.20 ± 1.08	3.48 ± 1.20	ns
Anti-GAD (%)	37.5 (3/8)	0.88 (1/113)	ns
Insulin treatment (%)	50 (4/8)	18.58 (21/113)	< 0.05

Note: Values represent the mean ± 2SD. ns = not significant.

Table 4. Prevalence of ICA in NIDDM patients with short duration and nonobese.

	Duration of disease < 3 years	Duration of disease ⩾ 3 years	p value
ICA(+)	11.11 (6/54)	2.90 (2/67)	< 0.05
	BMI < 24	BMI ⩾ 24	
ICA(−)	11.62(5/43)	3.64(3/78)	< 0.05
ICA(+)	16.12(5/31)	3.33(3/90)	< 0.01

result may be due to the large proportion of nonobese patients with NIDDM included in this study. Nonobese NIDDM patients and those with a shorter disease duration had ICA more frequently than those who were obese or with longer disease duration; and 50% of NIDDM patients with positive ICA required continuous insulin treatment within 1 year of diagnosis. We estimate that some ICA positive patients with nonobese NIDDM may be included in the questionable insulin dependency group. The pathogenesis in some ICA or anti-GAD positive nonobese NIDDM could be similar to that in IDDM: autoimmune destruction of pancreatic β cells.

References

1. Leslie RDG, Elliott RB. Early environment event as a cause of IDDM. Diabetes 1994;43: 843—850.
2. Atkinson MA, Maclaren NK. Islet cell autoantigens in insulin-dependent diabetes. J Clin Invest 1993;92:1608—1616.
3. Atkinson MA, Maclaren NK, Scharp DW, Lacy PE, Riley WJ. 64000Mr autoantibodies as predictors of insulin-dependent diabetes. Lancet 1990;335:1357—1367.
4. Baekkeskov S, Aanstoot HJ, Christgau S. et al. Identification of the 64K autoantigen in insulin dependent diabetes as the GABA-synthesizing enzyme glutamic acid decarboxylase. Nature 1990;347:151—156.
5. Clare Salzler MJ, Tobin AJ, Kaufman DL. Glutamate decarboxylase: an autoantigen in IDDM. Diabet Care 1992;15:132—135.
6. Chritina L, Vandewalle, Alerto F et al. High diagnotic sensitivity of glutamate decarboxylase autoantibodies in insulin-dependent diabetes mellitus with clinical onset between age 20 and 40 years. J Clin Endocrinol Metab 1995;80:846—851.
7. Tuomi T, Groop LC, Zimmet PZ, Rowley MJ, Knowles W, Mackay IR. Antibodies to glutamic acid decarboxylase reveal latent autoimmune diabetes mellitus in adults with a non-insulin-dependent onset of disease. Diabetes 1993;42:359—362.
8. Zimmet PZ, Tuomi T, Mackay IR, Rowley MJ, Knowles W, Cohen M. Latent autoimmune diabetes mellitus in adult (LADA): the role of antibodies to glutamic acid decarboxylase in diagnosis and prediction of insulin dependency. Diabet Med 1994;11:299—303.
9. Akira T, Ikuro M, Takayoshi T, Gen I, Shigenobu N, Yoshio I. Antibodies to GAD in Japanese diabetic patients: a multicenter study. Diabet Res Clin Pract 1995;28:191—199.
10. Zimmet PZ, Rowley MJ, Mackay IR et al. The ethnic distribution of antibodies to glutamic acid decarboxylase: present and level in insulin-dependent diabetes mellitus in European and Asian subjects. J Diab Comp 1993;7:1—7.
11. WHO Study Group. Definition, diagnosis, and classification: diabetes mellitus. In: World Health Organization Technical Report Series, 1985;727:9—20.

Macroangiopathy

Recent Advances on the Pathogenesis and Management of Diabetes Mellitus.
S.H. Shinn, M. Shichiri and K.-W. Kim, editors.

The GLN-ARG191 polymorphism of the human paraoxonase gene in Korean coronary artery disease patients with/without diabetes

Yoonju Cho, Yongsoo Park, Youhern Ahn, Taewha Kim, Mokhyun Kim, Jaewoong Lee, Kyungsoo Kim, Sunkil Kim, Jeongyeon Kim, Banghun Lee and Jungkyun Lee
Department of Internal Medicine, Hanyang University College of Medicine, Seoul, Korea

Abstract. *Background.* The human paraoxonase gene (PONA (paraoxonase/arylesterase)) is associated with HDL and possibly prevents LDL from oxidation by hydrolysing lipid peroxides. PONA is codominantly expressed as alleles A (glutamine) and G (arginine) at position 191 of the enzyme. This genetic polymorphism has been suggested to be associated with the predisposition to coronary artery disease (CAD).

Methods. We performed an association study of this polymorphism with CAD among 67 Korean CAD patients with and without diabetes. Patients were divided according to the results of coronary angiography as normal (n = 20), one-vessel (n = 34), two-vessel (n = 8) and three-vessel disease (n = 5). Forty-nine matched healthy subjects served as controls.

Results. The most common genotype both in the CAD patients (45%) and controls (55%) was AB. AA+AB isoform existed with high prevalence in CAD patients compared with controls, but this did not reach statistical significance. Even when we confined the patients to those with angiography proven CAD (n = 47), we could not find a significant difference.

Conclusions. In conclusion, the prevalence of the Gln-Arg 191 polymorphism of the PONA was not associated with CAD in Koreans.

Keywords: coronary artery disease, paraoxonase, polymorphism.

Introduction

There is increasing evidence that genetic factors play an important role in predisposition to atherosclerotic coronary artery disease (CAD) [1]. One gene that has been related to the pathogenesis of CAD is the human paraoxonase/arylesterase (PONA) gene [2]. The gene is codominantly expressed as alleles A and G. A allele (genotype A) codes for a PONA having glutamine at position 191, whereas the G allele (genotype B) codes for a protein with arginine at position 191 [3]. PONA is a Ca^{2+}-dependent glycoprotein that is associated with HDL and has been shown to prevent LDL oxidation in vitro [4]. Previous studies have shown that variation in PONA activity appears to be caused by polymorphism of the PONA gene. Individuals homozygous for the A allele have lower plasma PONA activity than those homozygous for the G allele. Several recent studies in which

Address for correspondence: Yongsoo Park MD, Department of Internal Medicine, Hanyang University Hospital, 249-1 Kyomun-dong, Kuri, Kyunggi-do, Seoul 471-020, Korea.

PONA allele frequencies were compared in CAD patients and in controls suggested that the two allelic variants of PONA were independent risk factors of CAD [5,6]. The aim of the present study was to evaluate whether this association also exists in Korean patients with CAD.

Materials and Methods

Forty-nine healthy subjects and 67 CAD patients were studied. The diagnosis of CAD was made when a patient complained of the typical chest pain and showed an ECG evidence of myocardial ischemia. All the patients with CAD had the opportunity of examining and visualizing their coronary arteries. Patients were divided according to the results of coronary angiography as normal (n = 20), one-vessel (n = 34), two-vessel (n = 8) and three-vessel disease (n = 5). Thirty-six of the 67 CAD patients also had NIDDM. The criteria for classification of NIDDM were determined by the National Diabetes Data Group. Thirty-seven were male, 30 were female; their mean age was 47 years (range: 35—65 years). Forty-nine nondiabetic healthy control subjects, matched for age and sex with no family history of diabetes had no symptoms of CAD or any other disease. Twenty-five were male and 24 were female (mean age: 45 years). Serum triglyceride and cholesterol levels were measured by automated enzymatic methods using Hitach 736 autoanalyzer. HDL cholesterol was measured after precipitation of the apoB-containing lipoproteins with magnesium chloride. All the patients and control subjects gave their informed consent to the study. Genomic DNA was obtained from all donors for the molecular typing of the PONA gene. The PONA gene polymorphism was identified by PCR-RFLP method using restriction enzyme Alw I [2]. Difference in the allelic distributions of the gene was determined using the χ^2 test with Yates' correction (two-tailed). When the expected frequency for one of the alleles was less than 5, Fisher's exact test was used.

Results

The frequency distribution of genotypes for both the controls and the CAD patients was compatible with Hardy-Weinberg equilibrium. The genotype frequencies did not differ significantly between the patients with CAD and controls (Table 1). The most common genotype in both the patients with CAD (45%) and controls (55%) was AB. AA+AB isoform existed with high prevalence in CAD patients compared with controls, but this did not reach statistical significance. Even when we confined the patients to those with angiography proven CAD (n = 47), we could not find a significant difference. The respective alleles G and A occurred at nearly the same frequency of 0.41 and 0.59 in both groups. The genotype frequencies did not differ between the CAD patients with NIDDM (n = 36) and without NIDDM (n = 31). When clinical and laboratory values were compared among genotypes in the patient group, no significant differences

Table 1. Human PONA genotypes and the frequency of alleles.

PONA gene	IDDM	Control
Genotypes		
AA	9 (19.1%)	7 (14.3%)
A/B	21 (44.7%)	27 (55.1%)
BB	17 (36.2%)	15 (30.6%)
Alleles		
A (Gln)	41.5%	41.8%
G (Arg)	58.5%	58.2%

were noted with regard to BMI or triglyceride, cholesterol or HDL-cholesterol levels.

Discussion

We performed an allelic association study, and determined the PONA genotypes in 67 patients with CAD and 49 healthy Korean control subjects matched for age and sex. Our results showed that AA+AB isoform existed with high prevalence in CAD patients compared with controls, but this did not reach statistical significance. Even when we confined the patients to those with angiography proven CAD, we could not find a significant difference. In conclusion, the prevalence of the Gln-Arg 191 polymorphism of the PONA gene was not associated with CAD in Koreans.

Human PONA gene is located on to chromosome 7q21-22 and codes for a protein of 355 amino acids. The protein contains two polymorphic sites; one at amino acid position 55 (Met/Leu) and the second at amino acid at position 191 (Gln/Arg). The latter polymorphism determines the activity of the enzyme [2]. Arginine at position 191 confers high activity and glutamine low activity to PONA. PONA is known to be associated with HDL and has been shown to prevent LDL oxidation in vitro [4]. Two previous studies in which PONA allele frequencies were compared in CAD patients and in controls suggested that the two allelic variants of PONA were independent risk factors of CAD [5,6]. In both studies patients with CAD had an increased frequency of the more active enzyme (G allele and the B genotype), which suggested that PONA was involved in atherosclerosis through a mechanism other than lipid oxidation. However, our results showed that the relative proportion of BB genotype in controls was rather high, so the difference in the frequencies between the patients and controls was not observed. That is to say that the polymorphism of PONA gene was not associated with Korean CAD and did not contribute to CAD susceptibility irrespective of diabetic status. One possibility is that the Korean gene pool is such that the association is lost. This difference between the Korean and Caucasian data may be a result of the differences in the genetic make-up of the control population or those in the patterns of linkage disequilibrium. This result, however, is not consistent with the study [7] of nearby Japanese NIDDM patients with CAD suggesting the association of CAD with AB+BB genotype. Another explanation for the discrepancy between these studies could be patient selection. However, even when we confined the patients to those with angiography proven CAD, we could still not find a significant difference. Therefore, further studies are needed to clarify whether the polymorphisms in PONA gene have less value as genetic markers for Korean IDDM.

References

1. Marenberg ME, Risch N, Berkman LF, Floderus B, de-Faire U. Genetic susceptibility to death from coronary heart disease in a study of twins. N Engl J Med 1994;330:1041–1046.
2. Humbert R, Adler DA, Disteche CM, Hassett C, Omiecinski CJ, Furlong CE. The molecular basis of the human serum paraoxonase activity polymorphism. Nature Genet 1993;3:73–76.
3. Adkins S, Gan KN, Mody M, La Du BN. Molecular basis for the polymorphic forms of human serum paraoxonase/arylesterase: glutamine or arginine at position 191, for the respective A or B allozymes. Am J Hum Genet 1993;52:598–608.
4. La Du BN. Human serum paraoxonase/arylesterase. In: Kallow W (ed) Pharmacogenetics of Drug Metabolism. New York: Pergamon Press, 1992;51–91.
5. Ruiz J, Blanche H, James RW, Blatter Garin M-C, Vaisse C, Charpentier G, Cohen N, Morabia A, Passa P, Froguel P. Gln-Arg192 polymorphism of paraoxonase and coronary heart disease in type 2 diabetes. Lancet 1995;346:869–872.
6. Serrato M, Marian AJ. A variant of human paraoxonase/arylesterase (HUMPONA) gene is a risk factor for coronary artery disease. J Clin Invest 1995;96:3005–3008.
7. Odawara M, Tachi Y, Sasaki K, Tada K, Yamashita K. Gln192Arg polymorphism in paraoxonase gene is associated with coronary heart disease in Japanese NIDDM.

Recent Advances on the Pathogenesis and Management of Diabetes Mellitus.
S.H. Shinn, M. Shichiri and K.-W. Kim, editors.

Effect of insulin on gene expression and synthesis of collagen in aortic smooth muscle cells cultured in normal and high glucose

Sung Woo Ha[1], Jung Guk Kim[1], In San Kim[2], Kun Young Sohn[2] and Bo Wan Kim[1]

Departments of [1]Internal Medicine, and [2]Biochemistry, School of Medicine, Kyungpook National University, Taegu, Korea

Abstract. To evaluate possible roles of hyperglycemia and hyperinsulinemia in the development of atherosclerosis in diabetes mellitus, we examined the effects of high glucose and insulin on gene expression and synthesis of collagen in aortic smooth muscle cells. The cells cultured in high glucose (25 mM) synthesized more collagen protein and expressed higher levels of $\alpha 1(I)$ procollagen mRNA, as compared to those cultured in normal glucose (5.5 mM) medium. Insulin increased collagen synthesis and $\alpha 1(I)$ procollagen mRNA level. The cells cultured in high glucose seemed to be more sensitive to insulin than those cultured in normal glucose. These results suggest hyperglycemic condition and hyperinsulinemia may accelerate the atherosclerotic process by stimulating vascular smooth muscle cells to produce more collagen.

Keywords: aortic smooth muscle cell, atherosclerosis, collagen, diabetes mellitus, high glucose, insulin.

Introduction

Diabetes mellitus is associated with a greater prevalence of atherosclerotic disease [1]. It is widely accepted that the accumulation of extracellular matrix such as collagen and smooth muscle cell accumulation increases in the arterial intima during the development of atherosclerosis [2,3]. It has been suggested that hyperglycemia and hyperinsulinemia in diabetes are important factors in the development of the diabetic complications [4,5]. To evaluate possible roles of hyperinsulinemia and hyperglycemia in the development of atherosclerosis in diabetes mellitus, we studied the effect of insulin on the synthesis and gene expression of collagen by rat aortic vascular smooth muscle cells cultured under normal and high glucose conditions.

Materials and Methods

An aortic smooth muscle cell line of rat, A-10 (CRL-1476), was obtained from ATCC. Cells were cultured in DMEM supplemented with 20% FBS. After the

Address for correspondence: Sung Woo Ha, Department of Internal Medicine, School of Medicine, Kyungpook National University, Taegu 700-422, Korea. Tel.: +82-53-420-5564. Fax: +82-53-426-2046. E-mail: swha@kyungpook.ac.kr

cells were grown to confluence, they were made quiescent by incubation for 24 h in fresh DMEM with a D-glucose concentration of 5.5 or 25 mM and added with different concentrations of insulin. After conditioning, the synthesis of collagen and noncollagenous protein (NCP) in the cells were measured by the collagenase digestion method. Percent collagen synthesis, which represents the relative rate of collagen synthesis as a percentage of total protein synthesis, was then calculated. Total cellular RNA was isolated with acid guanidinium thiocyanate-phenol-chloroform and followed by Northern blot hybridization. The cDNA probe used for hybridization was HF677, human α1(I)procollagen cDNA. Experimental data were analyzed by the Mann-Whitney test. A value of $p < 0.05$ was considered to be significant.

Results

Effect of insulin on the steady-state levels of α1(I) procollagen mRNA in aortic smooth muscle cells cultured in normal and high glucose condition

The steady-state levels of α1(I) procollagen mRNA from the cells grown in normal glucose with insulin were higher than those from the cells grown in normal (Fig. 1) or high (Fig. 2) glucose without insulin. Signal of 18 S rRNA was used as an internal control. There was a significant difference in the mRNA levels between cells grown in either normal or high glucose condition with insulin for 24 h (Fig. 3).

Effect of insulin on collagen synthesis in aortic smooth muscle cells cultured in normal and high glucose condition

Cells grown in high glucose medium synthesized more collagen and noncollagen protein compared to the cells grown in normal glucose medium under the same concentration of insulin (Fig. 4A,B). Insulin-stimulated collagen synthesis in the

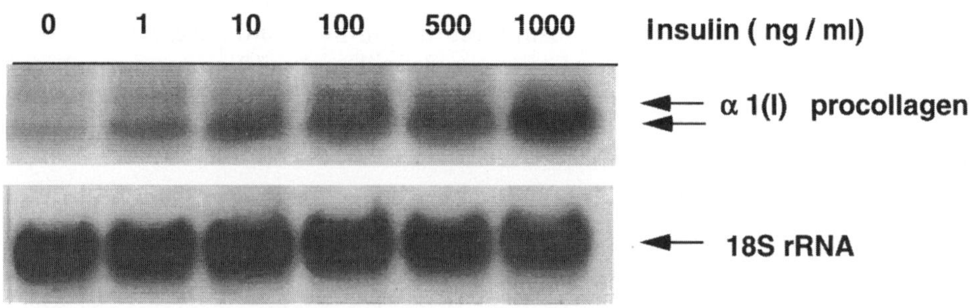

Fig. 1. Effect of insulin on the steady-state levels of α1(I) procollagen mRNA in vascular smooth muscle cells cultured in normal glucose media (5.5 mM). The α1(I) procollagen mRNA bands (4.3 kb) are standardized with the 18 S rRNA signal.

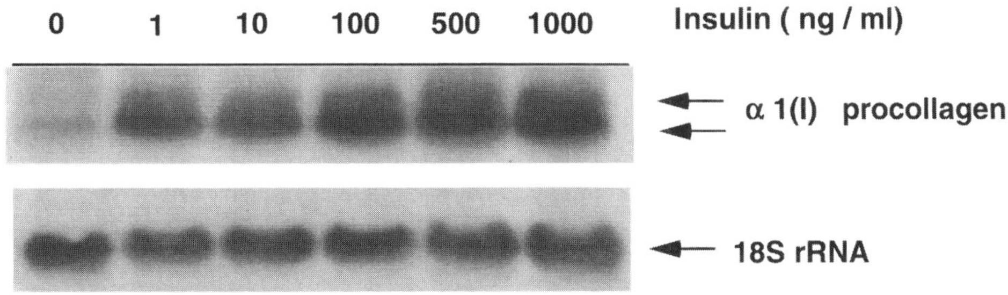

Fig. 2. Effect of insulin on the steady-state levels of α1(I) procollagen mRNA in vascular smooth muscle cells cultured in high glucose media (25 mM).

cells cultured in normal glucose in a dose-dependent manner (Fig. 4A). Percent collagen synthesis did not differ significantly in the cells grown in either normal or high glucose condition at any insulin concentration (Fig. 4C).

Discussion

The mechanism for accelerated atherosclerosis in diabetes and hyperinsulinemia is unclear, although diabetes mellitus and hyperinsulinemia is a known risk factor for atherosclerosis [1,2,6]. This study shows that aortic smooth muscle cells grown in high glucose condition with or without insulin synthesize more collagen and express more type 1 procollagen mRNA compared to the cells grown in the normal glucose condition. The aortic smooth muscle cells showed more sensitivity to insulin in high glucose than normal glucose condition. Previous investigators have demonstrated that high glucose concentration stimulates collagen

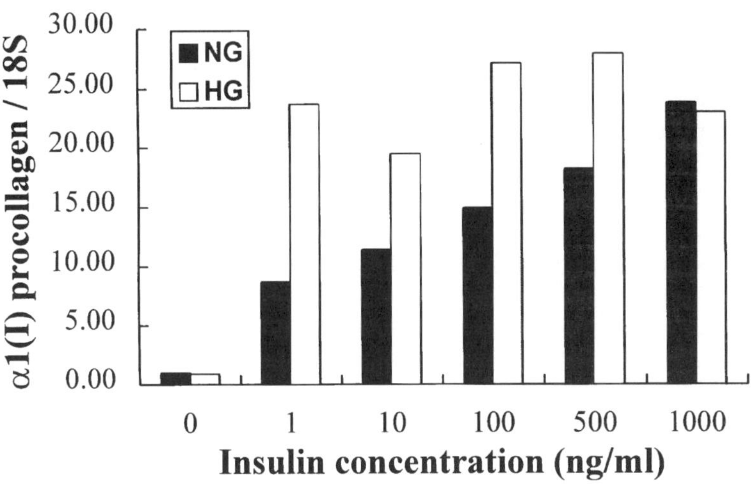

Fig. 3. Effect of insulin on the steady-state levels of α1(I) procollagen mRNA in vascular smooth muscle cells cultured in either normal or high glucose media. NG = normal glucose; HG = high glucose.

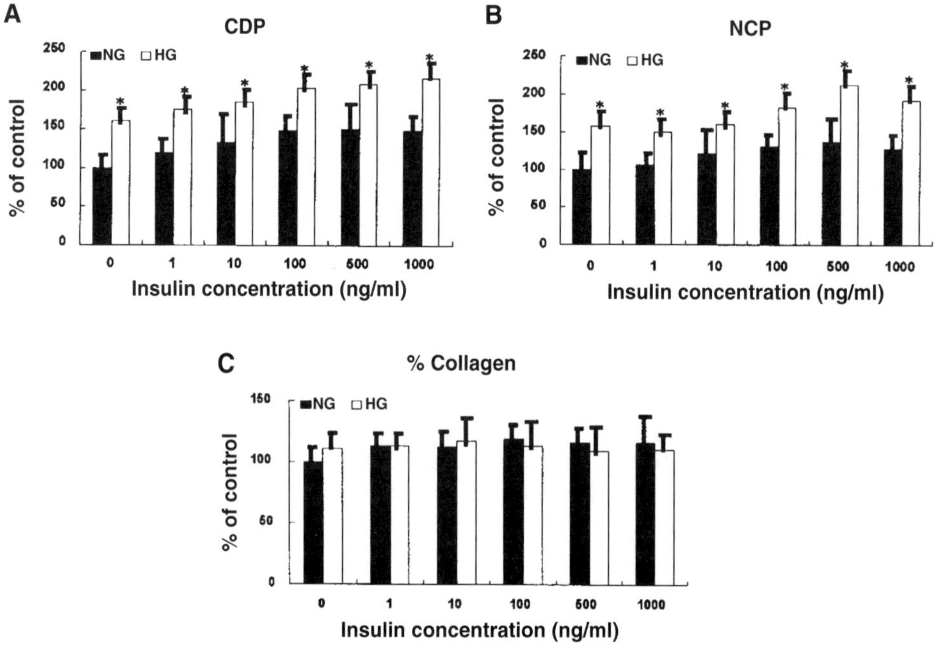

Fig. 4. Effect of insulin on the synthesis of collagen (**A**) and noncollagenous protein (**B**), and percent collagen synthesis (**C**) in vascular smooth muscle cells. Data are represented as mean ± SD of five measurements. Significantly different from cells grown in normal glucose ($p < 0.05$). CDP = collagenase digestible protein; NCP = noncollagenous protein; NG = normal glucose; HG = high glucose.

synthesis and increases procollagen mRNA levels [4,5]. Some investigators have reported that insulin stimulates proliferation of cultured primate arterial smooth muscle cells [6]. These results suggest that hyperinsulinemia and hyperglycemia in diabetes may accelerate the development of atherosclerosis by stimulating vascular smooth muscle cells to produce more collagen and also can be a possible mechanism of enhanced risk of atherosclerosis in diabetes.

Acknowledgements

This work was supported by a grant from the Korea Research Foundation.

References

1. Schwartz CJ, Valente AJ, Sprague EA, Kelley JL, Cayatte AJ, Rozek MM. Pathogenesis of the atherosclerotic lesion; Implications for diabetes mellitus. Diabetes Care 1992;15:1156–1167.
2. Ross R. The pathogenesis of atherosclerosis; A perspective for the 1990s. Nature 1993;362: 801–809.
3. O'Brien KD, Chait A. The biology of the artery wall in atherosclerosis. Med Clin N Am 1994; 78:41–67.

4. Spiro MJ, He Q, D'Autilia MLD. Effect of high glucose on formation of extracellular matrix components by cultured rat heart endothelial cells. Diabetologia 1995;38:430–436.
5. Ziyadeh FN, Sharma K, Ericksen M, Wolf G. Stimulation of collagen gene expression and protein synthesis in murine mesangial cells by high glucose is mediated by autocrine activation of transforming growth factor. J Clin Invest 1994;93:536–542.
6. Stout RW. Insulin and atheroma; 20-Yr perspective. Diabetes Care 1990;13:631–654.

Recent Advances on the Pathogenesis and Management of Diabetes Mellitus.
S.H. Shinn, M. Shichiri and K.-W. Kim, editors.

Oxygen free radical induced impairment of endothelium dependent relaxation in diabetic rat aortas

Jung-Guk Kim, Sung-Woo Ha and Bo-Wan Kim
Division of Endocrinology and Metabolism, Department of Internal Medicine, School of Medicine, Kyungpook University, Jung-Gu, Taegu, Korea

Abstract. *Background.* Macrovascular disease is responsible for more deaths in diabetic patients than all of the other causes of death put together. EDRF may play an important role in vascular smooth muscle relaxation and oxygen free radical (OFR)-induced vascular damage is one of major pathogenetic mechanisms developing atherosclerotic vascular changes.

Method. We used the thoracic aortas of diabetic and control rats and examined endothelium-dependent relaxation under the condition of OFR-induced injury.

Result. Endothelium-dependent relaxation was significantly impaired in diabetic rats and superoxide dismutase partially protected OFR-induced vascular damage.

Conclusion. Prolonged hyperglycemia and OFR altered vascular endothelial function and EDRF is the major site of impairment. Antioxidant, SOD, may protect OFR-induced vascular damage.

Keywords: EDHF, EDRF, lipopolysaccharide, oxygen free radical, SOD.

Introduction

Diabetes mellitus produces histological evidence of endothelial alterations as well as changes in vascular function in experimental animals [1–4]. Oxygen free radicals interfere with or destroy endothelium-dependent relaxation in normal and diabetic blood vessels [5,6]. The present study investigated whether the duration of diabetic state can affect the severity of impairment in endothelium-dependent relaxation and the sensitivity to oxygen free radical induced damage in diabetic rat vasculatures. Also, we studied the effect of lipopolysaccharide and potent free radical generating system in vascular dysfunction. Furthermore, the protective effect of antioxidants such as superoxide dismutase and catalase was also studied.

Material and Methods

Male Sprague-Dawley rats, 200–250 g in body weight, were divided randomly into two groups. One group (diabetic group) received a single intraperitoneal

Address for correspondence: Jung-Guk Kim, Division of Endocrinology and Metabolism, Department of Internal Medicine, School of Medicine, Kyungpook University, Sam-Duck 2 Ga, Jung-Gu, Taegu 700-721, Korea. Tel.: +82-053-420-5566. Fax: +82-053-426-2046. E-mail: jugkim@kyungpook.ac.kr.

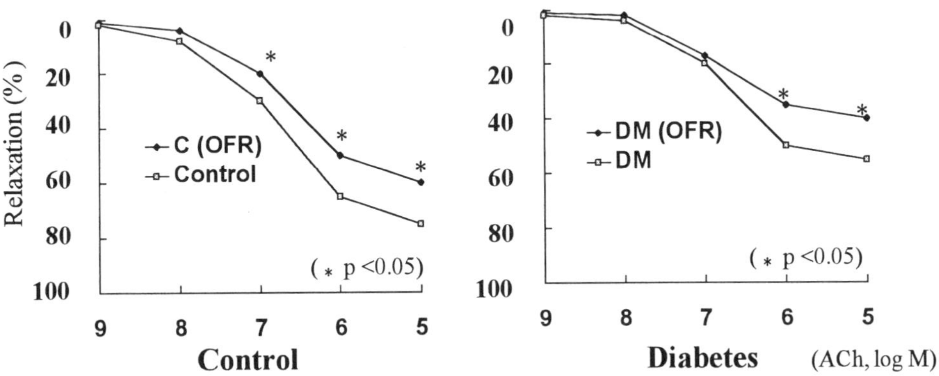

Fig. 1. Effect of OFR on ACh-induced relaxation in control and 3-week-old diabetic rat aortas.

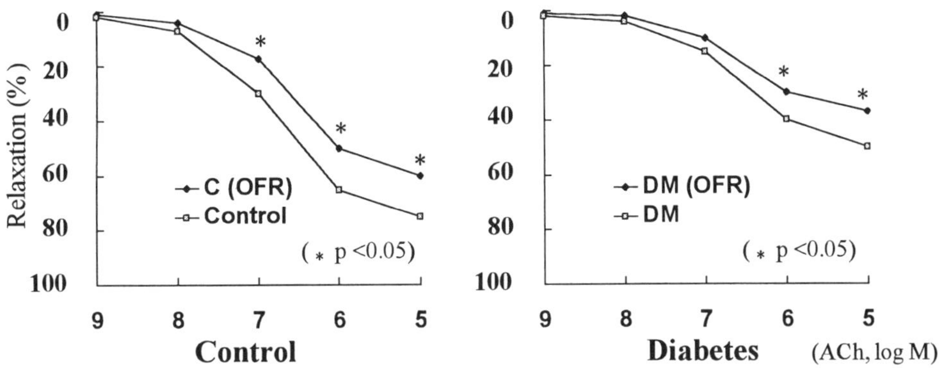

Fig. 2. Effect of OFR on ACh-induced relaxation in control and 10-week-old diabetic rat aortas.

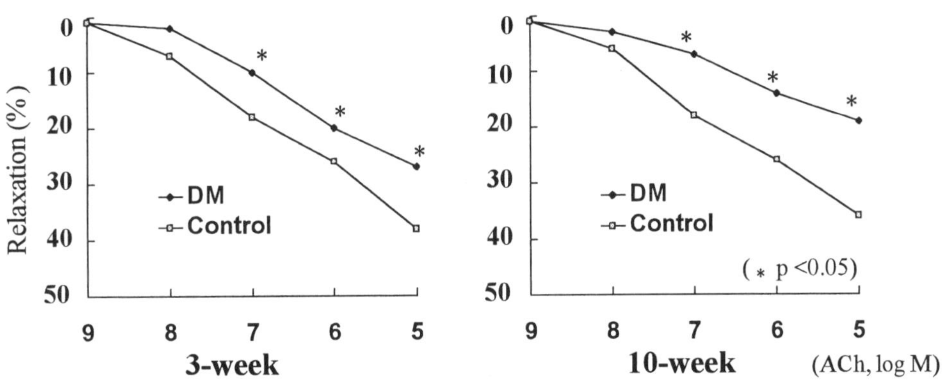

Fig. 3. Effect of EDRF on ACh-induced relaxation in control and diabetic rat aortas.

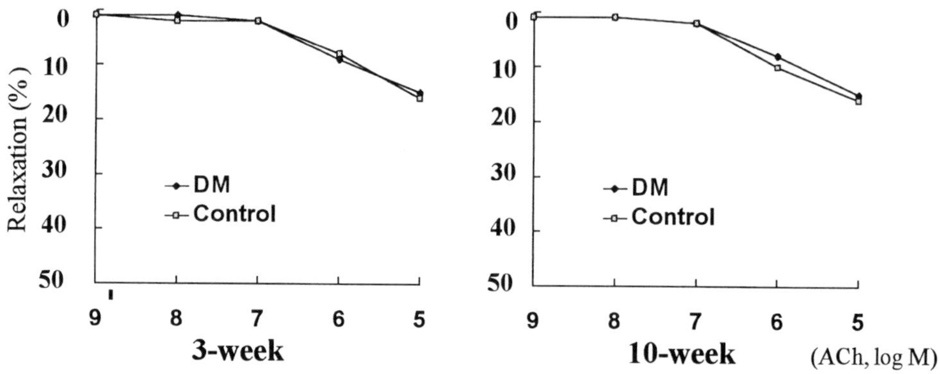

Fig. 4. Effect of EDHF on ACh-induced relaxation in control and diabetic rat aortas.

injection of streptozotocin 60 mg/kg to induce diabetes. Another group of rats were used as control. All animals were provided with food and water at libitum for 3—10 weeks before they were used for an isolated blood vessel experiment. On the day of each experiment, the rats were anesthetized with ketamine. Thoracic aortas were carefully removed and cut into rings of 4-mm long segments. The rings were suspended from strain gauges to measure circumferential isometric force and placed in organ chambers containing modified Henseleit solution. After several washings and re-equilibrations, contraction was evoked by submaximal concentration of norepinephrine. Contraction reached a plateau level and the relaxative response to ACh (10^{-9}, 10^{-8}, 10^{-7}, 10^{-6}, 10^{-5}) was examined in a single concentration effect manner. Relaxation responses were expressed as the percentage of decreased tension of contractile force. EDRF effect was blocked by L-NAME and high potassium solution for EDHF blocking effect. LPS, a free radical generator, was pretreated 6 h pre-experiment and we used antioxidants (SOD and catalase) in order to block free radical induced damage.

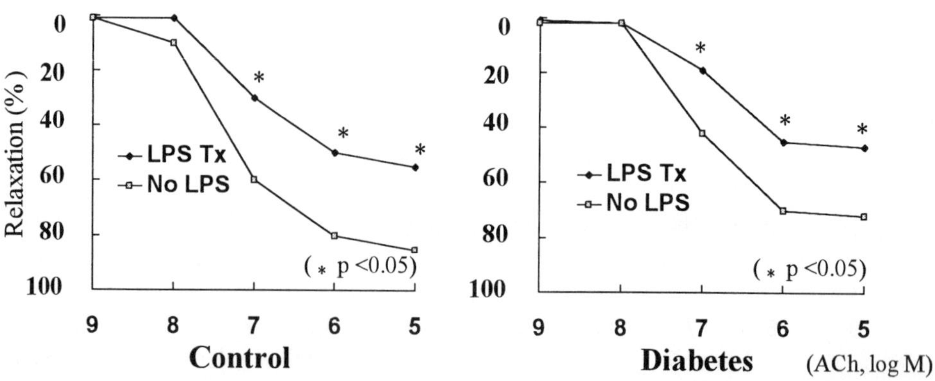

Fig. 5. Effect of LPS pretreatment on ACh-induced relaxation in control and diabetic rat aortas.

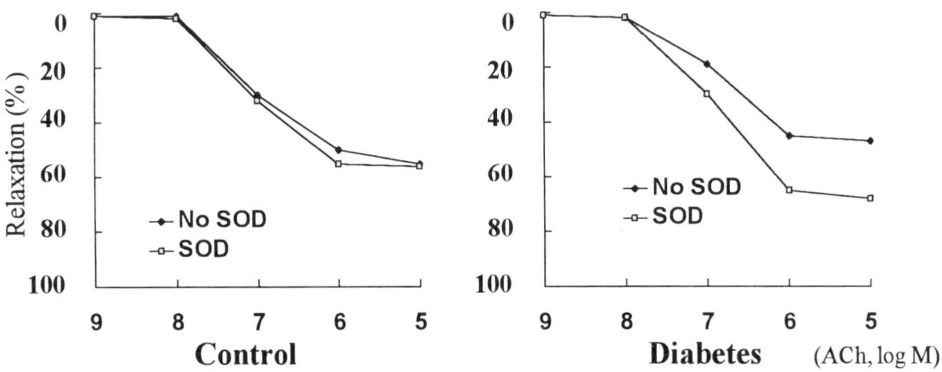

Fig. 6. Effect of SOD treatment on ACh-induced relaxation in control and diabetic rat aortas.

Results

The relaxative responses of aortic rings precontracted with norepinephrine in vitro to cumulative concentrations of ACh were significantly lower in both 3- and 10-week-old diabetic rats than in age-matched controls (Figs. 1 and 2). After H_2O_2 exposure, the impairments of relaxative response to ACh in 3- and 10-week-old diabetic rats' aortas was significantly greater than those in the control ones. However, the severity of H_2O_2-induced damage in 10-week-old diabetic rats' aortas was not different than that in 3-week-old rats (Figs. 1 and 2). EDRF-mediated relaxation was significantly lower in diabetic than control rats' aortas and the severity of impairment was greater in 10-week-old rats than in 3-week-old rats, however, EDHF-mediated relaxation was not different between diabetic and control rats (Figs. 3 and 4). After pretreatment of LPS, vasodilator response to ACh was significantly impaired in both control and diabetic rats' aortas. In contrast to control, the effect of LPS pretreatment on relaxative response to ACh in the diabetic rats' aortas were reversed, in part, by treatment with SOD (Figs. 5 and 6).

Discussion

In the diabetic rats' aortas, impairments of relaxative response to ACh could be greater in those with longer duration of diabetic state which were mainly due to damage in EDRF, not EDHF-mediated relaxation. However, the sensitivity to the impairment by OFR were not related to the duration of diabetes. Bacterial lipopolysaccharide induced impairments of relaxation of aortic rings to ACh were not different between diabetic and control rats. These impairments of relaxation of diabetic aortas to ACh were inhibited by treatment with superoxide dismutase (SOD), largely protecting EDRF-mediated reactivity. These results suggest that OFR could alter selectively EDRF-mediated relaxation of diabetic rats' aortas and these effects would be protected by SOD.

References

1. Meraji S, Jayakody L, Manohara PJ, Senaratne MPJ. Diabetes 1987;36:978–981.
2. Voorde VD, Leusen I. Am J Physiol 1986;250:711–717.
3. Furchgott RF, Zawadski JV. Nature (London) 1980;288:373–376.
4. Katama K, Miyata N, Kasuya Y. Br J Pharmacol 1989;97:614–618.
5. Rubany GM, Vanhoutte PM. Am J Physiol 1986;250:H815–821.
6. Pieper GM, Gross GJ. Am J Physiol 1988;255:H825–833.

Recent Advances on the Pathogenesis and Management of Diabetes Mellitus.
S.H. Shinn, M. Shichiri and K.-W. Kim, editors.

Blood pressure pattern of pregnancy complicated with impaired glucose tolerance

K.S. Oh[2], N.H. Cho[2], H.M. Kim[3], H.S. Kim[1], J.I. Yang[1], H.C. Kwon[1], H.S. Ryu[1], Y.S. Chung[3], K.W. Lee[3] and H.M. Kim[4]

Departments of [1] Obstetrics and Gynecology, [2] Preventive Medicine, and [3] Endocrinology, Ajou University School of Medicine, Paldal-Gu, Suwon; and [4] Department of Food and Nutrition, Sookmyung Women's University, Chungpa-Dong, Yongsan-Gu, Seoul, Korea

Abstract. *Background.* A pregnancy complicated with diabetes has an increased risk of pregnancy-induced hypertension (PIH). Therefore in this study we investigated the pattern of blood pressure during antepartum in three groups: normal (normal for gestational diabetes screening), IGT (single positive for gestational diabetes screening), and GDM (gestational diabetes mellitus).

Methods. A total of 856 (768 normal, 44 IGT, and 44 GDM) pregnant women's vital signs were evaluated during the 2nd and 3rd trimesters.

Results. We observed a positive correlation between glucose metabolism and blood pressure at the time of history taking (i.e., approximately 20 weeks of gestation). The frequency of PIH, defined by systolic $\geqslant$140 mmHg, and diastolic $\geqslant$90 mmHg, was significantly higher in GDM subjects. Four, 4.5, and 15.9% of hypertension was observed in the normal, IGT, and GDM groups, respectively. Furthermore, the odds ratio for GDM was 4.65 (95% CI 1.7–12, $p<0.001$) times greater when compared to the normal group. Therefore, we evaluated blood pressure patterns among the three groups during antepartum. A positive relationship was noted between the antepartum blood pressures (2 through 9 months) and glucose tolerance status. Both systolic and diastolic blood pressures were significantly higher in the GDM group, followed by the IGT and normal groups. Although the magnitude of the antepartum blood pressures was different among the three groups the pattern was similar. Since we found two potential confounders (i.e., BMI and maternal age), it was adjusted to determine the independent relationship between blood pressure and glucose tolerance status. These relationships were persistent even after controlling for the confounders.

Conclusion. This study suggests that both IGT and GDM sufferers should receive extra precaution for PIH and other obstetric problems related to hypertension.

Keywords: blood pressure, gestational diabetes mellitus, pregnancy.

Introduction

A pregnancy complicated with diabetes has an increased risk of pregnancy-induced hypertension (PIH) [1,2]. Therefore, in this study, we investigated the blood pressure pattern during antepartum among three groups who presented with a different level of glucose tolerance (i.e., normal, borderline based on gestational diabetes diagnostic criteria, and gestational diabetics).

Address for correspondence: K.S. Oh, Ajou University School of Medicine, #5 Wonchon-Dong, Paldal-Gu, Suwon 442-749, Korea.

Materials and Methods

All pregnant women who visited Ajou University Hospital between 1 February 1995 and 31 March 1997 for antepartum care underwent universal screening with a 50-g glucose load at 24—28 weeks gestational age. Those with a 1-h plasma glucose ⩾130 mg/dl underwent a 3-h, 100-g oral glucose tolerance test after 8 h of fasting but not exceeding 14 h. Subjects were considered to have GDM if at least two values, and IGT if at least one value, reached or exceeded the following: 105 mg/dl on fasting, 190 mg/dl at 1 h, 165 mg/dl at 2 h, and 145 mg/dl at 3 h [3]. Anthropometric and vital signs were measured every month. Blood pressure was measured after a 5-min rest in a sitting position. Multiple gestations, and patients with chronic medical conditions and hypertension were excluded from the study. PIH was defined by systolic ⩾140 mmHg, and diastolic ⩾90 mmHg during the pregnancy. Analysis of variance, χ^2 test, and repeated measures analysis were used to investigate the blood pressure patterns among the three study groups (normal, single positive and GDM).

Results

A total of 856 (768 normal, 44 single positive (IGT), and 44 GDM) pregnant women's vital signs were evaluated during the 2nd and 3rd trimesters. We observed a positive correlation between glucose metabolism and blood pressure at the time of history taking (i.e., approximately 20 weeks of gestation). The frequency of PIH was significantly higher in GDM subjects. Four, 4.5, and 15.9% of hypertension was observed in the normal, IGT, and GDM groups, respectively. Furthermore, the odds ratio for the GDM group was 4.65 (95% CI 1.7—12, p<0.001) times greater when compared to the normal group. Therefore, we evaluated blood pressure patterns among the three groups during antepartum.

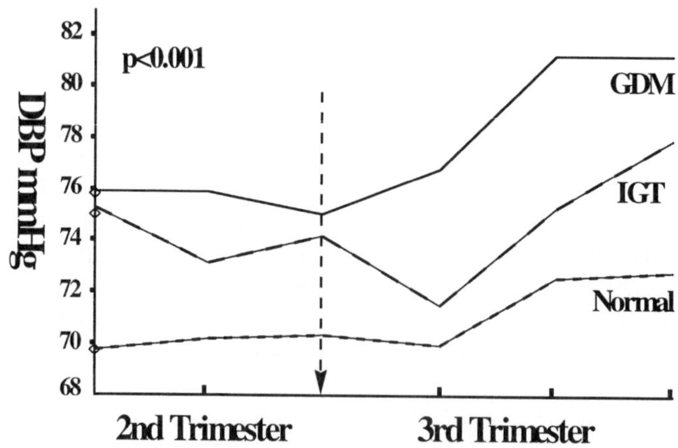

Fig. 1. Diastolic blood pressure.

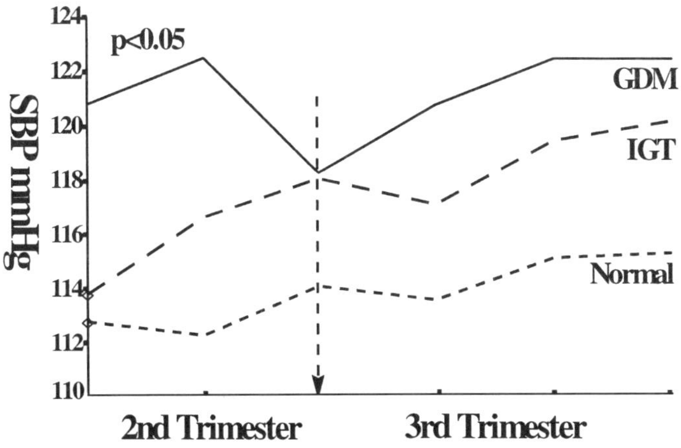

Fig. 2. Systolic blood pressure.

A positive relationship was noted between the antepartum blood pressures (2 through 9 months) and glucose tolerance status. Both systolic and diastolic blood pressures were significantly higher in the GDM group, followed by the IGT and normal groups. Although the magnitude of the antepartum blood pressures was different among the three groups the pattern was similar. Since we found two potential confounders (i.e., BMI and maternal age), it was adjusted to determine the independent relationship between blood pressure and glucose tolerance status. These relationships were persistent even after controlling for these confounders.

Discussion

In this study, we found an increased frequency of PIH in IGT and GDM subjects. Systolic blood pattern continued to increase during the pregnancy. However, a somewhat different diastolic blood pressure pattern was observed. Diastolic blood pressure decreased until the end of the 2nd trimester and started to increase at the beginning of the 3rd trimester (Fig. 1). Moreover, both the systolic (Fig. 2) and diastolic blood pressures were significantly elevated in IGT and GDM subjects compared to the normal subjects. Thus, this study suggests that women who experience glucose tolerance, both IGT and GDM, during pregnancy should be closely monitored for PIH and/or any sign of preeclampsia to prevent pregnancy complications.

References

1. Oren S, Golzman B, Reitblatt T, Turkot S, Kogan J, Segal S. Gestational diabetes mellitus and hypertension in pregnancy: hemodynamics and diurnal arterial pressure profile. J Hum Hypertens 1996;10(8):505–509.

2. Siddiqi T, Rosenn B, Mimouni F, Khoury J, Miodovnik M. Hypertension during pregnancy in insulin-dependent diabetic women. Obstet-Gynecol 1991;77(4):514–519.
3. National Diabetes Data Group. Classification and diagnosis of diabetes and other categories of glucose intolerance. Diabetes 1979;28:1039–1057.

Recent Advances on the Pathogenesis and Management of Diabetes Mellitus.
S.H. Shinn, M. Shichiri and K.-W. Kim, editors.

Relationship between carotid artery plaque measured by ultrasound and cerebral infarction in patients with non-insulin-dependent diabetes mellitus (NIDDM)

T.S. Park, K.H. Rhee, S.I. Choi, S.O. Lee, C.S. Lim and H.S. Baek
Department of Internal Medicine, Chonbuk National University College of Medicine, Chonju, Korea

Introduction

The frequency of cerebral infarction is significantly increased in diabetic patients [1]. The early detection of atherosclerotic lesions will prove useful in predicting and delaying the occurrence of cerebral infarction in diabetic patients [2]. The purpose behind the study was to investigate the relationships between extracranial carotid artery plaque and cerebral infarction using noninvasive B-mode ultrasonography, brain computed tomography and MRI in both NIDDM patients and cerebral infarction patients without DM.

Subjects and methods

The subjects involved were 55 patients with CVD (NIDDM: 27, non-DM: 28) and 37 NIDDM patients without CVD (Table 1).

Ultrasound high-resolution B-mode imaging of carotid arteries was conducted on cerebral infarction patients with NIDDM and also without NIDDM, in order to determine the amount of plaque presence on the carotid artery. Simultaneously, cholesterol and HbA1c were measured by standard laboratory techniques. Any history of hypertension and smoking was also noted. The measurement of the IMT begins from the leading edge of the 1st ectogenic line to the leading edge of the 2nd line of the thickest carotid bulb [3]. Carotid plaque thickness is defined as the IMT over 1.3 mm.

Results

The incidence of cerebral infarction was increased in relation to extracranial carotid artery plaque existence. The frequency of carotid artery plaque was higher than in NIDDM patients with cerebral infarction (63 vs. 35%, $p<0.05$, Table 2).

Address for correspondence: T.S. Park, Division of Endocrinology, Department of Internal Medicine, Chonbuk National University Medical School, 634-18 Keum-Am Dong, Chonju, Chonbuk 560-182, Korea.

Table 1. Basic characteristics of patients.

Group/Parameter	NIDDM		Non-DM	p value
	CVD (n=27)	Non-CVD (n=37)	CVD (n=28)	
Age (years)	65 ± 7.1	62 ± 10.3	61 ± 6.7	0.19[a]
BM[d] (kg/m^2)	24.0 ± 3.7	22.7 ± 3.3	23.7 ± 2.7	0.25[a]
Cholesterol (mg/l)	210 ± 57.5	180 ± 57.1	213 ± 40.2	0.02[a]
HbA_1c (%)	10.1 ± 3.1	10.2 ± 2.6		0.78[b]
Duration of DM (years)	10.3 ± 9.3	9.6 ± 8.0		0.90[b]
IMT[e] (mm)	0.89 ± 0.03	0.81 ± 0.04	0.78 ± 0.06	<0.01[a]
Hypertension[f]	16	10	19	0.002[c]
Smoking	10	7	14	0.03[c]
Male Sex	17	21	15	0.77[c]

[a]p value by ANOVA test; [b]p value by Student's t test; [c]p value by χ^2 test; [d]BMI (body mass index) mean ± SE; [e]IMT (intimal-medial thickness) mean ± SE; [f]hypertension, systolic >160 mmHg and diastolic pressure >90 mmHg.

Table 2. Prevalence of carotid plaque in 64 NIDDM patients with and without cerebral infarction.

	Plaque
Cerebral infarction (n = 27)	17 (63%)[a]
Noncerebral infarction (n = 37)	13 (35%)

[a]$p < 0.05$ vs. NIDDM patients without cerebral infarction.

Table 3. Prevalence of carotid plaque in cerebral infarction patients with and without NIDDM.

	Plaque
NIDDM (n = 27)	17 (63%)[a]
Non-DM (n = 28)	13 (46%)

[a]$p > 0.05$ vs. cerebral infarction patients without DM.

Table 4. Relations between risk factors and cerebral infarction in 64 NIDDM patients.

Risk factor	Regression coefficient	p value[a]
Age	0.009	0.25
Sex	0.098	0.52
Obesity	0.032	0.28
Smoking	0.269	0.32
Hypertension	0.295	0.006
Hypercholesterolemia	0.002	0.035
Plaque	0.185	0.041

[a]p value by multivariate regression analysis.

There was no significant difference in existence of carotid plaque between NIDDM patients and nondiabetic patients with cerebral infarction (Table 3). Multiple regression analysis showed that development of cerebral infarction in NIDDM patients was positively related to hypertension, hypercholesterolemia and carotid plaque (Table 4).

Discussion

As a result of this study there were two main findings. Firstly, cerebral infarction increased in relation to the existence of extracranial carotid artery plaque in NIDDM. However, there was no significant increase in the non-DM patients. Secondly, the development of cerebral infarction in NIDDM patients was positively related to hypertension, hypercholesterolemia and carotid plaque.

Conclusion

This study revealed that the existence of carotid plaque is very closely related to cerebral infarction in NIDDM patients. Therefore, it is extremely beneficial to use ultrasonography in the early detection of extracranial carotid plaque, as this will help predict cerebral infarction in NIDDM patients.

References

1. Kameyama M, Fushimi H, Udaka F. Diabetes mellitus and cerebral vascular disease. Diabet Res Clin Pact 1994;24(Suppl):S205–208.
2. Kwamori R, Hougaku H, Yamasaki Y, Maeda H, Nishizawa H, Matsumoto M, Nao. K, Kamada T. Prevalence of carotid atherosclerosis in diabetic patients. Ultrasound high resolution B-mode imaging on carotid arteries. Diabet Care 1992;15:1291–1294.
3. Pignoli P. Ultrasound B-mode imaging for arterial wall thickness measurement. Atherosclerosis 1984;12:177–184.

Recent Advances on the Pathogenesis and Management of Diabetes Mellitus.
S.H. Shinn, M. Shichiri and K.-W. Kim, editors.

The cerebral hemodynamic changes measured by transcranial Doppler in normotensive, hypertensive and diabetic patients

J.H. Nam, J.H. Lee, B.S. Cha, Y.D. Song, S.K. Lim, K.R. Kim, H.C. Lee and K.B. Huh

Division of Endocrinology, Department of Internal Medicine, Yonsei University College of Medicine, Seoul, Korea

Abstract. This study was designed to demonstrate cerebral hemodynamic changes as macrovascular complication related to diabetes mellitus and hypertension. We measured mean velocities (Vm), and pulsatility indices (PI) of the middle cerebral artery (MCA) and the internal carotid artery (ICA) in 37 stroke-free normotensive diabetic patients (DM, M:F = 15:22), 33 hypertensive diabetics (DMHT, M:F = 16:17), 51 nondiabetic hypertensive (HT, M:F = 25:26, duration $\geqslant$ 5 years) patients and 57 healthy controls (C, M:F = 26:31), using a three-dimensional transcranial Doppler (Transscan, EME, Uberlingen, Germany). The DM, DMHT and HT patients showed significantly higher PI of the MCA, and DMHT patients also had higher PI of the ICA than the C group. The PI of the MCA in DMHT patients was more elevated than in DM. These results showed that the cerebral hemodynamic changes in diabetes mellitus and hypertension affect pulsatility of cerebral arteries, especially small arteries. These atherosclerotic changes of cerebral arteries appear to be more aggravated in diabetes mellitus combined with hypertension.

Keywords: diabetes, hemodynamics, hypertension, small vessel disease, transcranial Doppler.

Introduction

Hypertension and diabetes mellitus (DM) are major risk factors for stroke. The major cerebrovascular changes related to hypertension and DM include arterial wall thickening and endothelial damage [1,2]. These changes may induce and accelerate atherosclerosis, which in consequence alter the cerebral blood flow (CBF) and eventually may produce a stroke [3,4]. Thus the early detection of CBF changes in hypertensive and DM patients could be helpful in evaluating the effect of antihypertensive therapy and DM control, as well as planning preventive strategies for stroke. Therefore, we evaluated hypertension and DM related cerebral hemodynamic changes by transcranial Doppler prior to stroke.

Subjects and methods

The study population consisted of 37 stroke-free normotensive diabetic patients (DM, M:F = 15:22), 33 hypertensive diabetics (DMHT, M:F = 16:17), 51 non-

Address for correspondence: Jae Hyun Nam MD, Department of Internal Medicine, Severance Hospital, Yonsei University College of Medicine, 134 Shinchon-Dong, Seodaemun-ku, Seoul 120-752, Korea. Tel.: +82-2-361-5410. Fax: +82-2-393-6884.

diabetic hypertensive (HT, M:F = 25:26, duration ⩾5 years) patients and 57 age- and gender-matched healthy volunteers (C, M:F = 26:31). The volunteers were selected from subjects visiting our medical center for a health screening program. All transcranial Doppler (TCD) studies were performed using a three-dimensional TCD mapping instrument (Trans-scan, Germany) according to examination techniques similar to those previously described [5,6]. Doppler signals from the main stem of the MCA were obtained with a 2 MHz probe attached to a stereotactic headpiece, through a transtemporal window, at a depth between 56—60 mm. Those from the cervical internal carotid artery were obtained with a 4 MHz hand-held probe below the mandible at a depth between 25 and 35 mm. For each artery, the mean, systolic and diastolic velocity were measured, and the Gosling pulsatility index (PI) was calculated automatically.

Results

The velocity measurements and Gosling pulsatility index in the four groups are shown in Table 1. The Gosling pulsatility index of MCA in DM, DMHT and HT patients were shown to be significantly higher than the control subjects, and DMHT patients also had a higher PI of ICA than the control subjects. The PI of MCA in DMHT patients was more elevated than in DM patients. The velocity measurements (mean, systolic and diastolic) in HT patients were significantly lower than in the control subjects. In the DMHT patients, however, the TCD examination revealed significantly lower diastolic velocity of MCA than in the control subjects.

Discussion

These results have shown patients with long-standing hypertension and DM manifest reduced flow velocity of MCA and increased pulsatility of both the MCA and ICA. The flow velocity of the cerebral artery is determined by the

Table 1. TCD measurements in the study subjects.

(cm/s)	C	DM	DMHT	HT
MCA				
Vm	54.23 ± 1.26	58.03 ± 2.99	52.90 ± 3.27	47.87 ± 1.50[a]
Vs	76.05 ± 1.79	85.00 ± 4.46[a]	79.71 ± 4.94	70.19 ± 2.33[a]
Vd	37.87 ± 0.98	38.63 ± 2.16	32.85 ± 2.30[a]	31.82 ± 0.02[a]
PI	0.71 ± 0.15	0.81 ± 0.21[a]	0.90 ± 0.04[ab]	0.80 ± 0.02[a]
ICA				
Vm	25.07 ± 0.63	25.37 ± 1.15	24.00 ± 0.97	23.70 ± 0.71
Vs	37.44 ± 0.88	39.28 ± 1.59	38.56 ± 1.80	36.45 ± 1.01
Vd	17.44 ± 0.53	17.44 ± 0.87	15.61 ± 0.64[a]	16.29 ± 0.58
PI	0.83 ± 0.02	0.88 ± 0.03	0.95 ± 0.03[a]	0.08 ± 0.03

[a]$p < 0.05$ compared with C; [b]$p < 0.05$ compared with DM.

volume flow and the vessel diameter. Thus reduced MCA flow velocity in hypertensive patients may reflect either decreased volume flow or an increased MCA diameter. Previous studies demonstrating reduced CBF in hypertensive patients favor the possibility of volume flow reduction. The cerebral artery flow velocity measured by TCD is well correlated with regional CBF in defined cerebral artery systems, although they cannot be compared simultaneously. However, DM patients did not show the reduced velocities. We believe that the number of subjects was too small, and that there might be diffuse stenotic lesions in DM and DMHT patients. The Gosling pulsatility index was designed to measure vascular resistance. A linear correlation between peripheral resistance and the pulsatility index was observed in the brachial artery of normal humans. The increased PI in hypertension and DM patients in the MCA, not in the ICA is presumably associated with increased vascular resistance in the distal branches. These results illustrated that the cerebral hemodynamic changes in diabetes mellitus and hypertension affect pulsatility of cerebral arteries, especially small arteries. These atherosclerotic changes of cerebral arteries appear to be more aggravated in diabetes mellitus combined with hypertension.

References

1. Sorteberg W, Lindegaard K-F, Rootwelt K, Dahl A, Russell D, Nyberg-Hansen R, Nomes H. Blood velocity and regional blood flow in defined cerebral artery systems. Acta Neurochir 1989;97:47–52.
2. Rodriguez G, Arvigo F, Marenco S, Nobili F, Romano P, Sandini G, Rosadini G. Regional cerebral blood flow in essential hypertension: data evaluation by a mapping system. Stroke 1987; 18:13–20.
3. Fujii K, Sadoshima S, Okada Y, Yao H, Kuwabara Y, Ichiya Y, Fujishima M. Cerebral blood flow and metabolism in normotensive and hypertensive patients with transient neurologic deficits. Stroke 1990;21:283–290.
4. Nobili F, Rodriguez G, Marenco S, De Carli F, Gambaro M, Castello C, Pontremoli R, Rosadini G. Regional cerebral blood flow in chronic hypertension. A correlative study. Stroke 1993; 24:1148–1153.
5. Gosling RG, King DH. Arterial assessment by doppler shift ultrasound. Proc R Soc Med 1974; 67:447–449.
6. Legarth J, Nolsoe C. Doppler blood velocity waveforms and the relation to peripheral resistance in the brachial artery. J Ultrasound Med 1990;9:449–453.

Recent Advances on the Pathogenesis and Management of Diabetes Mellitus.
S.H. Shinn, M. Shichiri and K.-W. Kim, editors.

Hemodynamic study of the feet of diabetic patients using a portable Doppler machine

Haewon Moon[1], Ilyung Lee[1], Jichan Chang[1], Hyunman Kim[2] and Yunseok Chung[2]
Departments of [1] Physical Medicine and Rehabilitation, and [2] Endocrinology and Metabolism, Ajou University School of Medicine, Suwon, Republic of Korea

Abstract. *Backgrounds.* The importance of neuropathy in the pathogenesis of foot lesions has been well-recognized. However, the circulation of limbs affected by peripheral neuropathy has received little attention.

Purpose. To discover the effects of somatic and autonomic nervous function in early change of blood flow of foot in diabetic patients.

Methods. We have studied 51 non-insulin-dependent diabetics. The evidence of neuropathy was screened by nerve conduction studies and sympathetic skin responses of both lower extremities. Blood flow of dorsalis pedis and posterior tibial arteries was measured by a portable Doppler machine and presented as a pressure index (ankle-to-arm systolic pressure ratio).

Results. The patients with sympathetic dysfunction showed a significant decrease in the pressure index compared to normal control, and to diabetic patients with normal sympathetic function.

Conclusion. The changes of the blood flow occur early in diabetic patients with sympathetic dysfunction.

Keywords: blood flow, diabetic foot, Doppler, peripheral neuropathy, sympathetic dysfunction.

Introduction

The importance of neuropathy in the pathogenesis of foot lesions has been well-recognized in diabetes mellitus [1, 2]. Although there has been a lot of blood flow studies for the ischemic limbs from peripheral vascular disease, little attention has been given to peripheral neuropathic limbs in diabetic patients.

In diabetic neuropathy, some studies have shown a remarkable increase in resting blood flow and vascularity, along with the loss of sympathetic regulation [3—5]. There is also some evidence that the neuropathy may lead to disturbances of blood flow without definite peripheral arterial disease [4—6]. The purpose of this study is to assess the effects of somatic and autonomic nerve function as early changes to blood flow in a diabetic foot.

Materials and Methods

Subjects

Fifty-one non-insulin-dependent (type II) diabetic patients (26 males and 25 females) were selected for study. They were all younger than 60 years old, and none of them had a history of hypertension or diabetic foot lesion. They also all had well palpable dorsalis pedis and posterior tibial arteries in both limbs. The average age was 48.8 (± 7.4) years and average % IBW was 112.7 (± 14.3). The control group consisted of 12 normal adults (5 males and 7 females) with average age of 47.2 (± 7.9) years and average % IBW 108.2 (± 9.4).

Grouping of subjects

The patients were divided into four groups as follows:
1. Group 1 (n = 8); normal somatic, normal sympathetic nerve functions.
2. Group 2 (n = 7); abnormal somatic, normal sympathetic nerve functions.
3. Group 3 (n = 14); normal somatic, abnormal sympathetic nerve functions.
4. Group 4 (n = 22); abnormal somatic, abnormal sympathetic nerve functions.

Electrodiagnostic study

The somatic nerve function was evaluated by electrodiagnostic study using sensory and motor nerve conduction studies of superficial peroneal, deep peroneal, sural, and posterior tibial nerves of lower limbs below the knee [7]. The sympathetic nerve function was evaluated by a sympathetic skin response recording at the soles, after contralateral median and posterior tibial nerves stimulation [8].

Hemodynamic study

The hemodynamic study of foot was performed by a portable Doppler machine (Haldeco, ES-1000sp) at the dorsalis pedis and posterior tibial arteries in both limbs. Ankle-to-arm systolic pressure ratios were calculated as a pressure index (PI).

Clinical features and statistics

The patients were examined and medical records were reviewed for age, duration of diabetes, serum cholesterol level, HbA1C level and percentage of IBW. For statistical analysis ANOVA, t-test and correlations were used.

Results

Table 1 illustrates the clinical features and pressure indices of four patient groups and a control group. Group 4 patients were older, and had a longer duration of diabetes. However, there was no significant correlation between the pressure index and age, duration of diabetes, serum cholesterol or HbA1C level. Only group 3 and 4 patients had significantly low values of pressure indices at the dorsalis pedis and posterior tibial arteries compared to the control group.

Table 1. Clinical features, laboratory results and pressure index of lower limbs.

	Control	Group 1	Group 2	Group 3	Group 4
No of limbs	24	16	13	28	45
Age (years)	47.2 ± 7.9	48.9 ± 4.7	49.8 ± 5.1	42.9 ± 8.2	52.2 ± 5.8
Duration (years)		5.5 ± 4.6	9.8 ± 4.0	3.8 ± 2.9	10.8 ± 5.6
Cholesterol (mg/dl)		189.1 ± 25.6	228.8 ± 23.6	201.8 ± 46.1	212.7 ± 45.9[a]
HbA1C (%)		8.2 ± 2.1	10.2 ± 2.5	7.8 ± 1.7	9.8 ± 2.2
% IBW	108.2 ± 9.4	117.6 ± 12.3	102.7 ± 8.2	111.5 ± 12.9	114.7 ± 15.8
PIDPA	1.065 ± 0.041	1.096 ± 0.142	1.092 ± 0.135	1.010 ± 0.109[a]	1.015 ±0.120[a]
PIPTA	1.124 ± 0.047	1.122 ± 0.111	1.133 ± 0.082	1.016 ± 0.110[a]	1.035 ± 0.100[a]

Notes: values are mean standard deviation. PIDPA: pressure index of dorsalis pedis artery. PIPTA: pressure index of posterior tibial artery. $^{a}p < 0.05$.

We regrouped the patients and analysed our data according to somatic nerve function (Table 2). The patients with abnormal somatic nerve function were older, had a longer duration of diabetes with a higher serum cholesterol and HbA1C level. Although the pressure indices of posterior tibial arteries were significantly lower than control, there was generally no significant difference of pressure indices between the two patient groups.

The patients were regrouped and analysed again, according to sympathetic nerve function (Table 3). There were no significant differences in age, duration of diabetes and other laboratory findings between the two patient groups. However, the pressure indices of both arteries in both lower limbs were significantly lower in patients with normal sympathetic function or in control groups.

Table 2. Clinical features, laboratory results and pressure index for nerve conduction studies of lower limbs.

	Control	Nerve conduction study	
		Normal	Abnormal
No of limbs	24	44	58
Age (years)	47.2 ± 7.9	45.1 ± 7.7	51.6 ± 5.7[b]
Duration (years)		4.4 ± 3.7	10.6 ± 5.2[b]
Cholesterol (mg/dl)		197.2 ± 40.1	216.3 ± 42.3[b]
HbA1C (%)		7.9 ± 1.9	9.9 ± 2.3[b]
% IBW	108.2 ± 9.4	113.7 ± 12.9	112.0 ± 15.3
PIDPA	1.065 ± 0.041	1.042 ± 0.128	1.033 ± 0.127
PIPTA	1.124 ± 0.047	1.055 ± 0.121[a]	1.058 ± 0.104[a]

Notes: values are mean standard deviation. PIDPA: pressure index of dorsalis pedis artery; PIPTA: pressure index of posterior tibial artery. $^{a}p < 0.05$ by t test between control and patient groups; $^{b}p < 0.05$ by t test between patient groups.

Table 3. Clinical features, laboratory results and pressure index for sympathetic skin responses of lower limbs.

	Control	Sympathetic skin response	
		Normal	Abnormal
No. of limbs	24	27	75
Age (years)	47.2 ± 7.9	48.9 ± 4.8	48.8 ± 8.1
Duration (years)		7.0 ± 4.7	8.2 ± 5.8
Cholesterol (mg/dl)		203.9 ± 0.6	209.6 ± 45.8
HbA1C (%)		9.0 ± 2.5	9.1 ± 2.2
% IBW	1.065 ± 0.041	1.091 ± 0.128	1.016 ± 0.122[a]
PIDPA	108.2 ± 9.4	111.5 ± 13.1	113.2 ± 14.7
PIPTA	1.124 ± 0.047	1.117 ± 0.114	1.034 ± 0.102[a]

Notes: values are mean standard deviation. PIDPA: pressure index of dorsalis pedis artery. PIPTA: pressure index of posterior tibial artery. [a]$p < 0.05$ by t test between patient groups.

Conclusion

The patients with abnormal sympathetic responses had significant low-pressure indices compared to patients with normal sympathetic responses and the control group. This finding suggests that changes in hemodynamics occur early in diabetic patients with abnormal sympathetic response despite well-preserved arterial pulse or absence of foot lesions.

References

1. Chew JTH, Tan SB, Sivathasan C, Pavanni R, Tan SK. Vascular assessment in the neuropathic diabetic foot. Clin Orthop 1995;320:95–100.
2. Oakley WG, Catterall RCF, Martin MM. Etiology and management of lesions of the foot in diabetes. Br Med J 1956;2:953–957.
3. Boulton AJM, Scarpello JHB, Ward JD. Venous oxygenation in the diabetic neuropathic foot: evidence of arteriovenous shunting? Diabetologia 1982;22:6–8.
4. Edmonds ME, Roberts VC, Watkins PJ. Blood flow in the diabetic neuropathic foot. Diabetologia 1982;22:9–15.
5. Christensen NJ. Spontaneous variations in resting blood flow, postischemic peak flow and vibratory perception in the feet of diabetes. Diabetologia 1969;5:171–178.
6. Partsch H. Vascular regulation disorders in the ulcerative and mutilating neuropathies of the lower extremities. VASA 1978;7:119–125.
7. Liveson JA, Ma DM. Laboratory reference for clinical neurophysiology. Philadelphia: FA Davis, 1992;237–262.
8. Kim JT, Cho MJ, Chun SI. Electrodiagnostic study of the sympathetic skin response (SSR). J Korean Academy Rehabil Med 1989;13:221–226.

Recent Advances on the Pathogenesis and Management of Diabetes Mellitus.
S.H. Shinn, M. Shichiri and K.-W. Kim, editors.

A study of the differentiated analysis of plethysmography in diabetes mellitus

H. Ueda[1,4], K. Suzuki[1], M. Ohishi[2], H. Ohyama[3], K. Ohnishi[3], K. Nobunaga[3], T. Miyauchi[3], Y. Ohyama[3] and H. Taniguchi[5]

Departments of [1]Diabetes and Endocrinology, [2]Ophthalmology, and [3]Division of Laboratory Medicine, Kobe Mahoshi Hospital; and [4]Second Department of Internal Medicine; and [5]Department of Metabolism and Community Health Science, Kobe University School of Medicine, Kobe, Japan

Abstract. We studied the usefulness of differentiated analysis of plethysmography in diabetes mellitus. Plethysmography was conducted in 52 diabetics and 40 healthy subjects using software for differentiation analysis of pulse wave development in our laboratory. The obtained plethysmogram was consecutively differentiated as much as three times, and arbitrary parameters were set up on the second and third derivative pattern of plethysmogram. The effect of autonomic blocking agents was also studied in healthy subjects. In the second derivative of plethysmogram of nondiabetic healthy subjects, the age was inversely related to b/a, C/B and (C+D)/(A+B). In healthy subjects taking β-sympathetic blocker, the parameter of C/B and (C+D)/(A+B) decreased in the second derivative of plethysmogram, but none of the three parameters changed in the third derivative. α-Sympathetic blocker raised b/a and (C+D)/(A+B) in the second and the third derivative of the plethysmogram, respectively. When compared with nondiabetics or diabetics without such complications, the diabetics with complications showed decrease of b/a and C/B in the third derivative of the plethysmogram.

It was suggested as a result of our present studies that b/a and C/B make new parameters irrelevant to the sympathetics to indicate the presence of diabetic complications.

Keywords: autonomic nerve system, diabetic complication, peripheral blood flow.

Background

A circulatory disorder has been reported in diabetes mellitus using the plethysmogram as well as its second derivative, i.e., the accelerated plethysmogram. However, it has not been investigated as to which factor or factors are abnormal among those influencing the formation of the pulse wave. In the following discussion we report new indices of diabetic complications previously supposed to be irrelevant to a sympathetic system.

Subjects and Methods

After a rest in a supine position for 15 min, plethysmography was carried out

Address for correspondence; H. Ueda MD, Department of Diabetes and Endocrinology, Kobe Mahoshi Hospital, Yamada-cho, Kita-ku, Kobe 651-12, Japan. Tel.: +81-78-582-0111. Fax: +81-78-581-8464.

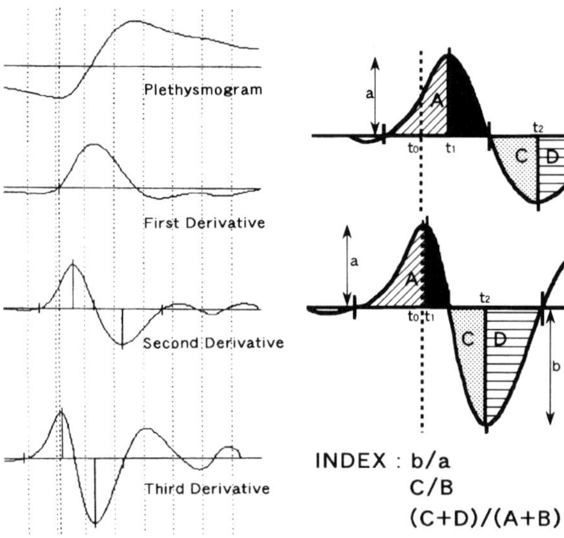

Fig. 1. A plethysmogram and indices of its components.

using a transducer applied on both forefingers which transduces analog signals of cardiac contraction obtained through ECG and pulse wave to an amplifier. These signals were transformed to digital signals and stored in a floppy disk. 100 pulses summed were differentiated to the third derivative using an analyzing software we developed at our laboratory.

A typical plethysmogram of a healthy 35-year-old man and its consecutively differentiated figures are illustrated in Fig. 1. The start of a pulse wave was indicated by null value of its first derivative. Some parameters of the second and the third derivative of a plethysmogram were set up arbitrarily as shown in Fig. 1. They were b/a, C/B and (C+D)/(A+B), where a and b is a maximum and a minimum height of the first positive and negative wave, respectively. The A and B param-

Table 1. Profile of subjects studied.

Number of subjects	
Total	92
Nondiabetics	40
Diabetics	52
Profile of diabetics	
Mean age (years)	61.8 ± 5.2
Duration of diabetes (years)	7.1 ± 7.2
Mean of HbA1c (%)	7.5 ± 1.8
Mode of therapy	
Diet	16
Hypoglycemic agents	20
Insulin	16

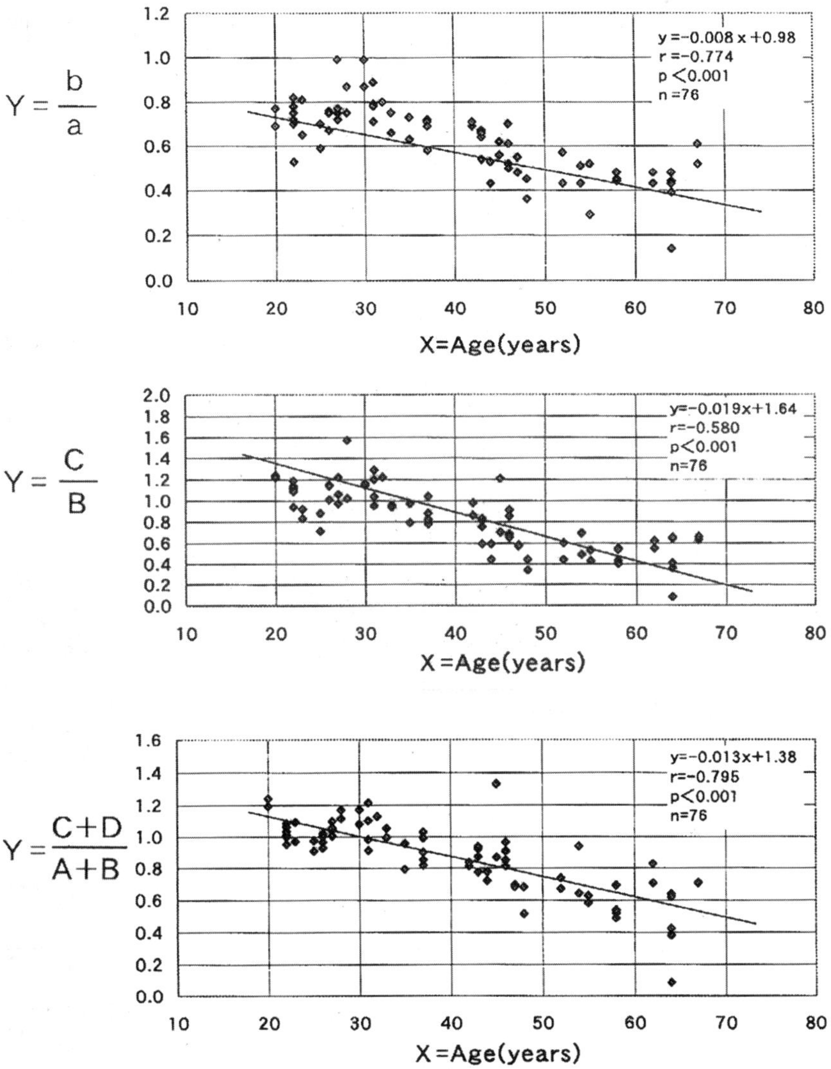

Fig. 2. Relationship between age and the three parameters of the accelerated plethysmogram in nondiabetic healthy subjects.

eters are the portion of an area before and after the time of obtaining a in the first positive wave, respectively. Similarly, C and D are the portion of an area before and after the time of obtaining b in the first negative wave, respectively.

Plethysmography was carried out in 40 nondiabetic and 52 diabetic subjects. The mean age of diabetics was 61.8 years and average duration of diabetes was 7.1 years. The other relevant clinical profiles are shown in Table 1.

For the analysis of the three parameters with relevance to the sympathetics, 10 healthy volunteers aged between 23 and 29 years were subjected to the plethys-

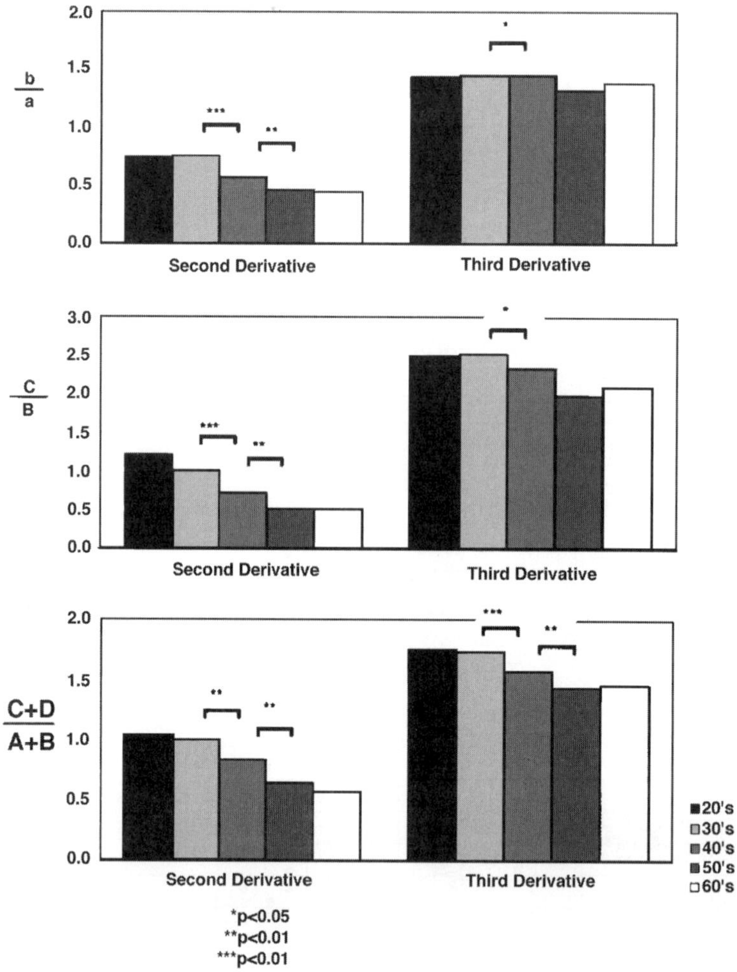

Fig. 3. Relationship between age and three parameters of the 2nd and 3rd differentiated plethysmogram in nondiabetic healthy subjects.

mographical examination at 0, 45 and 90 min after oral administration of 20 mg propranolol hydrochloride (β-blocker) and 3 mg doxazosin mesilate (α-blocker).

Results and Discussions

In the second derivative of the plethysmogram of nondiabetic healthy subjects, the age was inversely related to b/a, C/B and (C+D)/(A+B) (Fig. 2). This is consistent with observations hitherto reported, namely, the formation of a pulse wave being influenced not only by blood pressure and the rigidity of vessel wall, but also by age.

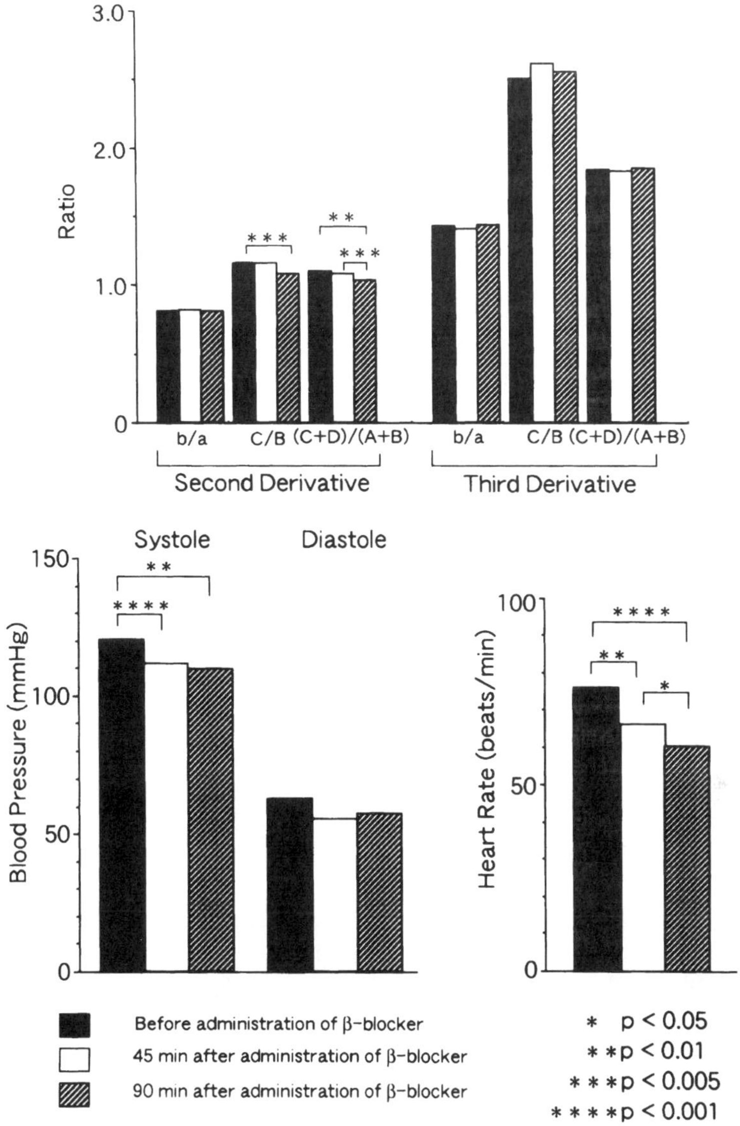

Fig. 4. Effect of β-blocker on plethysmogram, blood pressure and heart rate.

With regard to the second derivative of plethysmogram, the three parameters were the same between subjects at the age of 20—30 years, as well as those between the ages of 50 and 60 years. However, they were related to age in subjects at the 30- to 50-year age range. This was also the case with regard to (C+D)/(A+B) in the third derivative of the plethysmogram, although b/a and C/B are not so clearly related to age (Fig. 3).

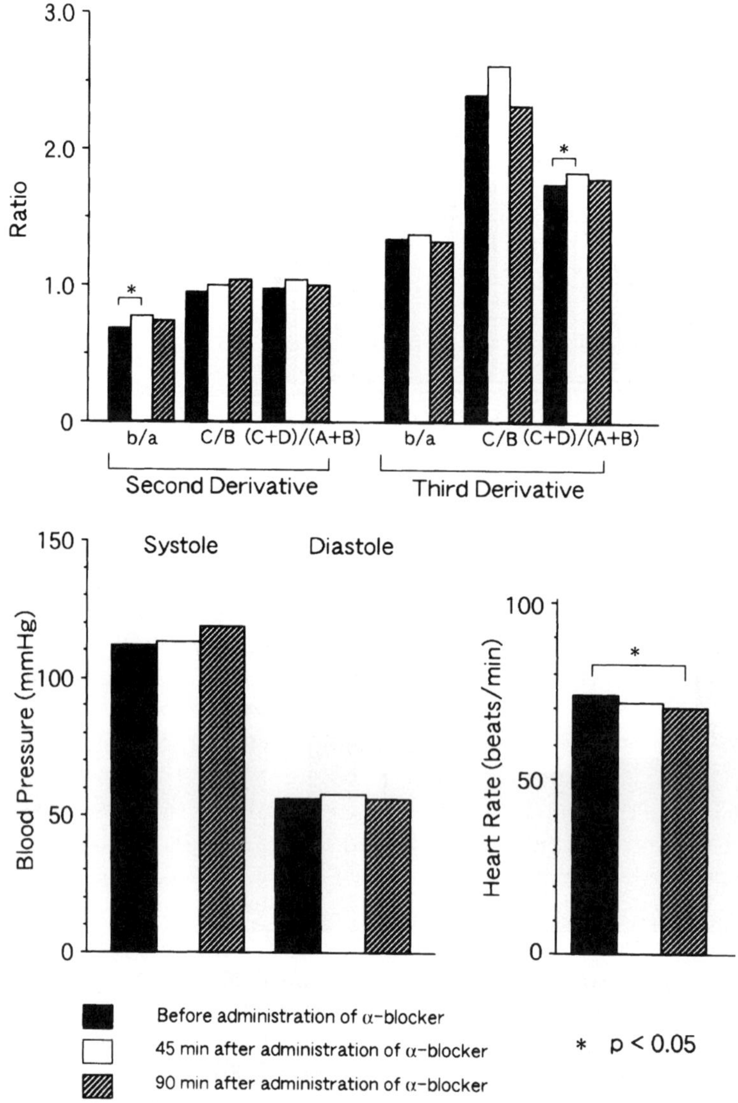

Fig. 5. Effect of α-blocker on plethysmogram, blood pressure and heart rate.

Systolic blood pressure as well as heart rate decreased in a time-dependent manner after the administration of propranolol hydrochloride. In parallel, the parameters of C/B and (C+D)/(A+B) decreased in the second derivative of the plethysmogram. However, in the third derivative none of the three parameters changed (Fig. 4). This indicates that the parameters of the third derivative are not influenced through change in the β-sympathetic function.

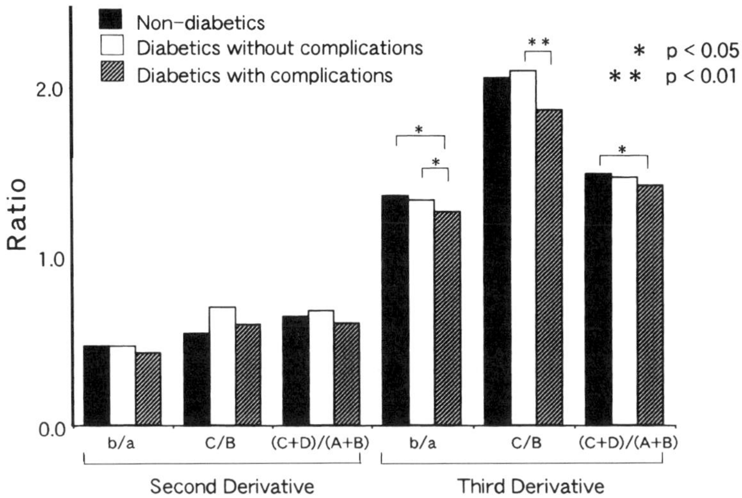

Fig. 6. Comparison of plethysmogram among nondiabetics and diabetics with and without complications.

Doxazosin mesilate did not cause any change in blood pressure and heart rate at 45 min postadministration, whereas b/a and (C+D)/(A+B) in the second and the third derivative of plethysmogram increased, respectively. These changes in the parameters might be due to the action of the α-blocker, except for the blood pressure and heart rate. At 90 min postadministration the heart rate decreased slightly. However, none of the three parameters altered (Fig. 5). These observations (together with those from the β-blocker) indicate that b/a as well as C/B in the third derivative of the plethysmogram are parameters that are influenced by change of blood pressure, heart rate and some other actions (if any) related to the sympathetics. b/a and C/B may create new parameters in terms of irrelevance to the sympathetics. There was no significant difference observed in the parameters among different modalities of treatment, and among the control state of blood glucose judged from mean value of HbA1c during 6 months before the examination (data not shown).

The three parameters were studied in 52 diabetics aged 50–60 years, and the age-matched nondiabetic subjects. The diabetics were divided into two groups, a group of subjects with retinopathy and/or nephropathy, and a group without these complications. When compared with nondiabetics or diabetics without complications, the diabetics with complications indicated decrease of b/a and C/B in the third derivative of the plethysmogram (Fig. 6). Therefore, the pulse wave generated through blood circulation shows some disturbances unrelated to the sympathetic nerve functions in the presence of diabetic complications.

In conclusion, as a result of our present studies it was suggested that b/a and C/B make new parameters irrelevant to the sympathetics in indicating the presence of diabetic complications.

Acknowledgements

We are grateful to Fukuda Denshi Co. Ltd. (Tokyo, Japan) for help in the development of software for the analysis of a plethysmogram.

Recent Advances on the Pathogenesis and Management of Diabetes Mellitus.
S.H. Shinn, M. Shichiri and K.-W. Kim, editors.

Effect of high glucose on function of cultured rabbit vascular endothelial cells

S.M. Son[1], S.D. Yoo[1], I.J. Kim[1], Y.K. Kim[1], C.D. Kim[2] and K.W. Hong[2]
Departments of [1]Internal Medicine, and [2]Pharmacology, College of Medicine, Pusan National University, Ami-Dong, Seo-Gu, Pusan, Korea

Introduction

Vascular disease accounts for the majority of the clinical complications of diabetes mellitus [1]. Changes in local control of vascular tone such as imbalanced production of relaxing and contracting factors by endothelium may be related to the initiation and maintenance of abnormal vascular reactivity characteristically seen in diabetic vascular complications [2]. There is evidence that leukocytes are involved in the pathogenesis of atherosclerosis, the earliest morphological evidence of the disease being the binding of neutrophils to endothelium [3]. Cytokines and growth factors released from injured endothelial cells, T-cells, and macrophages enhance atherogenesis. In this study, we examined nitric oxide (NO) and TNF-α released from cultured rabbit aortic endothelial cells (RAECs) under different glucose concentrations to investigate the relationship between high glucose and endothelial cell dysfunction and analyzed the effect of high glucose on the adhesion of neutrophils to endothelium.

Materials and Methods

The thoracic and abdominal aortae of rabbit (2 ~ 3 kg) were isolated and periadventitial connective tissue was carefully removed. Rabbit aortic endothelial cells in primary culture were prepared by the method of Schwartz [4] with modification. RAECs were grown to confluence in 25 cm^2 flask in DMEM supplemented with 20% fetal bovine serum (FBS), 150 μg/ml endothelial cell growth supplement, 90 μg/ml heparin, 100 U/ml penicillin and 100 μg/ml streptomycin at 37°C in humidified 5% carbon dioxide in air. For experiments, confluent cells were replaced in a 11-mm, 48-well plate containing the same medium composition. Cells were then incubated in the presence or absence of FBS for various times up to 48 h (time course) to evaluate the NO and TNF-α response to different glucose concentrations (0, 5.5, 11, 22 and 44 mmol/l). Cells were also incubated with various concentrations of acetylcholine (ACH) and 5-adenosine

Address for correspondence: S.M. Son, Department of Internal Medicine, College of Medicine, Pusan National University, Ami-Dong, 1 Ga-10, Seo-Gu, Pusan 602-739, Korea.

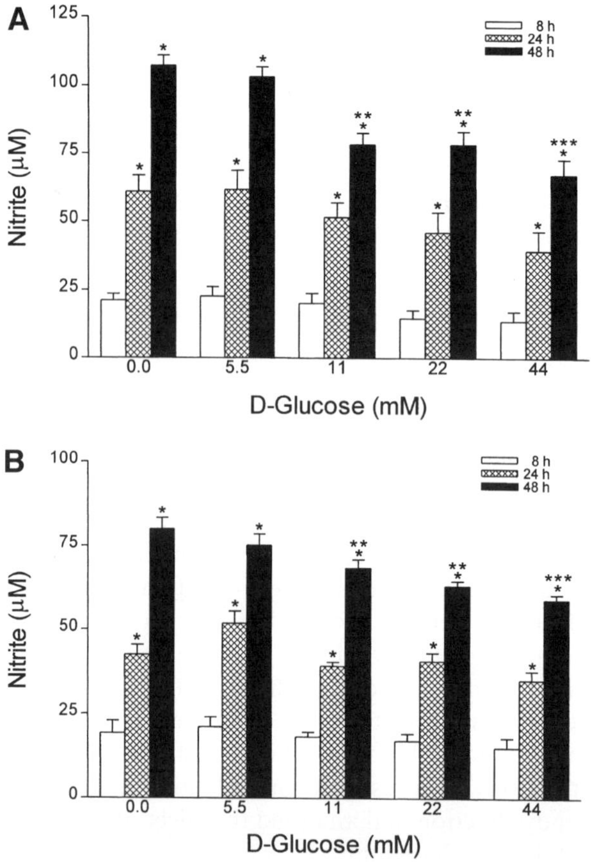

Fig. 1. Glucose and nitrite secretion; effects of glucose (0, 5.5, 11, 22 and 44 mmol/l) on nitrite secretion from cultured rabbit endothelial cells after 8, 24 and 48 h incubation. Values are given for cells incubated in the presence (**A**) or absence (**B**) of FBS. Data are given as the mean ± SD of five different glucose concentrations. *$p < 0.05$ vs. 8 h incubation; **$p < 0.05$; ***$p < 0.01$ vs. 0 mM of D-glucose.

diphosphate (ADP) (10^{-7}, 10^{-6}, 10^{-5} and 10^{-4} mol/l) and 10^{-4} mol/l of ACH or ADP with different glucose concentrations for 24 h to evaluate the stimulated effect of ACH and ADP on NO release. To evaluate the adhesion of neutrophils to endothelium, cells were incubated for 24 h to a different glucose concentration except 44 mmol/l, and then isolated rabbit neutrophils were incubated with monolayers of rabbit aortic endothelial cells for 1 h at 37°C.

Results

1. Total NO release from RAECs was significantly time-dependent. After 48 h incubation, the total secretion of NO was significantly higher in culture medium with FBS than without FBS.

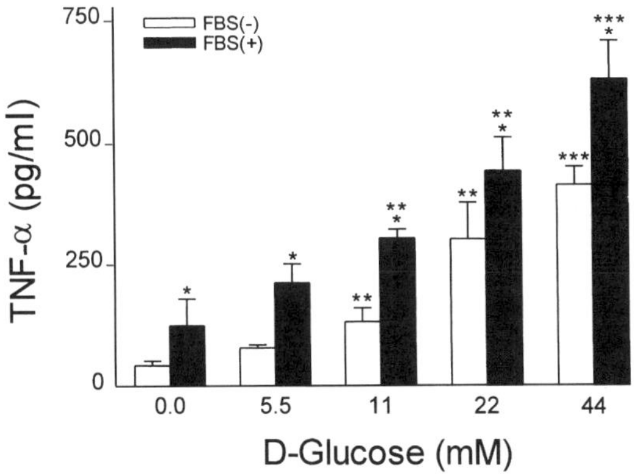

Fig. 2. Glucose and TNF-α secretion; effects of glucose on TNF-α release from rabbit endothelial cells after 24 h incubation in the presence or absence of FBS. Data are given as the mean ± SD. *$p<0.05$ vs. without FBS; **$p<0.05$; ***$p<0.01$ vs. 0 mmol/l D-glucose.

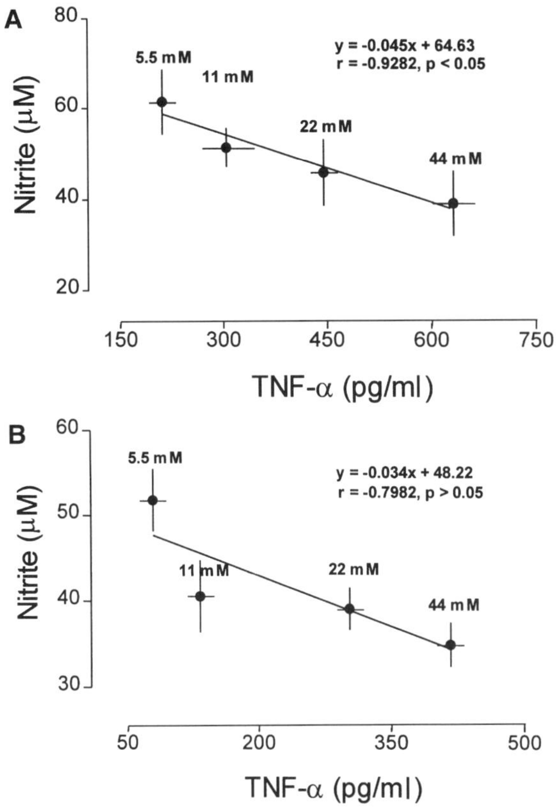

Fig. 3. Relationship between nitrite and TNF-α. Relationship between changes in TNF-α levels and corresponding changes in nitrite according to four different glucose concentrations with (**A**) or without (**B**) FBS after 48 h incubation. Data are given as mean ± SD.

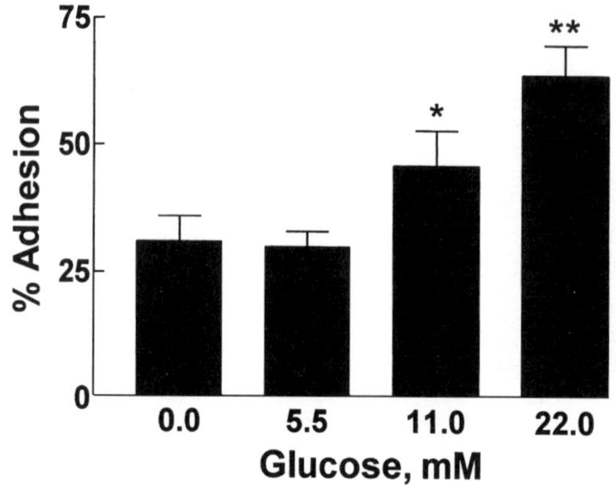

Fig. 4. Concentration-dependent effect of glucose on neutrophil adhesion to rabbit aortic endothelial cells. Confluent monolayers of endothelial cells were exposed to various concentrations of glucose (0—22 mM) for 23 h at 37°C, followed by assessment of neutrophil adherence. Results are averaged from five different paired experiments. $^{*}p < 0.05$; $^{**}p < 0.01$ vs. value of 5.5 mM glucose.

2. Glucose concentration resembling severe hyperglycemic conditions (22 and 44 mmol/l) significantly inhibited NO release from RAECs (Fig. 1).
3. Acetylcholine and ADP induced a clear dose-dependent NO release in RAECs.
4. Stimulation of acetylcholine and ADP on NO release according to a different glucose concentration was not significantly higher than NO release in culture medium with glucose alone.
5. The increment in TNF-α levels was associated with a significant increase at higher glucose concentration (Fig. 2).

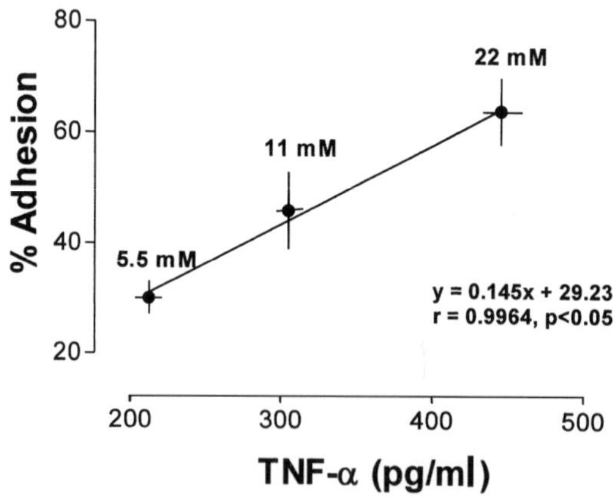

Fig. 5. Relationship between neutrophil adhesion and TNF-α. Relationship between changes in TNF-α levels and corresponding changes in neutrophil adhesion to endothelium according to three different glucose concentrations. Data are given as mean ± SEM.

6. There was a negative correlation between NO and TNF-α release in culture medium with FBS but not in culture medium without FBS (Fig. 3).
7. After 24-h incubation with various concentrations of glucose, neutrophil adherence to high concentration of glucose (11 and 22 mmol/l)-treated endothelium was significantly increased compared with adhesion to low concentration of glucose (0 or 5.5 mmol/l)-treated endothelium (Fig. 4).
8. There was a positive correlation between neutrophil adhesion and TNF-α release (Fig. 5).

Discussion

Our data show that decreased NO release and increased TNF-α release from RAECs were noted under high glucose concentration. High glucose concentration of glucose stimulated neutrophils adhesion to endothelial cells in association with increased production of TNF-α from endothelial cells. Such interaction could play a significant role in the development of diabetic vascular complication in hyperglycemic conditions.

References

1. Ruderman NB, Williamson JR, Brownee M. Glucose and diabetic vascular disease. FASEB J 1992;6:2905–2914.
2. Meraji S, Joykody L, Senaratne MP, Thomson ABR, Kappagoda T. Endothelium-dependent relaxation in aorta of BB rat. Diabetes 1986;36:978–981.
3. Ross R. The pathogenesis of atherosclerosis – an update. N Engl J Med 1986;314:488–500.
4. Schwartz SM. Selection and characterization of bovine aortic endothelial cells. In Vitro 1978; 14:966–980.

Recent Advances on the Pathogenesis and Management of Diabetes Mellitus.
S.H. Shinn, M. Shichiri and K.-W. Kim, editors.

The activation of PKC is involved in Ox-LDL-induced macrophage growth

Takeshi Matsumura[1], Masakazu Sakai[1], Shozo Kobori[1], Takeshi Biwa[1], Toru Takemura[1], Hirofumi Matsuda[1], Seikoh Horiuchi[2] and Motoaki Shichiri[1]
Departments of [1]Metabolic Medicine and [2]Biochemistry, Kumamoto University School of Medicine, Kumamoto, Japan

Abstract. Recent studies from our laboratory have demonstrated that oxidized low-density lipoprotein (Ox-LDL) induces macrophage growth in vitro. The present study was undertaken to elucidate the intracellular signaling pathways for macrophage growth. Ox-LDL initiated a rapid and transient rise in intracellular free calcium ion and induced activation of membrane protein kinase C. Pertussis toxin completely inhibited Ox-LDL-induced rise in free calcium ion and significantly inhibited macrophage growth. Moreover, protein kinase C inhibitors (calphostin C) significantly inhibited Ox-LDL-induced macrophage growth. Our results suggest that the intracellular signaling pathways through increased concentrations of intracellular calcium ion and activation of protein kinase C may play an important role in Ox-LDL-induced macrophage growth.

Keywords: atherosclerosis, G-protein, macrophage growth, oxidized LDL, PKC.

Introduction

One of the characteristic events in the development of atherosclerotic lesions in arterial walls is the growth of cellular components. In particular, proliferating foam cells found in the advanced or mature stages of atherosclerosis are derived from smooth muscle cells [1]. However, recent reports emphasized that a proportion of foam cells proliferating in the atherosclerotic lesions are also derived from macrophages [2,3]. Since macrophage-derived foam cells play an important role in the development of atherosclerotic lesions, it seems reasonable to expect that macrophage growth might be linked to atherosclerotic processes, probably by enhancing its progression.

Recently, we observed the capacity of Ox-LDL to stimulate the growth of macrophages [4—8]. These findings strongly suggest that in order to promote macrophage cell growth, Ox-LDL probably acts as a growth factor to macrophages by inducing certain intracellular signaling pathways. In the present study, we characterized Ox-LDL-induced intracellular signaling pathways for the growth of mouse resident macrophages. The results indicate that a rise in intra-

Address for correspondence: Takeshi Matsumura MD, Department of Metabolic Medicine, Kumamoto University School of Medicine, 1-1-1 Honjo, Kumamoto 860, Japan. Tel.: +81-96-373-5169. Fax: +81-96-366-8397.

cellular calcium ion and subsequent activation of protein kinase C (PKC) are two potential pathways involved in Ox-LDL-induced macrophage growth.

Materials and Methods

Lipoproteins and their modifications

Human LDL (d = 1.019—1.063 g/ml) was isolated by sequential ultracentrifugation of human plasma of normolipidemic subjects obtained after overnight fasting. Acetyl-LDL was prepared by chemical modification of LDL with acetic anhydride. To prepare Ox-LDL, LDL (0.1 mg/ml) was incubated for 20 h at 37°C with 5 μM $CuSO_4$, followed by the addition of 1 mM EDTA and cooling.

Cell culture

Peritoneal macrophages were collected from nonstimulated male C3H/He mice (25—30 g) and suspended in RPMI 1,640 medium (Nissui Seiyaku Co., Tokyo) supplemented with 10% heat-inactivated fetal bovine serum (Life Technologies, Inc.), streptomycin (0.1 mg/ml), and penicillin (100 units/ml). All cellular experiments were performed at 37°C in a humidified atmosphere of 5% CO_2 in air. Cell proliferation was determined by both tritiated thymidine incorporation assay and cell-counting assay [4]. Cytosolic free calcium concentration was determined by the method using Fura-2. PKC activity was determined by MESACUP Protein Kinase Assay Kit (Medical and Biological Laboratories, Japan).

Results

Effect of Ox-LDL on intracellular calcium concentration in macrophages

Addition of Ox-LDL, though not LDL or acetyl-LDL, to macrophages resulted in an instantaneous rise in $[Ca^{2+}]i$ followed by a return to the baseline level within 5 min (Fig. 1A). Even when the cells were pretreated with acetyl-LDL, a well-known ligand for the scavenger receptor to induce foam cell formation similar to Ox-LDL, Ox-LDL continued to cause a rise in $[Ca^{2+}]i$ in these macrophages (data not shown). These results suggested the possible involvement of a receptor(s) other than type I and II scavenger receptors in this phenomenon.

Ox-LDL-induced rise in $[Ca^{2+}]i$ was neither inhibited by calcium channel blockers nor by the addition of calcium chelater EGTA into the medium (data not shown), suggesting that the rise in $[Ca^{2+}]i$ might be derived from intracellular calcium store.

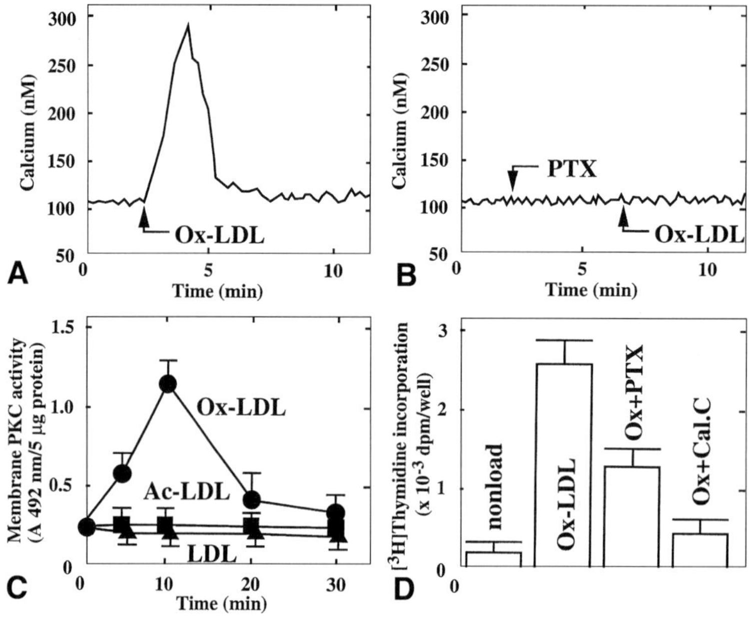

Fig. 1. Calcium concentration and PKC activity in Ox-LDL-induced macrophage growth. **A:** Mouse resident peritoneal macrophages (1×10^4 cells/well) were incubated at 37°C with 50 µg/ml of Ox-LDL. Arrow indicates the time of addition of Ox-LDL. Cytosolic free calcium concentrations were determined. **B:** Macrophages were preincubated at 37°C with 10 ng/ml of pertussis toxin (PTX), followed by the addition of 50 µg/ml of Ox-LDL. Cytosolic free calcium concentrations were determined. **C:** Macrophages (1×10^7 cells/well) were incubated for indicated time with 20 µg/ml of Ox-LDL, LDL or acetyl-LDL. The membrane PKC activity was determined. **D:** Macrophages (4×10^4 cells/well) were incubated for 6 days with 20 µg/ml of Ox-LDL in the absence or presence of calphostin C (200 nM) or PTX (10 ng/ml). [^{3}H]Thymidine uptake was determined.

Effect of pertussis toxin on intracellular calcium concentration and macrophage proliferation

Pretreatment of macrophages with 10 ng/ml of pertussis toxin inhibited Ox-LDL-induced [Ca^{2+}]i rise (Fig. 1B). As shown in Fig. 1D, pertussis toxin significantly inhibited Ox-LDL-induced increase in [^{3}H]thymidine incorporation by 50%. Parallel experiments with the cell-counting assay also showed that the increased cell numbers induced by 20 µg/ml of Ox-LDL was inhibited by 70% with 10 ng/ml of pertussis toxin.

Involvement of protein kinase C in Ox-LDL-induced macrophage growth

Figure 1C shows the time-course study of the effect of Ox-LDL on the membrane PKC activity. Following the addition of 20 µg/ml of Ox-LDL to these cells, the enzyme activity increased 5-fold above the basal level at 10 min, followed by a rapid decline close to the baseline level at 20 min. However, PKC seemed to be still activated to some extent even 30 min after the addition of Ox-LDL. Both LDL and acetyl-LDL failed to stimulate the membrane PKC activity in these cells (Fig. 1C).

To elucidate the role of PKC activation in Ox-LDL-induced macrophage growth, the effect of a PKC inhibitor, calphostin C, on Ox-LDL-induced macrophage growth was examined. The Ox-LDL-induced increase in [^{3}H]thymidine incorporation was significantly suppressed by calphostin C (Fig. 1D). To further confirm the results obtained by [^{3}H]thymidine incorporation assay, the effect of calphostin C on Ox-LDL-induced macrophage growth was also assessed by cell-counting. The increased number of cells induced by Ox-LDL was 2.0-fold above the basal level. When macrophages were cultured under the identical conditions but in the presence of calphostin C, the increase in cell numbers was only 1.2-fold above the basal level, indicating the effective suppression of cell growth by this drug. These results suggested a possible role of PKC in Ox-LDL-induced macrophage growth.

Discussion

The present study has clearly shown that two phenomena induced by Ox-LDL; the activation of PKC (Fig. 1C) and macrophage growth, were significantly inhibited in common by PKC inhibitor, calphostin C, (Fig. 1D), suggesting an important role of PKC in Ox-LDL-induced macrophage growth. This conclusion is supported by the results of Hamilton and Dientsman [9] demonstrating proliferation of mouse peritoneal macrophages by phorbol esters.

The present study showed that Ox-LDL stimulated a rapid increase in [Ca^{2+}]i (Fig. 1A). Since the addition of calcium channel blockers or EGTA to the medium did not affect Ox-LDL-induced calcium rise (data not shown), it is likely that the increased [Ca^{2+}]i is derived from intracellular calcium store. This notion was supported by Shackelford et al. [10] who demonstrated that Ox-LDL initiated a rapid increase in PIP2 hydrolysis into IP3 which in turn enhanced calcium release from the endoplasmic reticulum. Our results also showed that Ox-LDL-induced [Ca^{2+}]i rise was completely inhibited by pertussis toxin (Fig. 1D). Moreover, pertussis toxin inhibited Ox-LDL-induced macrophage growth by 50% (Fig. 1D). These results suggest that the rapid release of Ca^{2+} from the endoplasmic reticulum is likely to be involved in Ox-LDL-induced macrophage proliferation.

The inhibition by pertussis toxin of Ox-LDL-induced [Ca^{2+}]i rise and macrophage growth (Fig. 1A,D) suggests the presence of a G-protein coupled Ox-LDL receptor which initiates the intracellular signal(s) and finally leads to macrophage growth. Most G-protein-linked receptors identified so far have a common structure; seven membrane-spanning domains connected by extracellular and intracellular loops. According to a general model of chemokine-mediated signal transduction events in phagocytes, an appropriate ligand-receptor interaction causes the activation of a pertussis toxin-sensitive G-protein with subsequent induction of phospholipase C activity. This leads to the accumulation of both diacylglycerol and cytosolic inositol trisphosphate. The former directly stimulates PKC activity, whereas the latter in turn initiates mobilization of intracellular Ca^{2+} from the endoplasmic reticulum, leading to PKC activation [11].

Figure 2 is a schematic representation of the events that lead to macrophage growth. Binding of Ox-LDL to its receptor on plasma membranes of macrophages initiates activation of a pertussis toxin-sensitive G-protein and then induces phospholipase C activity, thereby activating PKC by diacylglycerol and increasing $[Ca^{2+}]i$ through IP3 (Fig. 2). Well-established as a major endocytic receptor, the macrophage scavenger receptors (type I and type II) [12] are also known to modulate a variety of macrophage activities such as endocytosis of modified proteins, cell adhesion and the release of lipoprotein lipase. However, intracellular signaling in response to the ligand binding to the scavenger receptors has not been well-established. Recently, Claus et al. [13] demonstrated that acetyl-LDL could activate PKC in P388D1 cells, but was inhibited by polyinosinic acid, suggesting that type I and II scavenger receptors could induce intracellular signals. However, acetyl-LDL did not initiate $[Ca^{2+}]i$ rise. Furthermore, our previous studies clearly showed that acetyl-LDL had no capacity to induce macrophage growth [5,7]. Thus, type I and II scavenger receptors are probably

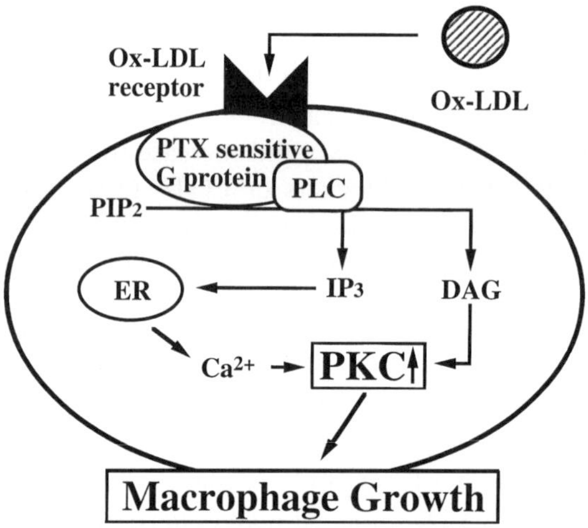

Fig. 2. Schematic representation of possible intracellular signaling pathways for Ox-LDL-induced macrophage growth. Ox-LDL first interacts with the G-protein coupled Ox-LDL receptor leading to the activation of pertussis toxin-sensitive G-protein and then activation of PLC. The latter results in accumulation of DAG and IP3 in the cytoplasm, DAG then directly activates PKC, whereas IP3 also activates PKC but indirectly by increasing the concentration of intracellular calcium through efficient mobilization of calcium from the endoplasmic reticulum. The activation of PKC plays a key role in Ox-LDL-induced macrophage growth, although the downstream pathway from PKC to macrophage proliferation is still not known. Ox-LDL = oxidized low-density lipoprotein; PLC = phospholipase C; PIP2 = phosphatidylinositol bisphosphate; IP3 = inositol trisphosphate; DAG = diacylglycerol; ER = endoplasmic reticulum; PKC = protein kinase C.

not involved in increased $[Ca^{2+}]i$ in Ox-LDL-induced macrophage growth. In addition to type I and II receptors, the presence of other scavenger receptors has also been reported. However, a 7-transmembrane domain, a characteristic feature of the G-protein coupled receptor, is not found in these receptors. Thus, further studies are necessary to determine the exact receptor that mediates the rise in $[Ca^{2+}]i$ for macrophage proliferation by Ox-LDL.

References

1. Ross R. The pathogenesis of atherosclerosis: a perspective for the 1990s. Nature 1993;362: 801–809.
2. Gordon D, Reidy MA, Benditt EP, Schwartz SM. Cell proliferation in human coronary arteries. Proc Natl Acad Sci USA 1990;87:4600–4604.
3. Rosenfeld ME, Ross R. Macrophage and smooth muscle cell proliferation in atherosclerotic lesions of WHHL and comparably hypercholesterolemic fat-fed rabbits. Arteriosclerosis 1990; 10:680–687.
4. Yui S, Sasaki T, Miyzaki A, Horiuchi S, Yamazaki M. Induction of murine macrophage growth by modified LDLs. Arterioscler Thromb 1993;13:331–337.
5. Sakai M, Miyazaki A, Hakamata H, Sasaki T, Yui S, Yamazaki M, Shichiri M, Horiuchi S. Lysophosphatidylcholine plays an essential role in the mitogenic effect of oxidized low density lipoprotein on murine macrophages. J Biol Chem 1994;269:31430–31435.
6. Sato Y, Kobori S, Sakai M, Yano T, Higashi T, Matsumura T, Morikawa W, Terano T, Miyazaki A, Horiuchi S, Shitiri M. Lipoprotein(a) induces cell growth in rat peritoneal macrophages through inhibition of transforming growth factor-b activation. Atherosclerosis 1996;125:15–26.
7. Sakai M, Miyazaki A, Hakamata H, Sasaki T, Yui S, Yamazaki Y, Shichiri M, Horiuchi S. Lysophosphatidylcholine potentiates the mitogenic activity of modified LDL for human monocyte-derived macrophages. Arterioscler Thromb Vasc Biol 1996;16:600–605.
8. Sakai M, Miyazaki A, Hakamata H, Kodama T, Suzuki H, Kobori S, Shichiri M, Horiuchi S. The scavenger receptor serves as a route for internalization of lysophosphatidylcholine in oxidized low density lipoprotein-induced macrophage proliferation. J Biol Chem 1996;271: 27346–27352.
9. Hamilton JA, Dientsman SR. Induction of macrophage DNA synthesis by phorbol esters. J Cell Physiol 1981;106:445–450.
10. Shackelford RE, Misra UK, Florine-Casteel K, Sheau-Fung T, Pizzo SV, Adams DO. Oxidized low density lipoprotein suppresses activation of NFkB in macrophages via a pertussis toxin-sensitive signaling mechanism. J Biol Chem 1995;270:3475–3478.
11. Pozzan T, Lew DP, Wollheim CB, Tsien RY. Is cytosolic ionized calcium regulating neutrophil activation? Science 1983;221:1413–1415.
12. Kodama T, Freeman M, Rohrer L, Zabrecky J, Matsudaira P, Krieger M. Type I macrophage scavenger receptor contains a helical collagen-like coiled coils. Nature 1990;343:531–535.
13. Claus R, Fyrnys B, Deigner HP, Wolf G. Oxidized low density lipoprotein stimulates protein kinase C (PKC) and induces expression of PKC-isotypes via prostaglandin-H-synthase in P388D1 macrophage-like cells. Biochemistry 1996;35:4911–4922.

Recent Advances on the Pathogenesis and Management of Diabetes Mellitus.
S.H. Shinn, M. Shichiri and K.-W. Kim, editors.

Lipoprotein(a) level and vascular complications in NIDDM

Ji Youn Kim, Mung Su Kim, Joung Min Kim, Jai Hong Park, Joung Hun Lee, Seung Won Yang, Dong Jin Chung, Min Young Chung and Tai Hee Lee
Department of Internal Medicine, Chonnam National University Hospital, Kwangju City, Korea

Abstract. *Background.* The contribution of Lp(a) to the increased risk for atherosclerosis and diabetic complications in subjects with diabetes is not well known. Therefore, we examined the relationship between Lp(a) levels and development of vascular complications, and the relationship between Lp(a) and other risk factors for vascular complications in NIDDM.

Methods. 152 NIDDM patients were evaluated. ECG, coronary angiography, brain CT/MRI, Doppler velocimetry, peripheral angiography, fundus camera, nerve conduction velocity, BBV, VPT, 24-h urine protein amount, Lp(a) level, and other risk factors for atherosclerosis were examined for this study.

Results. Lp(a) levels in subjects with ischemic heart disease, cerebrovascular disease and diabetic retinopathy, were significantly higher than those in subjects without the above-mentioned diseases. The ApoB/ApoA1 ratio and LDL-cholesterol levels in subjects with an Lp(a) level $\geqslant$ 30 mg/dl, were significantly higher than those in subjects with an Lp(a) level $<$ 30 mg/dl, and Lp(a) has a positive correlation with the ApoB/ApoA1 ratio and LDL-cholesterol in NIDDM patients with vasculopathy.

Conclusions. These results suggest that Lp(a) levels seem to be associated with macro- and microvascular complications in NIDDM.

Keywords: lipoprotein(a), macrovascular complication, microvascular complication, NIDDM.

Introduction

Lipoprotein(a) (Lp(a)) is an independent risk factor for atherosclerotic vascular disease in subjects without diabetes [1,2]. The contribution of Lp(a) to the increased risk for atherosclerosis and diabetic complications in subjects with diabetes is not well known.

In this report, we examined the relationship between Lp(a) levels and the development of vascular (macro- and/or micro-) complications, and the relationship between Lp(a) and other risk factors for vascular complications in subjects with NIDDM.

Material and Methods/Patients

For the study we evaluated 152 patients with NIDDM (72 women and 80 men). For determination of lipoproteins, blood samples were collected after an over-

Address for correspondence: Dr J.Y. Kim, Department of Internal Medicine, Chonnam National University Hospital, 8-Hakdong, Dong-ku, Kwangju City 501-757, Korea.

night fast. Lp(a) level was measured with an N-Latex Lp(a) reagent. Electrocardiography, coronary angiography, brain CT/MRI, Doppler velocimetry and peripheral angiography were carried out for the diagnosis of macrovascular complications. Fundus camera, nerve-conduction velocity, BBV (beat-to-beat variation), VPT (vibration perception threshold), and 24-h urine protein amounts were examined for diagnosis of microvascular complications. The results are expressed as mean values ± SE or median (Lp(a)). The significance of differences between the two groups was determined using the two-tailed t test with unpaired data or the Mann-Whitney U test (Lp(a)). Spearman's correlation coefficient was used for testing correlations between different variables. Values of $p<0.05$ were considered significant.

Results

Lp(a) levels in subjects with ischemic heart disease and cerebrovascular disease were significantly higher than those in subjects without (Table 1). Lp(a) levels in subjects with diabetic retinopathy were significantly higher than those in subjects without (Table 2). The ApoB/ApoA1 ratio and LDL-cholesterol levels in subjects

Table 1. Association of ischemic heart disease (IHD), cerebrovascular disease (CVD) and arteriosclerosis obliterance (ASO) with Lp(a), lipid profile, and other risk factors of vasculopathy in NIDDM.

	IHD		CVD		ASO	
	without (n = 133)	with (n = 19)	without (n = 129)	with (n = 23)	without (n = 146)	with (n = 5)
Mean age (years)	59 (0.9)	65 (1.8)[a]	58.9 (0.9)	63.9 (1.8)[a]	59.6 (0.9)	65.4 (4.9)
Gender (male:female)	69:64	11:8	70:59	10:13	74:72	5:0
DM duration (years)	10.5 (0.6)	10.5 (1.8)	9.9 (0.6)	13.7 (1.7)[a]	10.4 (0.6)	11.8 (3.7)
Body mass index (kg/m^2)	23.9 (0.4)	24.8 (1.0)	23.6 (0.3)	25.9 (1.4)[a]	24.0 (0.4)	23.7 (1.0)
ApoA1 (mg/dl)	109.4 (2.9)	94.8 (8.3)	110.2 (2.9)	93.0 (7.0)[a]	108.8 (2.8)	76.8 (7.1)[a]
ApoB (mg/dl)	102.0 (3.6)	98.8 (8.0)	99.3 (3.2)	115.2 (12.8)	101.6 (3.4)	106.2 (16.5)
ApoB/ApoA1 ratio	1.0 (0.04)	1.1 (0.11)	0.95 (0.03)	1.32 (0.14)[a]	1.00 (0.04)	1.38 (0.20)
Lp(a) (mg/dl)	22.6	31.0[a]	22.9	34.0[a]	23.0	31.0
LDL-cholesterol (mg/dl)	119.9 (4.1)	124.0 (7.8)	116.3 (3.9)	144.3 (9.5)[a]	120.5 (3.8)	119.6 (21.5)
HbA1c (%)	9.6 (0.3)	10 (0.7)	9.7 (0.3)	9.5 (0.7)	9.7 (0.3)	9.0 (1.0)

Notes: values are expressed as mean (± SE) or median (Lp(a)). Significant differences between the the groups were determined using the two-tailed t test with unpaired data or the Mann-Whitney U test (Lp(a)). IHD: ischemic heart disease; CVD: cerebrovascular disease; ASO: arteriosclerosis obliterance. [a]$p<0.05$ vs. without vasculopathy.

Table 2. Association of retinopathy, neuropathy and nephropathy with Lp(a), lipid profile and other risk factors of vasculopathy in NIDDM.

	Retinopathy		Neuropathy		Nephropathy	
	without (n = 47)	with (n = 71)	without (n = 10)	with (n = 80)	without (n = 76)	with (n = 57)
Mean age (years)	58.9 (1.6)	59.1 (1.1)	60.7 (3.5)	58.7 (1.2)	59.0 (1.3)	58.6 (1.1)
Gender (male:female)	26:21	36:35	3:7	43:37	39:37	33:24
DM duration (years)	7.4 (1.0)	12.5 (0.8)[a]	5.7 (1.4)	10.6 (0.8)[a]	9.5 (0.8)	11.3 (0.9)
Body mass index (kg/m^2)	23.6 (0.5)	24.2 (0.6)	23.9 (1.2)	23.3 (0.4)	23.7 (0.4)	24.1 (0.8)
ApoA1 (mg/dl)	113.7 (4.5)	107.7 (4.1)	110.2 (5.9)	111.8 (3.7)	112.3 (3.5)	105.6 (4.5)
ApoB (mg/dl)	98.2 (5.0)	107.4 (5.6)	105.6 (9.6)	100.6 (5.4)	98.1 (4.1)	110.1 (6.4)
ApoB/ApoA1 ratio	0.90 (0.05)	1.06 (0.06)	0.98 (0.11)	0.95 (0.05)	0.90 (0.03)	1.11 (0.07)[a]
Lp(a) (mg/dl)	20.0	30.0[a]	25.0	29.0	25.5	23.0
LDL-cholesterol (mg/dl)	117.6 (5.2)	126.3 (6.4)	118.0 (10.6)	122.1 (5.6)	117.9 (4.1)	125.8 (7.2)
HbA1c (%)	9.5 (0.5)	9.6 (0.3)	10.0 (1.1)	9.9 (0.4)	9.9 (0.4)	9.4 (0.4)

Notes: values are expressed as mean (±SE) or median (Lp(a)). Significant differences between the two groups were determined using the two-tailed t test with unpaired data or the Mann-Whitney U test (Lp(a)). [a]$p < 0.05$ vs. without vasculopathy.

Table 3. Association of Lp(a) level with lipid profile and other risk factors of vasculopathy in NIDDM.

	Lp(a)		p value
	< 30 mg/dl (n = 90)	30 mg/dl (n = 57)	
Mean age (years)	58.8 (1.1)	61.5 (1.2)	NS
Gender (male:female)	43:47	34:23	NS
DM duration (years)	9.3 (0.9)	11.6 (0.8)	NS
Body mass index (kg/m^2)	24.5 (0.5)	23.1 (0.5)	NS
ApoA1 (mg/dl)	106.8 (3.5)	109.1 (4.5)	NS
ApoB (mg/dl)	92.3 (3.4)	117.4 (6.3)	0.000
ApoB/ApoA1 ratio	0.94 (0.04)	1.14 (0.07)	0.013
LDL-cholesterol (mg/dl)	111.6 (4.1)	130.5 (7.7)	0.021
HbA1c (%)	7.3 (0.5)	8.3 (0.6)	NS
24 h urine protein (g/day)	0.52 (0.08)	0.83 (0.20)	NS
Smoking (pys)	8.7 (1.70	11.1 (2.7)	NS

Values are expressed as mean (± SE). NS: Not significant. Significant differences between the two groups were determined using the two-tailed t test for unpaired data.

with an Lp(a) level ⩾ 30 mg/dl were significantly higher than those in subjects with an Lp(a) level < 30 mg/dl (Table 3), and Lp(a) have a positive correlation with the ApoB/ApoA1 ratio and LDL-cholesterol in NIDDM patients with vasculopathy (Table 4).

Discussion

These results suggest that Lp(a) levels seem to be associated with macro- and microvascular (especially with retinopathy) complications in subjects with NIDDM and a high ApoB/ApoA1 ratio, LDL-cholesterol, and Lp(a) are associated with the development of vasculopathy in NIDDM patients. Velho et al. [3] noted increased Lp(a) levels in subjects with diabetes who had a history of myocardial infarction. In contrast, Haffner et al. [4] found no relationship between Lp(a) levels and ischemic heart disease-associated mortality in subjects with diabetes mellitus. Nobuhiro et al. [5] found that Lp(a) is an independent risk factor for retinopathy in the elderly, and probably also in the middle-aged, with NIDDM. The role of Lp(a) in the formation of neuropathy or nephropathy is controversial [6,7]. Prospective studies on a large scale will be required in order to reach a definitive conclusion about what role Lp(a) plays in the formation of diabetic complications.

Acknowledgements

We acknowledge the help of Dr B.J. Na with statistical analysis.

Table 4. Spearman's correlation coefficient between Lp(a), lipid profile, duration of diabetes, age and HbA1c in NIDDM.

	Lp(a)	B/A	LDL-C	Duration	Age	HbA1c
Retinopathy (n = 38)						
Lp(a)	1.0000					
ApoB/ApoA1 ratio	0.4097[a]	1.0000				
LDL-cholesterol	0.4198[a]	0.4964[a]	1.0000			
Duration of diabetes	0.0325	−0.0012	0.0424	1.0000		
Age	0.0597	0.0830	−0.0085	−0.0182	1.0000	
HbA1c	−0.1258	0.0076	0.2027	0.0868	−0.2586[a]	1.0000
Macrovasculopathy (n = 14)						
Lp(a)	1.0000					
ApoB/ApoA1 ratio	0.5687[a]	1.0000				
LDL-cholesterol	0.3386[a]	0.4899[a]	1.0000			
Duration of diabetes	−0.0387	0.4237[a]	−0.0338	1.0000		
Age	−0.2106	−0.3564[a]	−0.2782	−0.1556	1.0000	
HbA1c	−0.1322	0.1963	0.4750[a]	−0.0691	−0.4011[a]	1.0000

Notes: macrovasculopathy: IHD, CVD and/or ASO. B/A: ApoB/ApoA1 ratio. LDL-C: LDL-cholesterol. Duration: duration of diabetes. [a]$p < 0.05$.

References

1. Rhoads GG, Dahlen G, Berg K, Morton NE, Dannenberg AL. Lp(a) lipoprotein as a risk factor for myocardial infarction. JAMA 1986;256:2540–2544.
2. Armstrrong VW, Cremer P, Eberle E, Manke A, Schulze F, Wieland H. The association between serum Lp(a) concentrations and angiographically assessed coronary atherosclerosis: Dependence on serum LDL levels. Atherosclerosis 1986;62:249–257.
3. Velho G, Erlich D, Turpin E, Cohen D, Froguel P. Lipoprotein(a) in diabetic patients and normoglycemic relatives in familial NIDDM. Diabet Care 1993;16:742–747.
4. Haffner SM, Moss SE, Klein BE, Klein R. Lack of association between lipoprotein(a) in patients with diabetes mellitus. Diabet Care 1993;16:819–823.
5. Nobuhiro M, Koutaro Y, Jun T, Hidekuni I. Lipoprotein(a) is a risk factor for diabetic retinopathy in the elderly. JAGS 1994;42:965–967.
6. Michael MR, Monika L, Werner OR, Peter S. Lipoprotein(a) in diabetes mellitus. Clin Chim Acta 1993;214:45–54.
7. Gruden G, Veglio M, Cavallo-Perin P, Olivetti C, Mormile A. Lipoprotein(a) in non-insulin-dependent diabetic patients with normo- and microalbuminemia. Horm Metab Res 1994;26: 489–490.

Lipids and lipoproteins

Recent Advances on the Pathogenesis and Management of Diabetes Mellitus.
S.H. Shinn, M. Shichiri and K.-W. Kim, editors.

Acute effect of insulin on triglycerides clearance in nondiabetic normolipidemic female subjects

T. Goto[1], T. Onuma[2], T. Hinata[1] and T. Suda[1]
[1]*Third Department of Internal Medicine, Hirosaki University School of Medicine, Aomori-Ken; and* [2]*Department of Internal Medicine, Metabolism and Endocrinology, School of Medicine, Juntendo University, Japan*

Abstract. A decreased clearance rate of triglycerides (TG) plays a role in the development of dyslipidemia, manifested in the syndrome of insulin resistance. However, lipoprotein lipase (LPL) in skeletal muscle decreases in response to metabolic stimuli. In order to clarify the acute effect of insulin on TG clearance, 32 nondiabetic normolipidemic female subjects received euglycemic hyperinsulinemic clamps and an intravenous fat tolerance test (IVFTT) on separate days. IVFTT were again carried out on 16 of the subjects to compare the TG clearance rate in basal state (K_2b) to that during clamp procedure (K_2c). K_2b correlated negatively with BMI, WHR and TG levels and positively with the HDL-C and glucose infusion rate during the clamp test. K_2c was significantly smaller than K_2b and related to the suppression of plasma FFA levels during the clamp test. In addition, the decline in TG levels during the clamp procedure could be attributable to the reduction in TG production.

Keywords: dyslipidemia, FFA, hyperinsulinemia, LPL.

Background

Several studies have been performed to define the causal sequence between insulin resistance and dyslipidemia (i.e., increased VLDL-TG, decreased HDL-C and a preponderance of small dense LDL particles) [1,2]. Lipoprotein lipase (LPL), the key enzyme in hydrolysis of TG-rich lipoprotein particles, is insulin sensitive. A decreased clearance rate of TG, as a consequence of the impaired insulin action on LPL activation, has been regarded as playing a pivotal role in the development of dyslipidemia, manifested in the syndrome of insulin resistance [3]. Some previous studies, however, have shown that the LPL activity in skeletal muscle (the main route of TG clearance) remains unchanged or decreases in absorptive state [4,5], while insulin stimulates adipose tissue LPL activity in a dose-dependent manner [6]. Therefore, the effects of insulin on LPL activity in skeletal muscle and in adipose tissue are tissue-specific [7]. As humans spend the majority of their existence in the absorptive state, the change in TG clearance in response to metabolic stimuli is as important as that in the fasted state. In addition, the percentage of TG-derived fatty acids that are stored in adipose tissue, as opposed to being oxidised in muscle in response to insulin, has not been fully understood [4]. This study was performed to clarify the changes in overall TG clearance in response to insulin infusion. Furthermore, fuel requirements of fatty acids in the skeletal muscle is hypothesized to be responsible for the decrease in skeletal muscle LPL activity in response to metabolic stimuli [3,5]. Using the euglycemic and hyperinsulinemic clamp technique, we also investigated the possibility that the decline in FFA levels could be responsible for the delay in TG clearance in response to glucose/insulin infusion.

Subjects and Methods

Thirty-two female subjects were included in this study. Their clinical characteristics are presented in Table 1. None of the subjects were judged as diabetics by a 75-g oral glucose tolerance test (OGTT) and WHO criteria. Those with hypertriglyceridemia (i.e., fasting plasma TG levels were 200 mg/dl or more) were excluded. None of the females used medication that affects carbohydrate or lipid metabolism. Anthropometric measurements were performed to evaluate overall (BMI) and upper body (WHR) adiposity. Insulin secretion was measured from the plasma IRI levels during an OGTT. The glucoregulatory action of insulin was measured using 2 h of euglycemic hyperinsulinemic clamp technique performed under primed and continuous infusions of insulin at a rate of 40 mU/m^2/min, according to the method of DeFronzo. The glucose infusion rate (GIR) to maintain plasma glucose around fasting level during the last 30 min of the clamp test was used as an index of glucoregulatory insulin action. The decay of FFA during clamp was also determined.

On the above-mentioned separate day, after sampling for determination of serum lipids profile, intravenous fat tolerance tests (IVFTT) were carried out to evaluate the exogenous TG elimination. Samples for the IVFTT were collected before and every 5 min after the bolus injection of 10% intralipid (Otsuka pharmaceuticals, Japan), 0.1 g/kg body weight, according to the method of Rossner [8]. In each subject, the exponential decay of the incremental TG level in the basal state (K_2b) and during clamp procedure (K_2c) were determined as an index

Table 1. Clinical characteristics of the study subjects.

	Mean	Standard deviation
Age (years)	56.4	9.2
BMI (kg/m^2)	24.8	4.1
WHR	0.82	0.08
TC (mg/dl)	214	27
TG (mg/dl)	109	43
HDLC (mg/dl)	57.8	19.4
FFA (μEq/l)	935	303
FPG (mg/dl)	99	11
FIRI (μU/ml)	8.1	1.8
AUC_{PG} (mg/dl/h)	323	45
AUC_{IRI} (μ U/ml/h)	85	48
GIR (mg/kg/min)	7.0	2.5
FFA_{120} (μ Eq/l)	87	33

of TG clearance. All subjects received IVFTT in the basal state, and this test was also carried out in 16 of the subjects 2 h after the start of the clamp test, while the insulin infusion and glucose clamping were continued.

Results

As reported previously [9], there was a significant positive correlation between K_2b and GIR (Fig. 1). K_2b was also negatively correlated with TG ($r = -0.46$, $p < 0.01$), BMI ($r = -0.45$, $p < 0.01$), WHR ($r = -0.34$, $p < 0.10$) and positively correlated with HDL-C ($r = 0.46$, $p < 0.01$). The changes in TG clearance during clamp procedure from that in basal state is shown in Fig. 2. The mean K_2-value significantly declined to 1.59%/min during the clamp procedure from 1.96%/min in basal state. The relationship between FFA levels 2 h after the initiation of euglycemic clamp and K_2c is shown in Fig. 3. There was a significantly negative correlation between them, so the degree of plasma FFA suppression could be related to the decline in TG clearance during the euglycemic clamp procedure.

Conclusion

The constant rate of TG clearance in IVFTT (K_2) (validated to reflect the catabolism of endogenous TG-rich lipoproteins [8]) was delayed in response to acute glucose/insulin infusion, possibly as a consequence of decreased LPL activity in muscular tissue (the major route of TG clearance). Thus, although there was a close relationship between insulin resistance (glucoregulatory insulin action) and TG clearance in the basal state, acute insulin infusion may decrease

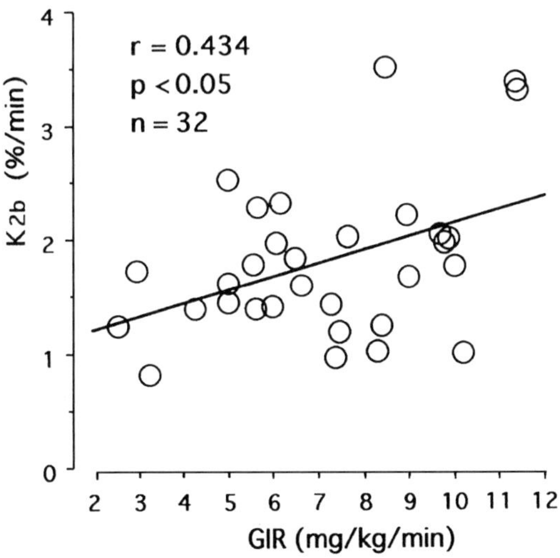

Fig. 1. Correlation between TG clearance rate in basal state (K_{2b}) and glucose infusion rate (GIR) during euglycemic clamp procedure.

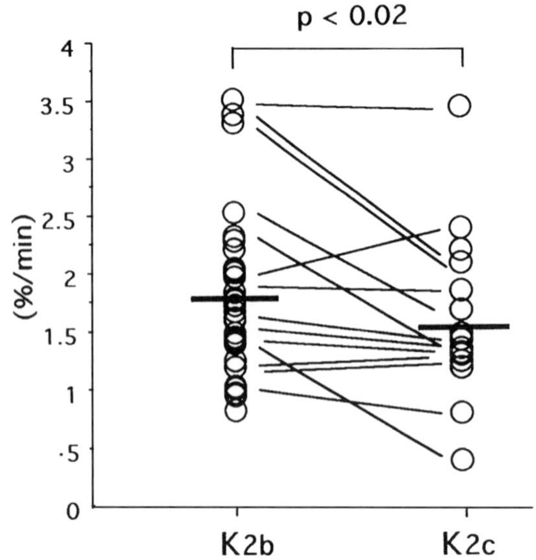

Fig. 2. Changes in TG clearance rate in basal state (K_{2b}) and during clamp procedure (K_{2c}).

the TG clearance. It has been hypothesized that the decline in LPL activity in muscular tissue in response to insulin is attributable to the degree of increased glucose uptake and suppressed plasma FFA levels, influencing tissue availability of fuel source. In cases with severe resistance to glucoregulatory insulin action or full suppression of FFA level, LPL may be activated sufficiently to meet sub-

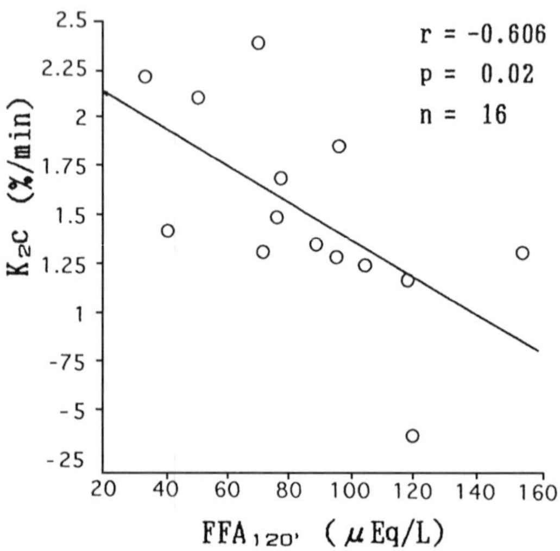

Fig. 3. Correlation between TG clearance rate during eugglycemic clamp procedure (K_{2c}) and plasma FFA levels 2 h after the start of the clamp (FFA_{120}).

strate demand in peripheral tissues. In the present study, the degree of decline in plasma FFA related to K_2c, although GIR did not, as Farese reported [4,9]. In addition, plasma TG levels declined 2 h after the initiation of the clamp procedure (105 ± 27 vs. 80 ± 30 mg/dl, M ± SD, $p<0.01$), which cannot be explained by the increased TG clearance, as the TG clearance was rather delayed. The suppression of hepatic TG secretion through the mechanism of insulin-induced suppression of FFA levels, or through the recently demonstrated direct inhibitory effect of insulin [10] would be involved.

References

1. Reaven GM. Diabetes 1988;37:1595.
2. Reaven GM et al. J Clin Invest 1993;92:141.
3. Taskinen M.-R. et al. Diabetes 1986;35:1268.
4. Farese KY et al. Metabolism 1991;40:214.
5. Kiens B et al. J Clin Invest 1989;84:1124.
6. Yki-Jarvinen N. Diabetologica 1984;27:364.
7. Pollare T et al. Arterioscl Thromb 1993;11:1192.
8. Rossner S. Acta Med Scan 1974;564(Suppl):1.
9. Ferraro RT et al. J Clin Invest 1993;92:441.
10. Lewis GF et al. J Clin Invest 1995;95:158.

Recent Advances on the Pathogenesis and Management of Diabetes Mellitus.
S.H. Shinn, M. Shichiri and K.-W. Kim, editors.

Plasma plant sterol levels and morphological markers of intestine in diabetes

H. Hidaka, H. Kojima, H. Matsumura, Y. Omoto, Y. Fujita, A. Kashiwagi and R. Kikkawa
Third Department of Medicine, Shiga University of Medical Science, Otsu, Shiga, Japan

Abstract. *Background.* In diabetic states, hypercholesterolemia may be caused by the increased intake of cholesterol. The dietary contribution can be estimated by the plasma levels of the exogenous sterols. Therefore, the plasma plant sterol levels were determined in diabetic rats and its relation to gut markers were analyzed.

Methods. Plasma levels of plant sterols and postheparin diamine oxidase (DAO) activity, a biological marker of intestine, were determined in streptozotocin-induced diabetic rats fed with 1% plant sterol-containing chow. The markers were also measured in IDDM subjects.

Results. In the diabetic rats, plasma plant sterol levels were increased compared with those in control rats. DAO activity and morphological markers of the gut were correlated with the plasma levels of plant sterols. These abnormalities were also observed in poorly controlled IDDM subjects, and insulin treatment improved these phenomena.

Conclusion. The abnormalities of intestine including increased sterol absorption efficacy play a role in the hypercholesterolemia in the insulin-deficient diabetic states.

Keywords: IDDM, phytosterol, sitosterol, sterol absorption.

Introduction

Mechanisms of hyperlipidemia in diabetes are reported to be due to the overproduction and/or decreased catabolism of lipoproteins [1]. The dietary contents of cholesterol are one of the important factors to regulate the plasma cholesterol levels. In diabetic animals, the plasma cholesterol concentrations were extremely elevated when the animals were fed with high cholesterol-containing chow [2].

Plant sterols such as sitosterol and campesterol are structurally very similar to the animal sterol, cholesterol. Though the mechanisms of absorption of the sterols from the gut have not been elucidated, the plasma concentrations of plant sterols, which are not synthesized in the mammalians, are reported to be used as a marker of cholesterol-absorption efficacy [3]. Therefore, we determined plasma levels of the sterols and gut markers to evaluate the exogenous sterol contribution to serum lipid levels in diabetic animals as well as in subjects with IDDM.

Address for correspondence: H. Hidaka, Third Department of Medicine, Shiga University of Medical Science, Seta-Tsukinowa-cho, Otsu, Shiga 520-21, Japan.

Methods

Sprague-Dawley rats were made diabetic by the intravenous injection of streptozotocin, and fed with experimental chow containing 1% plant sterols, 1% coconut oil, and 1% cholic acid for 2 weeks. After an overnight fasting, blood was drawn at 0, 10, 30 and 60 min after the injection of 5,000 U/kg BW heparin. Diamine oxidase (DAO) activities in the postheparin plasma were determined by the method of Okuyama and Kobayashi [4]. The morphological measurements were performed after removing the intestine. Wet weights and surface area of the small intestine were measured. Plasma plant sterol concentrations were determined by the high-performance liquid chromatography method [5] using desmosterol as an internal standard.

In subjects with insulin-dependent diabetes mellitus (IDDM), age- and sex-matched diabetic patients with good glycemic control or poor control were studied after obtaining informed consent. During overnight fasting, heparin was injected and DAO activity as well as plant sterol levels were determined in the plasma. For the control, the DAO activity and fasting plasma concentrations of the sterols were measured in age- and sex-matched healthy volunteers.

Results

Diabetic rats showed increased fasting plasma glucose levels and lower body weight (Table 1). Morphological markers of the gut were increased in diabetic rats compared with those in control rats, and the insulin treatment improved the abnormalities.

Plasma levels of plant sterols, sitosterol and campesterol in the diabetic rats were significantly elevated (Table 1). A half-life of the increased plasma plant sterols was similar in both diabetic and control rats. Good correlation between the gut surface area and the plasma plant sterol concentrations was observed (Fig. 1). Postheparin plasma diamine oxidase activity was increased in diabetic

Table 1. Plasma levels of plant sterols and gut morphological markers in diabetic rats.

	Control	Diabetes plus insulin	Diabetes
n	10	10	13
BW (g)	293 ± 20	282 ± 20	229 ± 20^{b}
FPG (mg/dl)	161 ± 19	361 ± 40^{b}	377 ± 40^{b}
Plasma sterol (mg/dl)			
Cholesterol	55 ± 20	91 ± 37	75 ± 32
Sitosterol	4.0 ± 1.2	6.3 ± 0.2^{b}	8.5 ± 3.7^{b}
Campesterol	7.9 ± 2.0	14.3 ± 4.3^{b}	17.8 ± 8.2^{a}
Morphological markers			
Wet weight (g)	8.1 ± 0.6	9.8 ± 0.7^{b}	11.3 ± 1.6^{b}
Area (cm^2)	120 ± 19	127 ± 10	157 ± 15^{b}

Results are expressed as mean ± SD. $^{a}p < 0.05$; $^{b}p < 0.01$ vs. control.

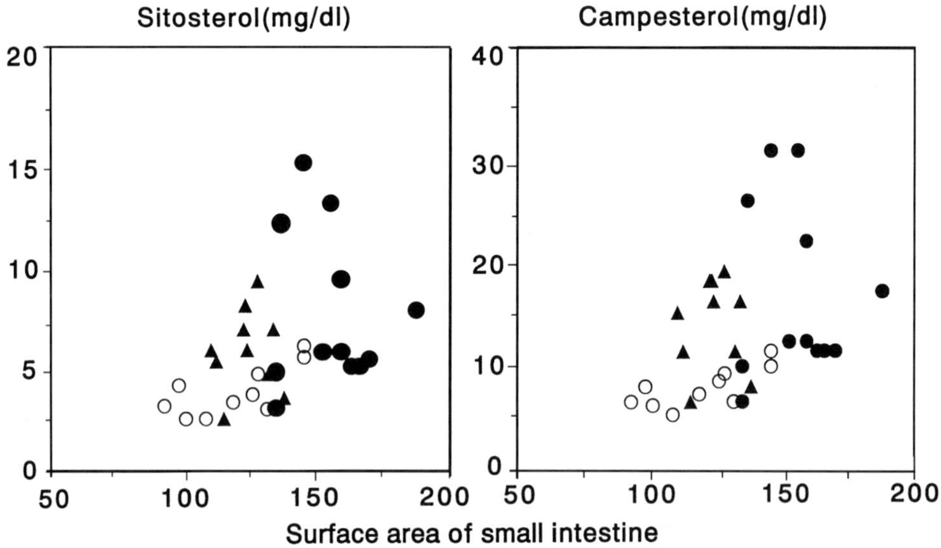

Fig. 1. Relation between gut surface area and plasma plant sterol levels in rats. Open circle: control rats; open triangle: diabetic rats with insulin treatment; closed circle: diabetic rats. Correlation coefficients are 0.80 in sitosterol and 0.82 in campesterol ($p < 0.001$).

rats, and decreased by the insulin treatment. The good correlation between the activity and the morphological markers of the gut as well as the plasma concentrations of the sterols were reported [6].

Plasma plant sterol levels were significantly elevated in IDDM subjects with poor glycemic control, and the levels in IDDM subjects with good control by the intensive insulin treatment were similar to the levels in control subjects. Plasma diamine oxidase activity after the injection of 30 U/kg BW of heparin was also significantly elevated in IDDM subjects with poor glycemic control, and the activity in IDDM subjects with good control was similar to those in control subjects.

Discussion

This study showed the increased plasma levels of plant sterols and the abnormalities of gut morphological and biological markers in diabetic rats. Insulin treatment improved these abnormalities. It has been known that plasma cholesterol concentrations are sensitive to dietary intakes of cholesterol [2]. This study confirmed the previous studies, and further indicated the importance of exogenous sterols in hypercholesterolemia in diabetes. Since the plasma plant sterol levels are markers of cholesterol absorption efficacy [3], the evidence also suggests that the absorption efficacy is increased in insulin-deficient diabetic states.

Plasma diamine oxidase is known to be localized in many tissues and to catalyze the degradation of histamine and putrescine. However, the postheparin plasma enzyme activity is exclusively released from the intestinal epithelial cells, and the postheparin enzyme activity is used to be a marker of the gut mucosal mass [7]. Since the increased activity in diabetic rats is proportional to the increase of morphological measurements of the gut, the postheparin plasma DAO activity might be used as a marker of the small intestine. The results that plasma plant sterol levels and diamine oxidase activity was increased in IDDM subjects with poor glycemic control, suggest that abnormalities of the gut function and morphology are also present in human insulin-deficient diabetes.

It is possible that the gut hypertrophy or hyperplasia as well as the increased plasma plant sterol levels might be due to overeating, since diabetic rats show hyperphagia. However, the morphological markers as well as the sterol concentrations were significantly higher than those in control rats, even when the diabetic rats were pair-fed with control rats (data not shown). Since the regulation of gut mucosal cell growth as well as the sterol absorption is not well-understood, the relation between the cell growth and the function, absorption of the nutrients, should be further studied in gut epithelial cells. The good relationships between the markers suggest that the hypertrophy of the gut itself might be related to the abnormality of the sterol absorption efficacy in diabetes.

In conclusion, these results indicate that hypercholesterolemia in diabetes is accounted for at least in part by the functional and morphological abnormalities of intestine, and suggest that the abnormalities may be related to hypertrophy or hyperplasia of the gut.

References

1. Howard BV. Pathogenesis of diabetic dyslipidemia. Diabet Rev 1995;3:423–432.
2. Matsubara K et al. Cholesterol lowering effects of melinamide in cholesterol-fed diabetic rats. Atherosclerosis 1988;72:199–204.
3. Miettinen TA et al. Serum plant sterols and cholesterol precursors reflect cholesterol absorption and synthesis in volunteers of a randomly selected male population. Am J Epidemiol 1990; 131:20–31.
4. Okuyama T, Kobayashi Y. Determination of diamine oxidase activity by liquid scintillation counting. Arch Biochem Biophys 1961;95:242–250.
5. Kasama T et al. Quantitative analysis of sterols in serum by high-performance liquid chromatography. J Chromatogr 1987;400:241–246.
6. Kojima H et al. Increased plasma post-heparin diamine oxidase activity and plant sterol levels in streptozotocin diabetic rat. Biochem Biophys Res Commun 1992;186:398–404.
7. Rokkas T et al. Postheparin plasma diamine oxidase in health and intestinal disease. Gastroenterology 1990;98:1493–1501.

Insulin synthesis and secretion

Recent Advances on the Pathogenesis and Management of Diabetes Mellitus.
S.H. Shinn, M. Shichiri and K.-W. Kim, editors.

Analysis of β-cell function in spontaneous diabetic NSY mice

Y. Hamada, H. Ikegami, E. Yamato, Y. Kawaguchi, T. Fujisawa, M. Hotta, H. Ueda, M. Shintani, K. Nojima, Y. Kawabata, N. Babaya, J. Fu, G.Q. Shen and T. Ogihara
Department of Geriatric Medicine, Osaka University Medical School, Suita, Osaka, Japan

Abstract. The NSY (Nagoya-Shibata-Yasuda) mouse is an inbred strain of mice with a spontaneous development of diabetes mellitus with moderate obesity. The cumulative incidence of diabetes is 98% in males at 48 weeks of age. Both insulin resistance and impaired insulin secretion in response to glucose contribute to the development of diabetes in NSY mice. To clarify the mechanisms of impaired insulin secretion in NSY mice, we examined the insulin response to glucose (5.6—27.8 mM) and arginine (20 mM) in isolated islets from male NSY and control C3H/He mice at 36 weeks of age by the batch incubation method. Insulin response to 5.6-mM glucose was not significantly different between NSY and C3H/He mice, however, insulin response to high concentration of glucose ($\geqslant$11.1 mM) and arginine was significantly lower in NSY mice than in C3H/He mice. These results suggest that insulin response to glucose and nonglucose stimuli in vitro is impaired in the NSY mouse, and that NSY mice are useful for studies on the pathogenesis of NIDDM with impaired insulin secretion.

Keywords: animal model, insulin secretion, NIDDM.

Background

Non-insulin-dependent diabetes mellitus (NIDDM) is a heterogeneous disorder, caused by an interaction of genetic and environmental factors [1]. This heterogeneity makes it difficult to clarify the pathogenesis of the disease. Animal models are helpful and necessary to understand the etiology of heterogeneous diseases such as diabetes. Several animal models for NIDDM have been described. Although recent studies have revealed impaired insulin secretion in GK rats [2], most of the animal models for NIDDM are characterized by obesity and insulin resistance [3].

The NSY (Nagoya-Shibata-Yasuda) mouse is an inbred animal model of NIDDM with moderate obesity that was established by selective breeding for glucose intolerance from an outbred Jcl:ICR mouse colony [4]. NSY mice spontaneously develop diabetes mellitus in an age-dependent manner. The cumulative incidence of diabetes is 98% in males and 31% in females at 48 weeks of age [5]. Previous in vivo studies suggested that both impaired insulin secretion in response to glucose and insulin resistance contribute to the development of diabetes in NSY mice [5]. These characteristics in NSY mice are similar to those in humans.

Address for correspondence: Dr Hiroshi Ikegami, Department of Geriatric Medicine, Osaka University Medical School, 2-2 Yamadaoka, Suita, Osaka 565, Japan.

In this study, we investigated the insulin secretion of NSY mice in vitro to clarify the mechanisms of impaired insulin secretion in NSY mice.

Methods

Male NSY and control C3H mice at 36 weeks of age were used in this study. Pancreatic islets were isolated by collagenase digestion [6]. Insulin secretory capacity in isolated islets was measured by the batch incubation method. DNA content was determined according to the fluorometric assay [7], and insulin secretion was normalized by DNA content of the islets.

To determine the site responsible for impaired insulin secretion in NSY mice, different concentrations (5.5, 8.3, 11.1, 16.7 and 27.8 mM) of glucose and 20 mM of L-arginine were used as secretagogues.

Results

Insulin response to glucose increased in a dose-dependent manner in both NSY and C3H mice. Insulin response to 5.5 mM of glucose was not significantly different between NSY and C3H mice. Insulin response to 8.3 mM concentration of glucose was slightly, but not significantly lower in NSY mice than in C3H mice (118 vs. 145% of basal). Insulin responses to 11.1 mM (129 vs. 199% of basal: $p<0.01$), 16.7 mM (138 vs. 212% of basal: $p<0.05$) and 27.8 mM (140 vs. 206% of basal: $p<0.05$) of glucose were significantly lower in NSY mice than in C3H mice. Insulin response to arginine was also impaired in NSY mice as compared with control C3H mice (146 vs. 214% of basal: $p<0.05$) to almost the same degree as that to 16.7 mM of glucose.

Conclusions

Previous reports indicated that most Japanese patients with NIDDM are characterized by impaired insulin secretion rather than insulin resistance, and this appears to precede the onset of diabetes [8,9]. NSY mice showed impaired insulin secretion in contrast to most other animal models for NIDDM with insulin resistance, making this strain a good animal model for NIDDM with impaired insulin secretion, as in the case of Japanese patients.

Most amino acids have been shown to stimulate insulin release. Arginine and leucine are the two most potent stimulators [10]. In this study insulin response to arginine was impaired in NSY mice as compared with control C3H mice. Considering the mechanism of insulin secretion in response to glucose, the site responsible for impaired insulin secretion in NSY mice is thought to be located at a voltage-dependent calcium channel or thereafter in the cascade of insulin secretion. Although insulin response to nonglucose stimuli, such as arginine, has been reported to be relatively preserved in human NIDDM patients as compared with that to glucose stimuli [11,12], insulin response to arginine in

NIDDM patients was reported to be lower than that in normal subjects. In this study insulin response to arginine was impaired in NSY mice as compared with control C3H mice to almost the same degree as that to 16.7 mM of glucose. We used NSY mice at 36 weeks of age, when most mice had established diabetes. Since glucose intolerance in NSY mice appears at around 12 weeks of age, glucose toxicity might worsen β-cell function at this age, which may have affected insulin response to arginine. Studies on in vivo insulin secretion of NSY mice at a young age will be necessary to clarify the primary defect in insulin secretion in NSY mice.

Acknowledgements

This work was supported in part by a Grant for Diabetes Research from the Ministry of Health and Welfare, Grants-in-Aid for Scientific Research from the Ministry of Education, Science, Sports and Culture, a Grant from the SANDOZ Foundation for Gerontological Research, and a Grant from the Kato Memorial Trust for Nambyo Research.

References

1. Hamman RF. Genetic and environmental determinants of non-insulin-dependent diabetes mellitus (NIDDM). Diabetes Metab Rev 1992;8:287–338.
2. Portha B, Serradas P et al. β-cell insensitivity to glucose in the GK rat, a spontaneous nonobese model of type II diabetes. Diabetes 1991;40:486–491.
3. Shafrir E. Animal models of non-insulin-dependent diabetes. Diabetes Metab Rev 1992;8: 179–208.
4. Shibata M, Yasuda B. New experimental congenital diabetic mice (N.S.Y. mice). Tohoku J Exp Med 1980;130:139–142.
5. Ueda H, Ikegami H, Yamato E et al. The NSY mouse: a new animal model of spontaneous NIDDM with moderate obesity. Diabetologia 1995;38:503–508.
6. Yamato E, Noma Y, Tahara Y et al. Suppression of synthesis and release of glucagon by glucagon-like peptide-1 (7-36 amide) without affect on mRNA level in isolated rat islets. Biochem Biophys Res Commun 1990;167:431–437.
7. Hinegardner RT. An improved fluorometric assay for DNA. Anal Biochem 1971;39:197–201.
8. Kadowaki T, Miyake Y, Hagura R et al. Risk factors for worsening to diabetes in subjects with impaired glucose tolerance. Diabetologia 1984;26:44–49.
9. Yoneda H, Ikegami H, Yamamoto Y et al. Analysis of early-phase insulin responses in nonobese subjects with mild glucose intolerance. Diabetes Care 1992;15:1517–1521.
10. Floyd JG, Fajans SS, Conn JW et al. Stimulation of insulin secretion by amino acids. J Clin Invest 1966;45:1487–1502.
11. Word WK, Bolgiano DC, McKnight B et al. Diminished B cell secretory capacity in patients with non-insulin-dependent diabetes mellitus. J Clin Invest 1984;74:1318–1338.
12. Pfeifer MA, Halter JB, Porte D. Insulin secretion in diabetes mellitus. Am J Med 1981;70: 579–588.

Recent Advances on the Pathogenesis and Management of Diabetes Mellitus.
S.H. Shinn, M. Shichiri and K.-W. Kim, editors.

Leptin directly stimulates basal insulin release from pancreatic β cells

Shigeru Okuya[1], Katsuya Tanabe[1], Yukio Tanizawa[1], Yasushi Inoue[1], Akira Matsutani[1], Ken Yaga[1], Yoshitomo Oka[1] and Toshio Kaneko[2]

[1]Third Department of Internal Medicine, Yamaguchi University School of Medicine, Ube, Yamaguchi; and [2]Yamaguchi Rosai Hospital, Onoda, Yamaguchi, Japan

Abstract. We examined a possible mechanism underlying the link between obesity and hyperinsulinemia, focusing on leptin. The leptin receptor isoforms (Ob-Ra and Ob-Rb) are present in the pancreatic β cell line MIN6 and in rat pancreatic islets, based on RT-PCR. Incubation with 1 nM recombinant mouse leptin, the concentration observed in obese subjects, stimulated basal (at 5 mM glucose) insulin secretion by approximately 40% in both MIN6 and rat islets. Stimulatory effects of leptin were dose-dependent and not observed without glucose, while 1 nM leptin did not induce an increase in insulin mRNA in the presence of 5 mM glucose. Thus, leptin acts directly on pancreatic β cells, and this stimulatory mechanism may account in part for the fasting hyperinsulinemia observed in obese subjects.

Keywords: hyperinsulinemia, leptin receptor (Ob-R), MIN6, obesity, rat pancreatic islets.

Introduction

Leptin plays an important role in regulating body weight through the satiety center of the brain [1,2]. There are strong positive correlations among the percentage of body fat, plasma leptin levels and fasting plasma insulin levels [3,4]. The action of leptin is mediated by a specific receptor (Ob-R), expressed in several isoforms by alternative splicing [5,6]. Although the leptin receptor is expressed abundantly in the brain, it is also expressed in a wide variety of other tissues [5—8]. However, to date few studies have been reported regarding direct effects of leptin on peripheral tissues [9,10].

In order to test the hypothesis that leptin is a direct signal from adipose tissue to pancreatic β cells of increased insulin demand associated with obesity, we examined the expressions of leptin receptor isoforms in pancreatic β cells and assessed the direct effects on insulin secretion.

Address for correspondence: Shigeru Okuya MD, Third Department of Internal Medicine, Yamaguchi University School of Medicine, 1144 Kogushi, Ube, Yamaguchi 755, Japan. Tel.: +81-836-22-2251. Fax: +81-836-22-2342. E-mail: okuya@po.cc.yamaguchi-u.ac.jp

Materials and Methods

RT-PCR

Pancreatic islets were isolated from 10-week-old male Wistar rats by the collagenase digestion method. Total cellular RNA was extracted from MIN6 cells, RINm5F cells, mouse epididymal adipose tissue, mouse brain and isolated rat pancreatic islets. The primers for Ob-Ra and Ob-Rb isoforms (Ob-R forward, Ob-Ra reverse and Ob-Rb reverse) were synthesized as reported [6]. The primer sequences are as follows: Ob-R forward: 5′-aca ctg tta att tca cac cag ag-3′; Ob-Ra reverse: 5′-agt cat tca aac cat agt tta gg-3′; Ob-Rb reverse: 5′-tgg ata aac cct tgc tct tca-3′. First strand cDNA was synthesized by incubation at 45°C for 60 min, 5 μg of total RNA (MIN6, RINm5F, adipose tissue and brain) or total RNA from 50 islets, in a 40-μl reaction mixture containing oligo dT, reverse transcriptase, etc. Then 1 μl of the incubation mixture was used for PCR for 40 cycles. The products were subjected to 2% agarose gel electrophoresis.

Insulin secretion

Insulin secretion from MIN6 cells and isolated rat islets were determined using a static incubation method in 5% CO_2 and 95% air for MIN6 cells or in 5% CO_2 and 95% O_2 for rat islets at 37°C as previously described [11]. After 2-h incubation at 37°C in HEPES-balanced Krebs-Ringer bicarbonate buffer supplemented with 0.5% BSA (HEPES-KRB) and various concentrations of glucose and mouse recombinant leptin (R&D Systems, Minneapolis, MN), the media were collected and assayed for immunoreactive insulin by RIA using rat insulin as a standard.

Insulin mRNA expression

After 2-h incubation at 37°C in HEPES-KRB and 5 mM glucose with or without 1 nM leptin, total RNA was isolated from 100 islets treated with each condition and hybridized to ^{32}P-labeled rat insulin I cDNA probe. RNA loading was normalized with a riboplobe for β actin.

Statistics

All the data are expressed as means ± standard error. The results were analyzed by Student's unpaired t test.

Results

We first analyzed which isoform (Ob-Ra, Ob-Rb or both) is expressed. Complimentary DNAs for the Ob-Ra and Ob-Rb were specifically amplified by RT-PCR using a common forward primer (Ob-R forward) and isoform-specific reverse primers (Ob-Ra reverse and Ob-Rb reverse). Specific products corresponding to Ob-Ra and Ob-Rb isoforms were detected in the β cell lines and isolated rat pancreatic islets (Fig. 1). The PCR products were directly sequenced.

These results prompted us to examine the effects of leptin on insulin secretion from pancreatic β cells. In the presence of 5 mM glucose, incubation of MIN6 cells with 1 nM leptin for 2 h increased insulin secretion by 36 ± 13% (mean ± s.e.m., n = 7, $p<0.05$; Fig. 2A). At 25 mM, glucose increased insulin secretion by approximately 3.5-fold as compared with 5 mM glucose, but the addition of 1 nM leptin did not further stimulate insulin secretion (data not shown). Essentially the same effects were observed in rat pancreatic islets; the basal insulin secretion (at 5 mM glucose) was increased by 37 ± 9% (mean ± s.e.m., n = 10, $p<0.01$) but no stimulatory effects were observed at 25 mM glucose (Fig. 2B). The stimulatory effects of leptin on basal insulin secretion (at 5 mM glucose) were dose-dependent and the maximal effects were achieved at around 1 nM in MIN6 cells (data not shown). However, no stimulation of insulin secretion by leptin was observed in rat pancreatic islets in the absence of glucose (Fig. 3). Finally we measured the insulin mRNA after 2-h incubation with 1 nM leptin in rat islets, but no significant change was observed (Fig. 4).

Discussion

According to the results of RT-PCR, Ob-R mRNA was demonstrated in both the pancreatic β cell line and isolated rat islets, strongly suggesting the presence of Ob-R in pancreatic β cells. It is noteworthy that not only the short (Ob-Ra) but also the long isoform (Ob-Rb), which presumably functions in mediating signals, is present in pancreatic β cells (Fig. 1).

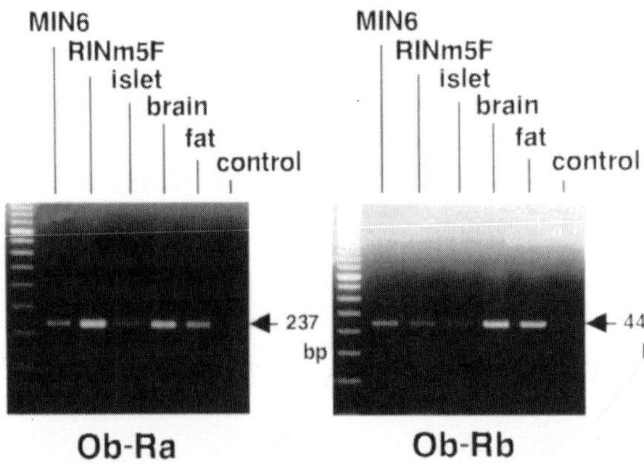

Fig. 1. The presence of leptin receptor a and b isoforms in pancreatic β cell lines and rat pancreatic islets. Reverse transcriptase-polymerase chain reaction (RT-PCR) revealed the presence of leptin receptor (Ob-R) isoforms a and b in the murine pancreatic β cell line MIN6, the rat pancreatic β cell line RINm5F and rat islets. The results in brain and adipose tissues are also shown as positive controls. The results obtained without RNA (control) are shown in the last lane.

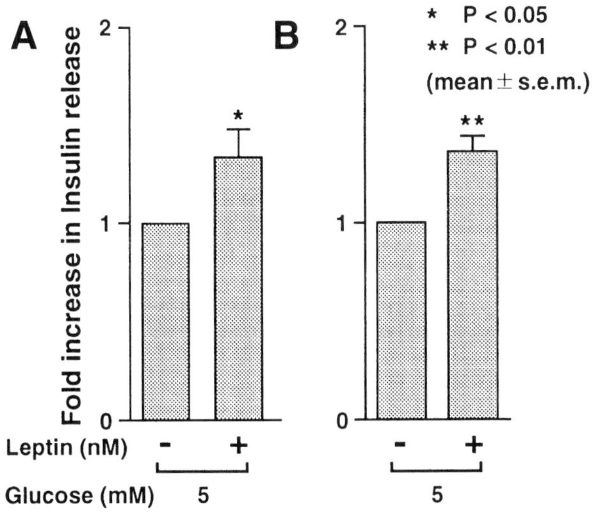

Fig. 2. Effects of leptin on insulin secretion. **A:** Incubation of MIN6 cells with 1 nM leptin for 2 h significantly increased basal insulin secretion (at 5 mM glucose). The results expressed as fold-increases above the value obtained at 5 mM glucose without leptin, are the mean ± s.e.m. of seven experiments, with each measurement performed in triplicate. **B:** Incubation of isolated rat islets with 1 nM leptin exerted effects essentially the same as those seen in MIN6 cells. The results (fold-increase) are expressed as the mean ± s.e.m. of 10 experiments, with each measurement performed in triplicate.

In the presence of 5 mM glucose, a 2-h incubation with 1 nM leptin stimulated insulin secretion by about 40% in both MIN6 and rat islets (Fig. 2), and the stimulatory effects were dose-dependent. This dose-dependency of leptin effects

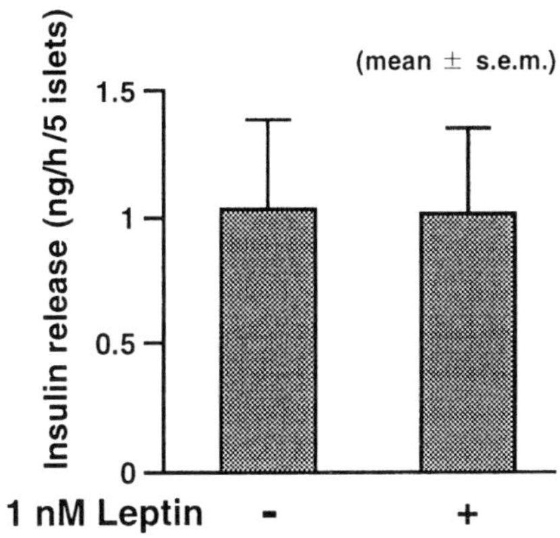

Fig. 3. Glucose-dependency of leptin effects on insulin release. In the absence of glucose, no stimulation of insulin secretion by 1 nM leptin was observed in isolated rat islets. The insulin secretion from five islets are expressed as the mean ± s.e.m. of nine experiments, with each measurement performed in triplicate.

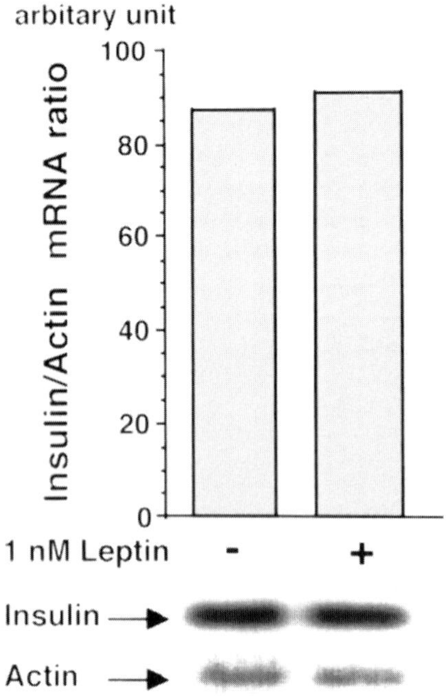

Fig. 4. Effects of leptin on insulin mRNA expression in isolated rat islets. No significant difference in insulin mRNA was observed after incubation with 1 nM leptin for 2 h. RNA loading was normalized with a riboprobe for actin. Northern blot was shown below.

on basal insulin secretion is consistent with the effects being mediated through binding to the Ob-R, considering the Kd value of 0.6—1.0 nM reported for the Ob-R [5,12]. In contrast to the effect on basal insulin secretion, 1 nM leptin had no significant effects on the maximal glucose-stimulated insulin secretion at 25 mM glucose. The leptin effects were not observed without glucose (Fig. 3), while 1 nM leptin did not induce an increase in insulin mRNA even in the presence of 5 mM glucose (Fig. 4). Further studies are needed to elucidate the molecular mechanisms underlying the stimulation of basal insulin secretion by leptin.

It is of great interest from the clinical point of view that leptin, at concentrations observed in obese subjects [3], directly stimulates basal insulin secretion. Hyperinsulinemia associated with obesity, in which the plasma leptin level is elevated, is usually attributed to the compensatory response to insulin resistance. Our results indicate that there is also a direct relationship between leptin and fasting (basal) insulin levels.

In conclusion, leptin is an adipose tissue sensor, which not only regulates appetite and thus food intake but also mediates pancreatic β cell adaptation to increased insulin demand. The direct effects exerted by leptin may account in part for the “missing link” between obesity and fasting hyperinsulinemia.

References

1. Zhang Y, Proenca R, Maffei M, Barone M, Leopold L, Friedman JM. Positional cloning of the mouse obese gene and its human homologue. Nature 1994;372:425–432.
2. Pelleymounter MA, Cullen MJ, Baker MB, Hecht R, Winters D, Boone T, Collins F. Effects of the obese gene product on body weight regulation in ob/ob mice. Science 1995;269:540–543.
3. Considine RV, Sinha MK, Heiman ML, Kriauciunas A, Stephens TW, Nyce MR, Ohannesian JP, Marco CC, McKee LJ, Bauer TL, Caro JF. Serum immunoreactive-leptin concentrations in normal-weight and obese humans. N Engl J Med 1996;334:292–295.
4. Dagogo-Jack S, Fanelli C, Paramore D, Brothers J, Landt M. Plasma leptin and insulin relationships in obese and nonobese humans. Diabetes 1996;45:695–698.
5. Tartaglia LA, Dembski M, Weng X, Deng N, Culpepper J, Devos R, Richards GJ, Campfield LA, Clark FT, Deeds J, Muir C, Sanker S, Moriarty A, Moore KJ, Smutko JS, Mays GG, Woolf EA, Monroe CA, Tepper RI. Identification and expression cloning of a leptin receptor, OB-R. Cell 1995;83:1263–1271.
6. Lee G-H, Proenca R, Montez JM, Carroll KM, Darvishzadeh JG, Lee JI, Friedman JM. Abnormal splicing of the leptin receptor in diabetic mice. Nature 1996;379:632–635.
7. Ghilardi N, Ziegler S, Wiestner A, Stoffel R, Heim MH, Skoda RC. Defective STAT signaling by the leptin receptor in diabetic mice. Proc Natl Acad Sci USA 1996;93:6231–6235.
8. Kieffer TJ, Heller RS, Habener JF. Leptin receptors expressed on pancreatic β-cells. Biochem Biophys Res Commun 1996;224:522–527.
9. Cohen B, Novick D, Rubinstein M. Modulation of insulin activities by leptin. Science 1996; 274:1185–1188.
10. Muller G, Ertl J, Gerl M, Preibisch G. Leptin impairs metabolic actions of insulin in isolated rat adipocytes. J Biol Chem 1997;272:10585–10593.
11. Ishihara H, Asano T, Tsukuda K, Katagiri H, Inukai K, Anai M, Kikuchi M, Yazaki Y, Miyazaki J-I, Oka Y. Pancreatic beta cell line MIN6 exhibits characteristics of glucose metabolism and glucose-stimulated insulin secretion similar to those of normal islets. Diabetologia 1993; 36:1139–1145.
12. Baumann H, Morella KK, White DW, Dembski M, Bailon PS, Kim H, Lai C-F, Tartaglia LA. The full-length leptin receptor has signaling capabilities of interleukin 6-type cytokine receptors. Proc Natl Acad Sci USA 1996;93:8374–8378.

Recent Advances on the Pathogenesis and Management of Diabetes Mellitus.
S.H. Shinn, M. Shichiri and K.-W. Kim, editors.

Comparison of GLUT2 expression and glucokinase activity between D11 and its parent RINm5F cells

Tai-Wook Yoon
Biotechnology Research Center, Boryung Research Institute, Kunpo, Korea

Abstract. D11 cells showing in vitro 5.6 mM and ex vivo 16.7 mM glucose-responses appear to have a much more active GLUT2 (liver type glucose transporter) than RINm5F cells showing ex vivo 5.6 mM glucose-response and no in vitro glucose-response. The former also showed a higher V_{max} of glucokinase and lower V_{max} of hexokinase.

Consequently, a higher level of glucose uptake and glucose metabolism occurs in D11 cells than in RINm5F cells, proving that the former can elicit an improved glucose-response compared to the latter. The magnitude of glucose-response is therefore closely coupled to the combination of active GLUT2 expression and glucokinase activity.

Keywords: D11 cells, glucokinase, GLUT2, RINm5F cells.

Introduction

Glucose-response in the pancreatic β cells depends on both glucose uptake [1] and glucose metabolism [2]. Glucose uptake occurs via facilitated diffusion which is mediated by GLUT2 [3–5]. GLUT2 is glycoprotein [6]. Active GLUT2 is 54 kDa [7]. Glucose binds to the extracellular loop in its outward-facing conformation. Then the GLUT2 undergoes conformational change and glucose is released within the cells [8,9]. Once entered, the glucose is metabolized to produce ATP via glycolysis and the TCA cycle. The ATP increases insulin secretion via a cascade of insulin-secretion processes [10–12]. The first irreversible rate-limiting step in the glucose metabolism is the conversion of glucose to glucose-6-phosphate by glucokinase (GK) [13], which subsequently passes the glycolysis and oxidative cycle, enhancing insulin secretion [14]. Consequently, GLUT2 and glucokinase are key factors in determining the level of glucose-induced insulin secretion.

Immortal pancreatic β cells, including RINm5F cells have much less glucose-response when compared with normal pancreatic β cells. The reason was found to have originated from little or no expression of GLUT2 [3] and negligible GK activity [15]. Instead, the cells showed increased GLUT1 expression [3] and hexokinase (HK) activity. These changes led the immortal β cells to have much less glucose-response compared to normal pancreatic β cells. In this regard, immortal rat pancreatic β cell lines (called RINm5F cells) and D11 cells will be com-

Address for correspondence: Tai-Wook Yoon, Life Science Lab, Seoul Branch of Korea Basic Science Institute, 126-16, Anam-dong 5-ga, Seoul 136-701, South Korea.

pared (Table 1).

D11 cells were generated from the modification of RINm5F cells [16]. Both lines showed quite different glucose-responses [17,18]. RINm5F cells have no in vitro glucose-response and ex vivo 16.7 mM glucose-response, but showed an ex vivo 5.6 mM glucose-response [17]. D11 cells responded to ex vivo 16.7 mM glucose and in vitro 5.6 mM glucose but not to ex vivo 5.6 mM glucose [17]. The different glucose-responses could stem from the differences in the glucose-uptake and glucose metabolism: GLUT2 and GK.

For this reason, GLUT2 expression and GK activity are investigated in both cell lines to identify the relationship between GLUT2 expression, GK activity and glucose-response.

Materials and Methods

Visualization of glucose transport protein

Cell harvesting

The cells were scraped from tissue culture flasks (using a scraper) into phosphate-buffered saline (PBS) containing EDTA. The cell suspension was centrifuged at 80 g for 10 min at 30°C.

Extraction of cellular component

Cells were washed in PBS and collected by centrifugation at 2,000 g for 2 min. The pellet containing approximately 40×10^6 cells was resuspended in an equal volume of a solution containing 0.2% (w/v) sodium deoxycholate (SDC) and 10 mM Tris-HCl (pH 8.0) at 20°C. The cell membranes were dissolved rapidly and nuclei were pelleted by centrifugation in an Eppendorf microcentrifuge at 9,000 g for 2 min. The cytoplasmic fraction and the dissolved membrane were removed and stored at −20°C until use. A protease inhibitor, such as phenylmethylsulfonylfluoride (PMSF) at 2 mM or aprotinin at 0.1 μM, was included in the extraction procedure.

Electrophoresis

Sodium dodesyl sulfate-polyacrylamide gel electrophoresis (SDS-PAGE) was performed in two 10% (w/v/) slab gels using the LKB vertical gel apparatus. This was run at a 30 mA constant current until pyronine Y dye had passed through

Table 1. Activities (μU/mg protein) of GK and HK in RINm5F and D11 cells.

Cell line	GK	HK
RINm5F cells	$V_{max} = 0.38$ $K_m = 0.047$	$V_{max} = 13.812$ $K_m = 0.001$
D11 cells	$V_{max} = 1.30$ $K_m = 7.82$	$V_{max} = 0.78$ $K_m = 0.02$

the stacking gel, and then at 60 mM until the dye front had travelled about 8.5 cm into the seperating gel.

Immunoblotting
SDS-PAGE gels were subjected to electrophoretic transfer in a 25 mM Tris buffer containing 192 mM glycine (pH 8.3, containing 20% methanol) using the trans-blot system (Bio-Rad Laboratories). Proteins and glycoproteins were transferred to nitrocellulose membrane filters (Schleicher and Schuell, Gmbh, Dassel, Germany). They were then blocked for 30 min with 1% (v/v) bovine serum albumin (BSA) in PBS, containing in addition 0.4 M NaCl and 0.2% Tween 20 (PNT). After rinsing in DW, the membrane was incubated for 30 min in the primary antibody solution, containing 25 μg/ml of rabbit antiglucose transporter in Tris-buffered saline which had 0.2% (v/v) Tween 20 (TBST). The bound antibody was located by probing with a radioiodinated second antibody followed by autoradiography. After being washed three to four times in TBST buffer, the membrane was incubated for 30 min in a radioiodinated second antibody, ^{125}I-labelled goat antirabbit serum. Excess radioactivity was washed off with 0.1% (w/v) SDS in PBS. Following staining with amido black (Sebia), the membrane was dried and exposed to X-ray film (Genetic Research Instrument Ltd., UK) at −70°C for 48 h.

Measurement of GK and HK activities

Glucose phosphorylation was measured by the method of Liang et al. [19]. The 2×10^6 cells were placed in 300 μl of buffer (1 mM EDTA, 20 mM K_2HPO_4, 5 mM dithiothreitol (DTT), 110 mM KCl) and homogenized on ice by 25 strokes of a machine-driven Teflon pestle in a Kontes glass homogenizer. Following a 10 min centrifugation at 12,000 g to remove mitochondrial-bound HK, glucose phosphorylation was assayed in the supernatant as NADH generation from NAD^+ by exogenous glucose-6-phosphate dehydrogenase. Homogenate was added to 100 μl reaction buffer (50 mM HEPES/HCl, pH 7.6, 100 mM KCl, 15 mM β-mercaptoethanol, 7.4 mM $MgCl_2$, 0.5 mM NAD^+, 0.7 U/ml glucose-6-phosphate dehydrogenase, 5 mM ATP, and 0.05% BSA). After 90 min at 30°C, the reaction was stopped with 2 ml of 500 mM $NaHCO_3$ (pH 9.4). Samples were completed in triplicate at multiple glucose concentrations (0.03, 0.06, 0.125, 0.5 and 1.0 for HK activity; 6.25, 12.5, 25, 50 and 100 M for GK activity). Reagent blanks without homogenate were included for all glucose concentrations. Tissue blanks consisted of homogenate and reaction buffer without glucose. A standard curve was constructed using a reaction buffer containing 100 mM glucose, no homogenate, and glucose-6-phosphate standards (0.3−500 nM; fluorometer excitation 350 nM/emission 460 nM). GK and HK V_{max} were calculated by linear regression from an Eadi-Scatchard plot (V/[S] vs. V) and corrected 10 times using the method of Spears et al. [20], after extrapolating the data assuming a Q10 of 2 [21].

Results

The autoradiograph (Fig. 1) shows that D11 cells have more normal 54 kDa liver type GLUT2 than RINm5F cells. However, RINm5F cells have much more 51 kDa erythrocyte type GLUT1 than D11 cells.

The cells were cultured in culture medium including 11 mM glucose. Glucose phospholylation was measured by a fluorometer in cytoplasmic fraction.

RINm5F cells showed lower activity of GK than D11 cells and there is statistical difference in HK between RINm5F and D11 cells (Table 1).

Discussion

GLUT is known as glycoprotein [6]. Much less and overglycosylated GLUT is the inactive form. Active GLUT2 and GLUT1 have 54 kDa and 51 kDa, respectively. Inactive GLUT have less or none of this function. RINm5F cells showed much less expression of active GLUT2 and high expression of active GLUT1 [3]. Based

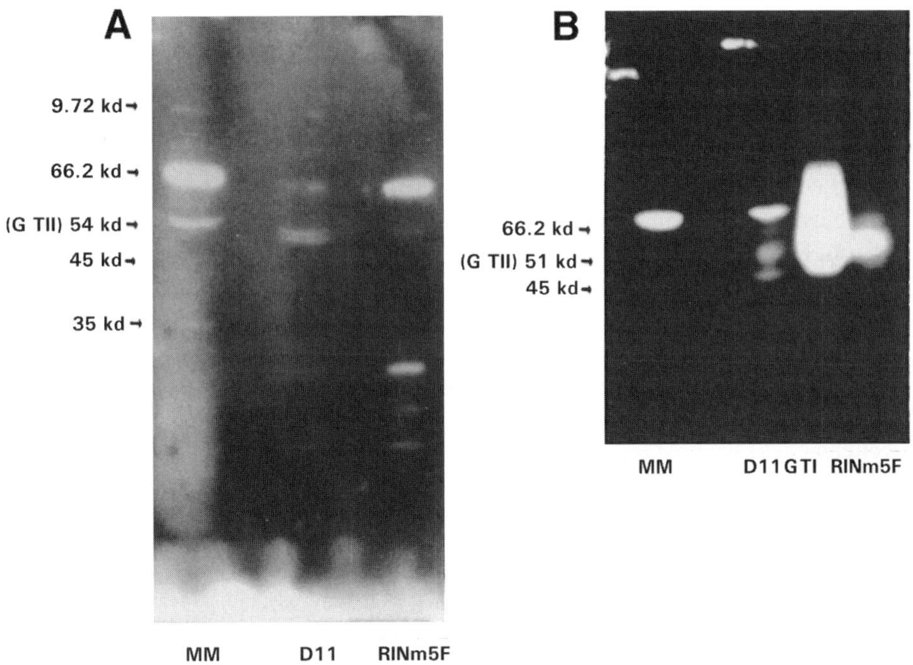

Fig. 1. Immunoblot analysis for GLUT. The membranes were prepared from RINm5F and D11 cells. The membrane proteins (100 μg) were separated by SDS-PAGE and transferred to a nitrocellulose membrane. The detection of the GLUT was carried out with a polyclonal antipeptide antibody directed against whole peptides of (**A**) liver-type GLUT and (**B**) erythrocyte-type GLUT. The position of protein markers (66.2, 54 and 35 kDa) are shown in the first track (M) of each photograph. GT2 (54 kDa) is the liver type GLUT. GT1 (51 kDa) is the erythrocyte type GLUT. GT1 in the third track of the photograph (**B**) is pure erythrocyte type GLUT.

upon the results, glucose-uptake is taking place in the presence of low glucose due to active GLUT1 and does not occur in the presence of high glucose owing to no active GLUT2 in RINm5F cells. However, glucose uptake could occur in the presence of high glucose, but not at low glucose in D11 cells. A higher level of glucose-uptake occur in D11 cells than in RINm5F cells, however, glucose response results from the combination of active GLUT2 expression and GK activity. Only with GLUT2 expression can D11 cells be expected to show a higher glucose-response than RINm5F cells. However, GK activity must be additionally taken into consideration to compare glucose-response more precisely.

RINm5F cells have low GK activity and high HK activity, whereas D11 cells have high GK and HK activities. This means that glucose is metabolized more actively in D11 cells than in RINm5F cells. Thus, more glucose-uptake and glucose metabolism occurs in D11 cells than in RINm5F cells. This evidence indicates that D11 cells elicit more glucose-response than RINm5F cells. In fact, D11 cells have ex vivo 16.7 mM glucose response and in vitro 5.6 mM glucose response, though RINm5F cells have an ex vivo 5.6 mM glucose response and no in vitro glucose response, despite the fact that both are immortal rat pancreatic β cell lines. One question is why D11 cells do not have ex vivo 5.6 mM glucose response even when they have active GLUT1 and HK.

It could be suggested that the expression of certain types of GLUT and activation of certain enzymes are selected by a certain machinery which is influenced by many factors such as islet cell interaction and in vivo conditions. This remains to be studied in the future.

In conclusion, immortal pancreatic β cell lines have a different GK activity and expression of active GLUT2. The degree of GK activity and active GLUT2 expression is related closely to that of glucose response. In this respect, D11 cells have a much better glucose response than RINm5F. Furthermore, the function of pancreatic β cells and insulin-producing cells is influenced by many factors such as islet cell interaction and in vivo conditions.

References

1. Miyazaki J et al. Establishment of a pancreatic β cell line that retains glucose-inducible insulin secretion: special reference to expression of glucose transporter isoforms. Endocrinol 1990; 127:127–132.
2. Sandler S, Andersson A. The partial protective effect of the hydroxyl radical scavenger dimethyl urea on streptosotocin-induced diabetes in the mouse in vivo and in vitro. Diabetologica 1982; 23:374–378.
3. Thorens B, Sarker JK et al. Cloning and functional expression in bacteria of a novel glucose transporter present in liver intestine, kidney and pancreatic islet cells. Cell 1988;55:281–290.
4. Thorens B, Charron MJ, Lodish HF et al. Molecular physiology of glucose transporter. Diabet Care 1990;13:209–218.
5. Oka Y Asano T, Shibasaki Y et al. C-terminal truncated glucose transporter is locked into an inward-facing form without transport activity. Nature 1990;345:550–553.
6. Johnson JH, Newgard CB, Milburn JL et al. The high K_m glucose transporter of islet of Langerhans is functionally similar to the low-affinity transporter of liver and has an identical primary

sequence. J Biol Chem 1990;265:6548–6551.

7. Davies A, Ciardelli TL, Lienhard GE et al. Site specific as probes of the topology and function of the human erythrocyte glucose transporter. Biochem J 1990;266:799–808.
8. Barnett JEG, Holman G, Chalkley RA et al. Evidence for two asymmetric conformational states in the human erytorocyte sugar-transport system. Biochem J 1975;145:417–429.
9. Kasanicki MA, Pilch PF. Regulation of glucose transporter function. Diabet Care 1990;13: 219–226.
10. Malaisse WJ. Insulin release. Metabolism 1979;28:373–386.
11. Chance B, William GR. Respiratory enzymes in oxidative phosphorylation. J Biol Chem 1985; 21:383–393.
12. Jacobus WE. Respiratory control and the integration of heart high energy phosphate metabolism by mitochondrial creatine kinase. Ann Rev Physiol 1985;4:707–727.
13. Megassen MD, Matschinsky FM. Pancreatic islet glucose metabolism and regulation of insulin secretion. Diabetes Metab Rev 1986;2:163–214.
14. Shimizu T, Parker JC, Najafi H et al. Control of glucose metabolism in pancreatic β cells by glucokinase, hexokinase and phosphofructokinase. Diabetes 1988;37(11):1524–1530.
15. Shimizu T, Knowles BB, Matschinsky FM. Control of glucose phosphorylation and glucose usage in clonal insulinoma cells. Diabetes 1988;37b:563–568.
16. McClenaghan NH, Barnett CR, Ah-Sing E et al. Characterization of a novel glucose-responsive insulin-secreting cell line BRIN-BDII, produced by electrofusion. Diabetes 1996;45(5): 1132–1140.
17. Yoon TW, Kwon O et al. In vitro and in vivo functions of rat pancreatic β cell lines. Kor J Biochem 1995;27(2):63–71.
18. McClenaghan NH, Gray AM, Barnett CR, Flatt PR. Hexose recognition by insulin-secreting BRIN-BDII cells. Biochem Biophys Res Commun 1996;223(3):724–728.
19. Liang Y, Najafi H, Matschinsky FM. Glucose regulates glucokinase activity in cultured islets from rat pancreas. J Biol Chem 1990;265:16863–16866.
20. Spears G, Sneyd GT, Loten EG. A method for deriving kinetic constants for two enzymes acting on the same substrate. Biochem J 1971;125:1149–1151.
21. Saleas J, Slas M, Vinuela E, Siks A. Glucokinase of rabbit liver. J Biol Chem 1965;240: 1014–1018.

Treatment

Recent Advances on the Pathogenesis and Management of Diabetes Mellitus.
S.H. Shinn, M. Shichiri and K.-W. Kim, editors.

Effects of troglitazone on hyperglycemia-induced insulin resistance

M.-K. Lee[1], K.A. Kim[1], Y.S. Kim[1], K.J. Ahn[1], J.H. Chung[1], Y.K. Min[1], M.-S. Lee[1], K.W. Kim[1], P.G. Miles[2] and J.M. Olefsky[2]
[1]*Department of Medicine, Samsung Medical Center, Sungkyoonkwan University, Seoul, Korea; and* [2]*University of California, San Diego, California, USA*

Abstract. *Background.* Troglitazone is a new class of oral hypoglycemic agent and improves insulin action both in NIDDM and nondiabetic insulin resistance such as fructose-fed rats. We performed this study to examine the effects of troglitazone on the nongenetic hyperglycemia-induced insulin resistance.

Methods. Male Sprague-Dawley rats were divided into three groups and were fed normal rat chow and chow admixed with troglitazone (0.2%) for 2 weeks. Rats were infused with normal saline or 30% dextrose for 6.5 h with somatostatin (8 μg/kg/min) followed by euglycemic hyperinsulinemic clamp study.

Results. 1) There was no significant difference in body weight among the three groups of rats. 2) Basal plasma glucose levels were significantly elevated in the hyperglycemia group and the troglitazone-treated group ($p < 0.05$). 3) There was no significant difference in basal insulin level among the three groups of rats. 4) Maximal GDR was significantly decreased in the hyperglycemia group compared to the control- and troglitazone-treated group, respectively. 5) Steady-state plasma free fatty acid concentration was significantly elevated in the hyperglycemia and troglitazone groups, however, there was no significant difference between the hyperglycemia group and the troglitazone-treated group.

Conclusion. These results suggest that a 6.5-h glucose infusion leads to significant insulin resistance and prior troglitazone treatment restores insulin action to near normal.

Keywords: clamp study, free fatty acid, glucose, hyperglycemia, insulin resistance, troglitazone.

Introduction

Thiazolidinediones are a new class of antidiabetic agents which potentiate insulin action in vitro and improve insulin resistance in both insulin-resistant animal models as well as NIDDM subjects. Troglitazone, one of the thiazolidinediones, has been shown to decrease plasma glucose levels in both insulin-resistant animal models and NIDDM subjects [1–4]. It also decreased serum insulin and triglyceride levels, insulin resistance and blood pressure. Insulin resistance is induced by the hyperglycemia in persons and animals without genetic susceptibility. Hyperglycemia is a cause of the diabetic complications, suppresses insulin secretion from pancreatic β cells and also inhibits insulin action, which lead to the

Address for correspondence: Moon-Kyu Lee MD, Division of Endocrinology, Department of Medicine, Samsung Medical Center, 50 Ilwon-dong, Kangnam-ku, Seoul 135-710, Korea.

emergence of concept of glucose toxicity [5]. We undertook this study to investigate whether troglitazone has any effects on insulin resistance induced by the nongenetic hyperglycemia.

Materials and Methods

Male Sprague-Dawley rats (body weight (BW) 1,250—1,150 g) were purchased and divided into two groups after a 1-week period of acclimation. Group 1 (n = 16) rats were fed normal animal chow in powder form and group 2 rats (n = 8) were fed normal chow admixed with troglitazone (0.2% w/w) for 2 weeks ad libitum, respectively. After 1-week feeding cathers were inserted into the right jugular veins and left carotid arteries under general anesthesia. One week postcannulation, after overnight fasting, rats were put into metabolic cages and cathers were extended using a tether device. Group 1 rats were divided into two groups. One group (n = 8) of rats were infused with 0.9% saline solution and somatostatin (8 μg/kg/min) for 6.5 h and were used as controls. The other group (n = 8) of rats were infused with 30% dextrose solution and somatostatin to induce hyperglycemia. Group 2 rats (n = 8) were infused with 30% dextrose and somatostatin for 6.5 h. Plasma glucose levels were checked every 2 h and the glucose infusion rate adjusted to maintain plasma glucose higher than 300 mg/dl. After 6.5 h euglycemic hyperinsulin clamp studies were started. Insulin infusion rate was 40 mU/kg/min, somatostatin was also infused during glucose clamp studies and studies were done for 90 min. During glucose clamp studies, plasma glucose levels were measured every 5—10 min and infusion rate of 20% dextrose solution was adjusted to maintain euglycemia. Steady-state glucose disposal rate (GDR) was calculated as the glucose infusion rate during the last 30 min of the glucose clamp study. After completion of the 90-min glucose clamp study plasma insulin and free fatty acid levels were measured. Plasma glucose was measured by glucose oxidase method using Beckman glucose analyzer II and insulin was measured by double antibody radioimmunoassay using rat insulin as standard. Plasma free fatty acid level was measured by enzymatic method. All values are expressed as mean ± standard deviation, and statistical analysis was done by two-way ANOVA for unbalanced data (SAS) with statistical significance for those with $p<0.05$.

Results

After 2-week feeding of respective diets there was no significant difference in body weights among the three groups of rats (control, 261 ± 9 g; hyperglycemia group, 270 ± 8 g; and hyper + troglitazone group, 267 ± 10 g, respectively). Basal plasma glucose levels of hyperglycemia group (20.0 ± 0.7 nM) and hyper + troglitazone group (18.5 ± 0.8 mM) were significantly ($p<0.05$) higher than the control group (8.4 ± 0.2 mM). There was no significant difference in basal plasma insulin levels among the three groups of rats (control 144 ± 36 pM, hyperglycemia 194 ± 57 pM, and hyper + troglitazone 201 ± 65 pM). GDR was significantly lower in the hyperglycemia group (139 ± 11 μmol/kg/min) compared to control (240 ± 6 μmol/kg/min) and hyper + troglitazone group (206 ± 6 μmol/kg/min, Fig. 1). Steady-state plasma free fatty acid levels were significantly higher in hyperglycemia group (0.59 ± 0.05 mM) and hyper + troglitazone group (0.62 ± 0.05 mM) compared to the control group (0.40 ± 0.03 mM).

Discussion

It is well known that hyperglycemia can induce insulin resistance as well as inhibit insulin secretion from pancreatic β cells. Hyperglycemia can cause post-receptor insulin signalling defects, can inhibit the glucose transporter translocation, and inhibit glycogen synthase activity, which can produce insulin resistance. Troglitazone[(+)-5-{4-(6-hydroxy-2,5,7,8-tetramethylchroman-2-methyloxy)benzyl}-2,4-thiazolidinedione] is a new class of antidiabetic agent which improves insulin action in the peripheral tissues without affecting insulin secretion from pancreatic β cells. It has been shown to increase glycogen synthase activity, to decrease gluconeogenesis, and recently peroxisome proliferator-activated receptor (PPARr) has been shown to be a thiazolidine-dione receptor [6]. In this study, somatostatin was infused with either 30% dextrose or 0.9% saline solution to block endogenous insulin secretion from pancreatic islets so as to see the effects of hyperglycemia, per se, without causing hyperinsulinemia. A period of 6.5 h of hyperglycemia induced severe insulin resistance, though this was prevented by troglitazone pretreatment. We assumed hepatic glucose production

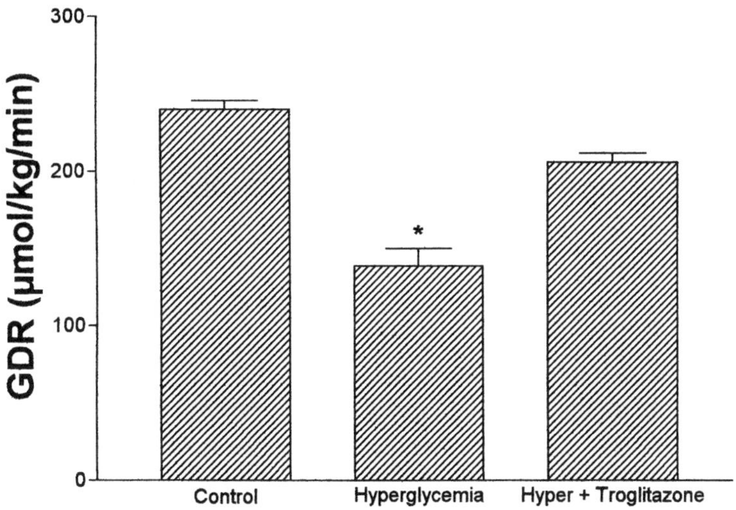

Fig. 1. Glucose disposal rate (GDR) during euglycemic hyperinsulinemic clamp study in control, hyperglycemic and hyperglycemia + troglitazone treated groups of rats, respectively. Values are expressed as mean ± SD. *$p<0.05$ vs. control and hyperglycemia + troglitazone group, respectively.

rate (HGP) was totally suppressed under maximal insulin stimulation, however, if one examined the effects on the liver and peripheral tissues separately, then ^{3}H-glucose should also be infused to measure hepatic glucose production rate. As elevated plasma free fatty acid level was not changed with troglitazone treatment, we can tell that changes in free fatty acids do not play any significant role in the improvement of hyperglycemia-induced insulin resistance by troglitazone treatment. In conclusion, 6.5 h of glucose infusion induced a state of insulin resistance in normal rats and troglitazone pretreatment restored insulin action to near normal.

Acknowledgements

We wish to express our deepest thanks to Dr Hiroyoshi Horikoshi of Sankyo Co., for providing us with the valuable troglitazone.

References

1. Ciaraldi TP, Gilmore A, Olefsky JM, Goldberg M, Heindenreich KA. In vitro studies on the action of CS-045, a new antidiabetic agent. Metabolism 1990;39:1056–1062.
2. Suter SL, Nolan JJ, Wallace P, Gumbiner B, Olefsky JM. Metabolic effects of new oral hypoglycemic agent CS-045 in NIDDM subjects. Diabetes Care 1992;15:193–203.
3. Fujiwara T, Yoshioka S, Yoshioka T, Ushiyama I, Horikoshi H. Characterization of new oral antidiabetic agent CS-045. Studies in KK and ob/ob mice and zycker fatty rats. Diabetes 1988; 37:1549–1558.
4. Lee M-K, Miles PG, Khoursheed M, Gao K-M, Moossa AR, Olefsky JM. Metabolic effects of troglitazone on fructose-induced insulin resistance in the rat. Diabetes 1994;43:1435–1439.
5. Rossetti L, Giaccari A, DeFronzo RA. Glucose toxicity. Diabetes Care 1990;13:610–630.
6. Lehmann JM, Moore LB, Smith-Oliver TA, Wilkinson WO, Wilson TM, Kliewer SA. An antidiabetic thiazolidinedione is a high affinity ligand for peroxisomal proliferator-activated receptor gamma. J Biol Chem 1995;270:12953–12956.

Recent Advances on the Pathogenesis and Management of Diabetes Mellitus.
S.H. Shinn, M. Shichiri and K.-W. Kim, editors.

Effects of long-term administration of an α-glucosidase inhibitor on the development of macroangiopathy in OLETF rats

Y. Mori[1], Y. Murakawa[1], S. Hata[3], S. Katoh[3], J. Yokoyama[3], N. Tajima[3], Y. Ikeda[4] and M. Nishimura[2]

[1]Department of Internal Medicine, National East-Utsunomiya Hospital, Utsunomiya; [2]Institute for Experimental Animals, Hamamatsu University School of Medicine, Hamamatsu; [3]Department of Internal Medicine (III), the Jikei University School of Medicine; and [4]Department of Preventive Medicine, Center for General Health Care, the Jikei University School of Medicine, Tokyo, Japan

Abstract. We investigated the effects of a long-term administration of acarbose, an α-glucosidase inhibitor on visceral fat accumulation and arteriosclerotic lesions in OLETF rats modeling obesity of the visceral fat accumulation type. Male OLETF rats, at the age of 4 weeks, were fed with an experimental diet containing acarbose at a concentration of 0 (control), 20, or 40 mg/100 g diet (n = 20 for each), and the course of the animals was observed. Weight gains in the acarbose-treated groups were significantly lower than that of the control group. Oral glucose (2 g/kg) tolerance tests performed at the age of 30 weeks revealed significantly milder impairment of glucose tolerance and significantly lower blood IRI in the acarbose-treated animals than in the controls. As for body-fat distribution, significant decreases were observed in the visceral fat. In the histopathological examination of the coronary arteries removed at the age of 81 weeks, the control animals showed a slight degree of intimal irregularity and intimal hypertrophy. On the other hand, the acarbose-treated animals never showed such intimal changes. In conclusion, long-term administration of this α-glucosidase inhibitor prevented the development of arteriosclerotic lesions in large vessels in OLETF rats modeling obesity of the visceral fat accumulation type.

Keywords: α-glucosidase inhibitor, accumulation, macroangiopathy, OLETF rats, visceral fat.

Introduction

We previously reported that long-term ingestion of dietary fiber delays the progress of glucose tolerance impairment in OLETF rats [1,2], an animal model of obesity of visceral fat accumulation type [3]. We suggested that dietary fiber inhibited postprandial hyperglycemia and accompanying insulin hypersecretion, and consequently reduced body fat increases and lowered insulin resistance in peripheral tissues. Acarbose, a recently developed oral hypoglycemic agent, moderately inhibits α-amylase, and markedly inhibits α-glucosidase which is localized in the epithelial cell membrane of the small intestine and is involved in the digestion and absorption of sugars. Thus, acarbose blunts postprandial increases in blood glucose by delaying the digestion and absorption of sugars taken in meals. In addition, this blunted postprandial hyperglycemia suppresses postprandial

Address for correspondence: Y. Mori, National East-Utsunomiya Hospital, 2160 Shimookamoto, Kawachi-Machi, Kawachi-Gun, Tochigi 329-11, Japan.

hypersecretion of endogenous insulin and lowers insulin resistance. Acarbose is further expected to correct abnormal metabolism of sugars and lipids, and this may contribute to the prevention and treatment of hypertension and arteriosclerosis. In the present study, we investigated effects of long-term administration of this α-glucosidase inhibitor on visceral fat accumulation and arteriosclerotic lesions in OLETF rats modeling obesity of the visceral fat accumulation type.

Methods

Male OLETF rats at 4 weeks of age were fed with an experimental diet containing acarbose at a concentration of 0 (control), 20, or 40 mg/100 g diet (n = 20 for each), and the subsequent courses of the animals were observed. At 30 weeks of age, 10 animals from each dose group were tested for oral glucose tolerance (2 g glucose per kg body weight) (OGTT), and the distribution of body fat and histopathological features of the pancreas were examined. In order to determine the body fat distribution, we removed and weighed fat tissues from the mesenterium, unilateral retroperitoneum, peripheral region of the unilateral epididymis, and subcutaneous area of the unilateral abdomen. The subcutaneous fat to be removed was defined according to the method described by Krotkiewski and Bjorntorp [4]. The amount of visceral fat was defined as the total weight of the fat tissues from the above-mentioned sites except the subcutaneous area of the abdomen. The remaining rats were further fed until they reached the age of 81 weeks, and then were used for histopathological examination of the coronary arteries.

Statistical analysis

Values were expressed as the mean ± SD, and analyzed using the unpaired t test. Differences at the level of $p < 0.05$ were considered to be statistically significant.

Results

The food consumption in the acarbose-treated groups showed a tendency of dose-dependent increases as compared with the control (Fig. 1). Weight gains of the acarbose-treated animals were significantly inhibited from the control in a dose-dependent manner (Fig. 2).

Oral glucose tolerance tests performed at the age of 30 weeks revealed significant lowering of glucose tolerance and significant decreases in the plasma insulin level in all acarbose-treated groups. The fasting blood glucose/insulin ratio, as an insulin resistance parameter, increased significantly in the acarbose-treated groups, suggesting an insulin resistance lowering effect of acarbose (Table 1). Fasting plasma total cholesterol as well as plasma triglyceride in all acarbose-treated groups, were significantly lower than the corresponding control values (Table 1). In the age-matched comparison of body fat distribution, visceral fat

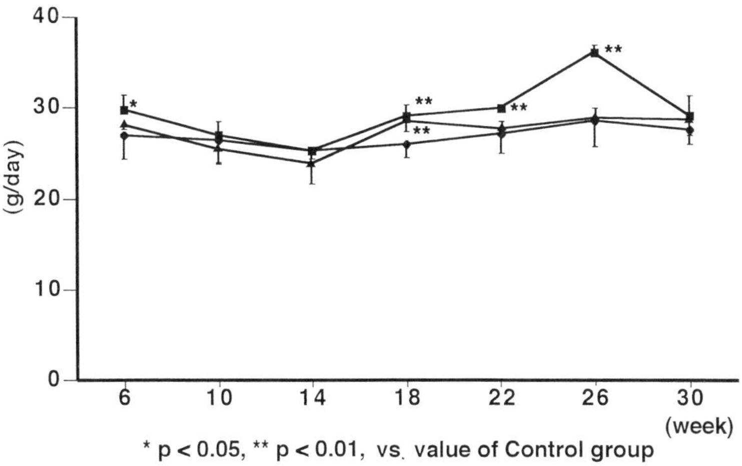

Fig. 1. Time courses of food consumption. ■—■: acarbose-treated group (40 ppm). ▲—▲: acarbose-treated group (20 ppm). ●—●: control group.

weights were significantly lower in the acarbose-treated groups than in the control, however, subcutaneous fat weights were significantly higher in the acarbose-treated groups. As a result, the visceral/subcutaneous fat ratio which reflects relative changes in the visceral fat amount was significantly lower in the acarbose-treated groups (Table 1). The age-matched histopathologic examination of the pancreas revealed enlargement and fibrosis of Langerhans islets in the control

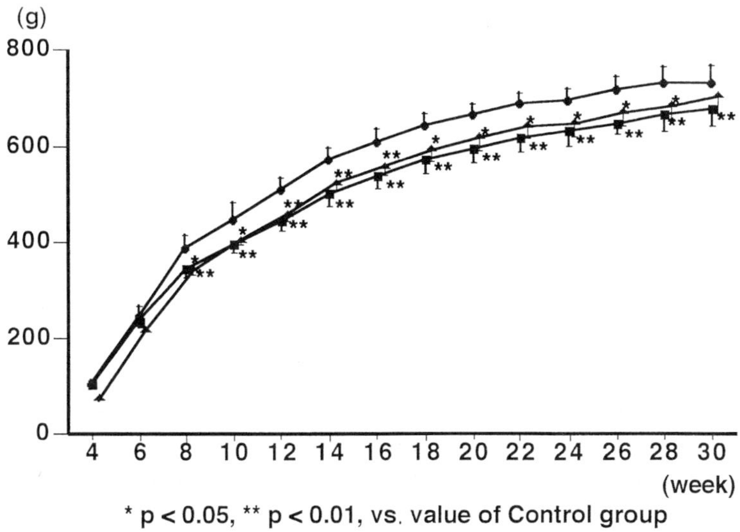

Fig. 2. Time courses of body weight. ■—■: acarbose-treated group (40 ppm). ▲—▲: acarbose-treated group (20 ppm). ●—●: control group.

Table 1. Results of oral glucose tolerance tests, plasma lipid and body fat distribution in the acarbose-treated and control groups.

		Acarbose-treated group (40 ppm)	Acarbose-treated group (20 ppm)	Control group
2 g/kg OGTT				
Glucose (mg/dl)	0′	226.9 ± 22.7	222.1 ± 32.7	230.4 ± 20.1
	30′	531.3 ± 56.2	525.1 ± 42.5	523.3 ± 29.0
	60′	538.0 ± 67.6[a]	560.9 ± 80.9	613.0 ± 34.2
	120′	405.0 ± 36.0[a]	378.5 ± 89.4[a]	483.0 ± 82.6
IRI (ng/ml)	0′	5.41 ± 1.27[b]	6.30 ± 2.53	8.54 ± 2.38
	30′	5.78 ± 2.66	5.83 ± 2.10	8.21 ± 3.55
	60′	3.21 ± 1.82[a]	3.49 ± 0.91[a]	6.98 ± 3.37
	120′	4.18 ± 2.02	4.71 ± 2.00	6.78 ± 3.21
Fasting glucose/IRI ratio		4.53 ± 1.47[a]	4.20 ± 1.90	2.95 ± 0.98
Lipid	TC (mg/dl)	153.7 ± 33.0[b]	168.8 ± 32.4[a]	200.2 ± 16.6
	TG (mg/dl)	258.7 ± 97.5[a]	295.8 ± 81.6[a]	408.6 ± 128.5
	FFA (mg/dl)	1.79 ± 0.38	2.15 ± 0.23	1.88 ± 0.26
Body fat distribution				
Visceral fat (V) weight (g/100 gBW)		5.24 ± 0.51[b]	5.35 ± 0.47[b]	6.45 ± 0.33
Subcutaneous fat (S) weight (g/100 gBW)		1.50 ± 0.25[a]	1.53 ± 0.19[b]	1.28 ± 0.13
V/S ratio		3.61 ± 0.81[b]	3.53 ± 0.55[b]	5.08 ± 0.60

[a]$p < 0.05$; [b]$p < 0.01$, vs. value of control group.

animals, but these changes were distinctly inhibited in the acarbose-treated groups.

In the histopathological examination of the coronary arteries at the age of 81 weeks, the control animals showed a slight degree of intimal irregularity and intimal hypertrophy (Fig. 3A). In addition, there was some evidence suggesting partial cell infiltration in the subendothelial tissue. On the other hand, the acarbose-treated animals did not show such intimal changes as noted in the controls (Fig. 3B).

Discussion

It is a question of great interest throughout the world why the progress of arteriosclerosis is accelerated in NIDDM. In the progress of NIDDM, especially of an obese type, there is a notable phase showing insulin resistance and hyperinsulinemia. Another interesting finding has been reported from the West: arteriosclerosis, unlike microangiopathy, often develops as early as diabetes and is still latent in the form of impaired glucose tolerance. These facts suggest that some unknown factors which do not necessarily behave in relation with hyperglycemia, contribute to the progress of arteriosclerosis. Reaven [5] proposed that a syn-

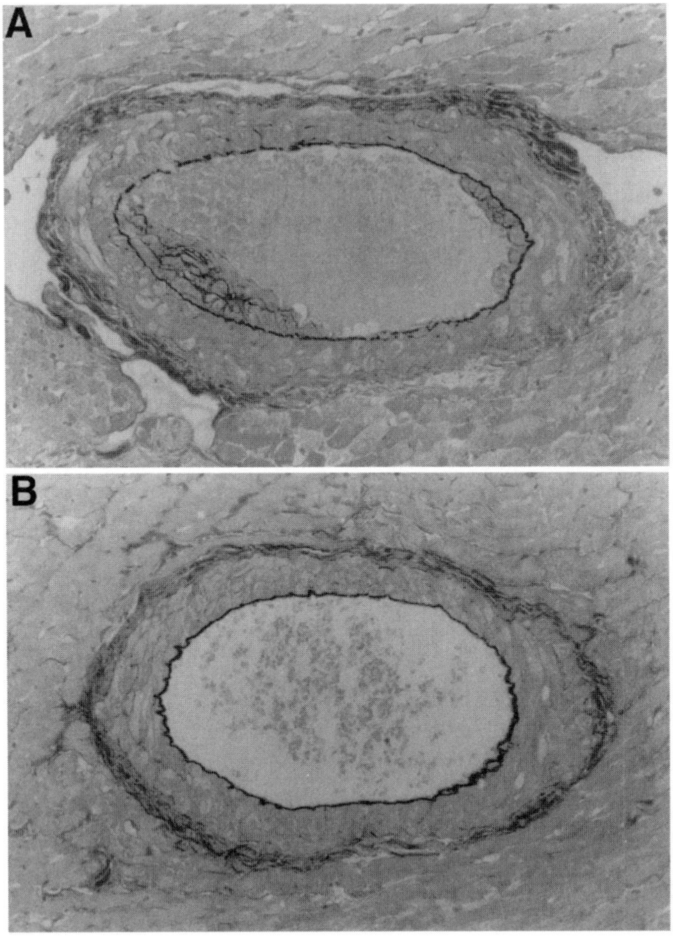

Fig. 3. Histological features of coronary arteries from OLETF rats at the age of 81 weeks (EVG staining). **A:** Control group. **B:** Acarbose-treated group.

drome X which occurs in some cases of NIDDM and shows insulin resistance, impaired glucose tolerance, hyperinsulinemia, increased VLDL triglycerides, decreased HDL cholesterol and hypertension. Kaplan [6] considered that obesity in the upper half of the body, impaired glucose tolerance, hypertriglyceridemia and hypertension, comprise the "deadly quartet". Nakamura et al. [7] considered that visceral fat accumulation is the core factor of arteriosclerosis around which various other risk factors cluster one after another, and they have proposed the concept of visceral fat syndrome characterized by visceral fat accumulation, impaired glucose tolerance (insulin resistance), hypertension and hypertriglyceridemia. Thus, they reported that visceral fat accumulation plays an important pathogenetic role in the onset of arteriosclerotic diseases. The presently observed sclerotic lesions in the coronary arteries of OLETF rats with visceral fat type obesity were very similar to those observed in the thoracic aorta of VMH-lesioned GK rats [8], and seemed to correspond to the initial stage of arteriosclerotic lesions in humans. In these rats, a close relationship was found between visceral fat accumulation and arteriosclerotic lesions as reported for humans.

However, a doubt arises: it may have been a defect in the conventional drug therapy of diabetes, that the basically important factors such as visceral fat accumulation, insulin resistance, hyperinsulinemia and hyperlipidemia had been left out of consideration. Under a hypoglycemic treatment without correction for hyperinsulinemia, the increase in arteriosclerotic risks seems to be unavoidable. In Japan, where the obese NIDDM population was small, hyperinsulinemia was previously not an important problem. At present, however, patients with obese NIDDM have been increasing in number as in the West, and the frequency of insulin therapy for NIDDM has also been increasing. Hyperinsulinemia in NIDDM should be more seriously considered in the future.

Sulfonylureas, which have been the mainstream of drug therapy for NIDDM, stimulate β cells to secrete insulin, and thereby reduce blood glucose. Because of this mechanism of action, some investigators are suspicious about the long-term treatment of obese NIDDM patients with sulfonylureas. We already pointed out the possibility that sulfonylureas may promote visceral fat accumulation and insulin resistance in NIDDM patients [9], and also reported that sulfonylureas promoted visceral fat accumulation in OLETF rats [10]. Thus, it is likely that drugs of this class may ultimately aggravate arteriosclerotic lesions. Recently developed acarbose, an oral hypoglycemic agent, delays digestion and absorption of carbohydrates by inhibiting α-glucosidase in the intestinal epithelium, and inhibits postprandial hypersecretion of endogenous insulin as well as postprandial hyperglycemia. Thus, acarbose would reduce insulin resistance, and is also expected to contribute to the prevention and treatment of arteriosclerosis. In the present study, long-term treatment of OLETF rats with acarbose was shown to reduce hyperglycemia, hypersecretion of endogenous insulin, visceral fat accumulation, insulin resistance and plasma lipids. As the possible mechanism by which long-term administration of acarbose prevented the histological development of arteriosclerosis, the following were considered: inhibition of glycation through reduced hyperglycemia, inhibition of lipid synthesis, and inhibition of arterial smooth muscle cell growth through correction of hyperinsulinemia.

References

1. Kawano K, Hirashima T, Mori S et al. Spontaneous long-term hyperglycemic rat with diabetic complications Otsuka Long-Evans Tokushima fatty (OLETF) strain. Diabetes 1992;41: 1422–1428.
2. Mori Y, Yokoyama J, Nemoto M et al. Characterization of a new genetically obese hyperglycemic OLETF rat. Jikeikai Med J 1992;39:349–359.
3. Mori Y, Yokoyama J, Nemoto M et al. Effect of dietary fiber on glucose tolerance and body fat store in OLETF rats. Matsushita Med J 1993;32:131–136 (in Japanese).

4. Krotkiewski M, Bjorntorp P. The effect of progesterone and of insulin administration on regional adipose tissue cellularity in the rat. Acta Physiol Scand 1976;96:122–127.
5. Reaven NM. Role of insulin resistance in human disease. Diabetes 1988;37:1595–1606.
6. Kaplan NM. The deadly quartet. Upperbody obesity, glucose intolerance, hypertriglycemia, and hypertension. Arch Int Med 1989;149:1514–1520.
7. Nakamura T, Tokunaga K, Shimomura I et al. Contribution of visceral fat accumulation to the development of coronary artery disease in non-obese men. Atherosclerosis 1994;107:239–246.
8. Nishida M, Tokunaga K, Miyagawa J et al. Macroangiopathy in male spontaneous non-insulin-dependent diabetic (Doto-Kakizaki) rats with VMH lesions. Ann Japan Soc Res Diab Complicat 1993;6:309–314 (in Japanese).
9. Katoh S, Mori Y, Yokoyama et al. Effect of long-term acarbose and glibenclamide treatment on visceral fat accumulation in patients with NIDDM. Diabetologia 1996;39(Suppl 1):A44.
10. Katoh S. Long-term effects of oral hypoglycemic agents on fat distribution and glucose tolerance in OLETF rats. Tokyo Jikeikai Med J 1996;111:919–926 (in Japanese).

Insulin action

Recent Advances on the Pathogenesis and Management of Diabetes Mellitus.
S.H. Shinn, M. Shichiri and K.-W. Kim, editors.

Effect of pertussis and cholera toxins on insulin receptor recycling in isolated fat cells of rats

Sang-Ah Chang, Yu-Bae Ahn, Ki-Ho Song, Soon-Jib Yoo, Jong-Min Lee, Hyun-Sik Son, Bong-Yun Cha, Kwang-Woo Lee, Ho-Young Son and Sung-Ku Kang

Department of Internal Medicine, Catholic University Medical College, Seoul, Korea

Abstract. *Background.* The mechanism is still not fully understood when the association of a guanine nucleotide binding protein (G-protein) to its receptor is coupled to its subsequent action. Consequently, in order to study the effects of G-protein on insulin action in peripheral insulin target tissue, we examined the effect of pertussis and cholera toxins. These alter the function of G-proteins on insulin binding, the internalization of the insulin-receptor complex and recycling of insulin receptors in isolated adipocytes of rats.

Methods. Adipocytes were isolated from male Wister rats and incubated with or without toxin. The study of insulin binding, insulin-insulin receptor internalization and insulin receptor recycling was carried out with ^{125}I-insulin and unlabeled insulin.

Results. 1. Incubation of adipocytes with pertussis toxin decreased the insulin binding significantly compared with that of control. However, cholera toxin did not affect the insulin binding. 2. Pertussis and cholera toxins have no effect on the internalization of the insulin-insulin receptor complex. 3. Pertussis toxin inhibited the recycling of the insulin receptor significantly compared with that of control. Nevertheless, the cholera toxin did not affect the recycling of the insulin receptor.

Conclusion. In view of the fact that pertussis toxin inhibits the insulin binding and recycling of an insulin receptor, a suggestion is made that pertussis toxin sensitive G-protein is closely associated with the insulin receptor, and modulates on the multiple steps of insulin binding.

Keywords: cholera toxin, G-protein, insulin receptor recycling, pertussis toxin.

Introduction

Guanine nucleotide binding proteins (G-protein) are linked to a number of surface membrane receptors and they mediate the regulation of a variety of effectors by hormones and neurotransmitters. It has been suggested that there is a possible role for G-protein in insulin action. For example, G-protein is an affinity regulator for insulin binding on insulin receptors, and regulates insulin receptor tyrosine kinase activity and insulin binding [1]. Recently it has been reported that G-proteins binding with insulin receptors were analyzed [2].

Thus we examined the effect of pertussis and cholera toxins which alter the function of G-protein on insulin binding, internalization of the insulin receptor complex and insulin receptor recycling in isolated adipocytes of rat.

Address for correspondence: Ho-Young Son MD, Department of Internal Medicine, Catholic University Medical College, 505 Banpodong, Seochoku, Seoul 137-040, Korea.

Materials and Methods

Animals

We used male Wister rats and their weight was between 120 and 140 g.

Materials

The following chemicals were obtained from commercial sources: procine monocomponent insulin from Novo-Nordisk, Denmark; ^{125}I-insulin (371 μCi/μg) from New England Nuclear, Boston, Mass; bovine serum albumin, collagenase (type II) and cholera toxins from Sigma Chemical Co., St. Louis, MO; and pertussis toxin from Cambell, CA.

Methods

Isolation of adipocytes in the rat
Adipocytes from epididymis in rat were isolated by Rodbell methods [3].

Insulin-binding study
Adipocytes were made 15% lipocrit by added HEPES buffer. The lipocrit was then incubated at 37°C for 30 min with 100 pM of ^{125}I-insulin and varying amounts (0—10 μM) of unlabeled insulin. Then, 100 μl of the incubated lipocrit were transferred to a microcentrifuge tube with silicone oil and centrifuged at 5,000 rpm for 1 min. After centrifuging, the tubes were frozen immediately at − 70°C. The tubes were sliced at the silicone layer and the radioactivity measured by γ-counter. The 10 μU of insulin was used for the nonspecific insulin binding. The pertussis and cholera toxin treated groups were made by incubation of isolated adipocytes with pertussis (0.5 μg/ml) or cholera toxin (1.0 μg/ml) at 37°C for 3 h with 95% O_2 and 5% CO_2 gas. The percentage of specific binding was calculated by subtraction of the percentage of nonspecific binding from the percentage of total binding.

Insulin receptor internalization and recycling
Adipocytes were incubated with or without pertussis (cholera) toxins at 37°C for 3 h with gas. Incubated adipocytes were made (15% lipocrit) adding HEPES buffer. For internalization, adipocytes were incubated at 37°C for 15 min in the presence of 100 ng/ml insulin and then ^{125}I-insulin binding was determined after incubation at 12°C for 120 min. Other aliquots of cells were warmed at 37°C for 15 and 30 min after an initial washing procedure, i.e., insulin receptors were allowed to recycle, and ^{125}I-insulin binding was determined after incubation at 12°C for 120 min.

Results

Insulin binding

The time course of specific ^{125}I- insulin binding to adipocytes revealed the results shown in Fig. 1.

In the control and cholera-toxin-treated group, there are no significant differences on insulin binding, but in the pertussis-treated group, insulin binding is significantly decreased compared to that of the control group.

Insulin-insulin receptor internalization and insulin receptor recycling

The percentage of insulin-insulin receptor internalization in the control group was 18.1%, in the cholera-toxin-treated group 16% and in the pertussis-toxin-treated group 21.4%. There were no significant differences among the three groups (Fig. 2). However, with the insulin receptor recycling, although there was no significant difference between the control and cholera-toxin-treated group, the insulin receptor recycling in pertussis-toxin-treated group was significantly decreased compared to that of the control group (Fig. 3).

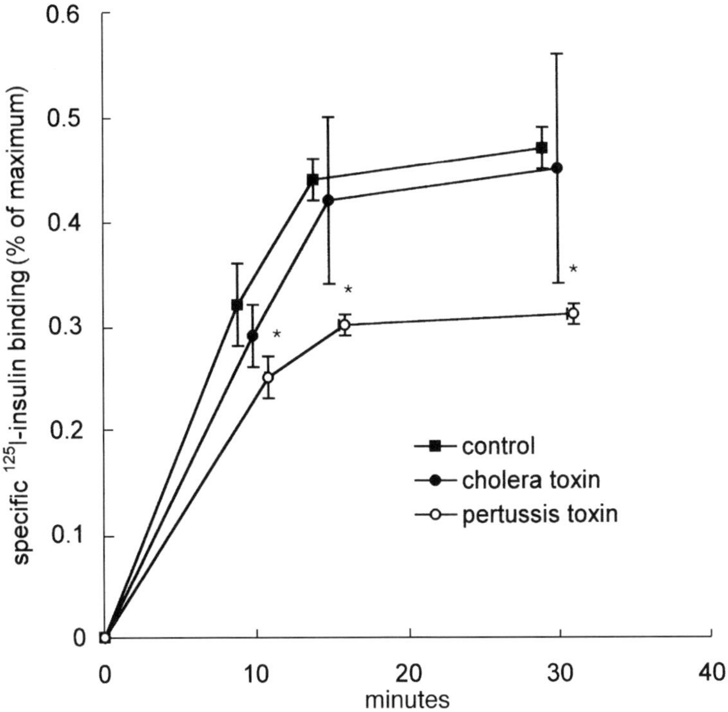

Fig. 1. Time course of specific ^{125}I-insulin binding to adipocytes at 37°C (mean ± SEM). $^{*}p<0.05$.

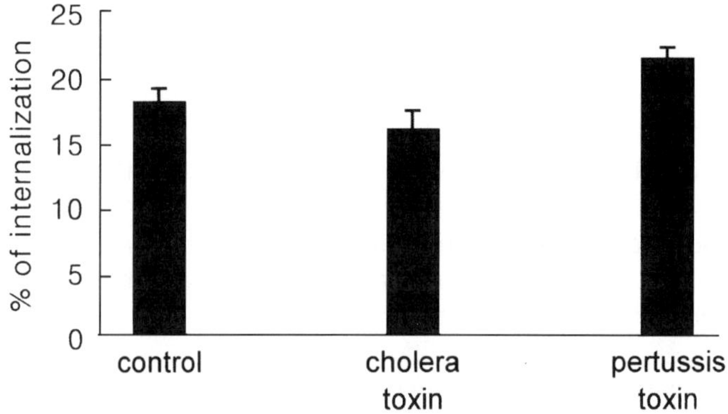

Fig. 2. Percentage of internalization of insulin-insulin receptor complex (mean ± SEM).

Discussion

The incubation of adipocytes with pertussis toxin decreased the insulin binding to insulin receptor.

This result was similar to the study of Ciaraldi et al. [4]. It has been reported that pertussis toxin modulates the affinity of insulin to insulin receptor, thus the insulin binding is decreased. However, cholera toxin did not affect the insulin

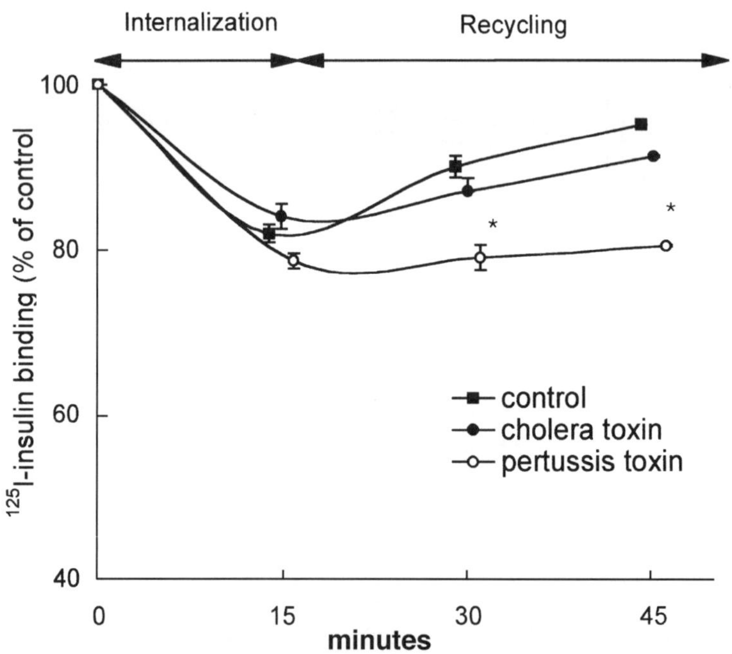

Fig. 3. Results of insulin receptor internalization and recycling in adipocytes (mean ± SEM). $*p < 0.05$.

binding, and pertussis and cholera toxin did not affect internalization of the insulin-insulin receptor. In the insulin receptor recycling, pertussis toxin inhibited the recycling of the insulin receptor. This finding suggests that cyclic AMP is not related to the insulin receptor recycling process because cholera and pertussis toxin both elevate cyclic AMP levels. However, the fact that only pertussis toxin influenced the recycling process means there are other pathways to influence the process by pertussis toxin. We do not exclude the effect of pertussis toxin on ADP ribosylation of Gi proteins that inhibit the insulin receptor kinase and autophospholylation. It may influence the insulin receptor recycling. Another suggestion is that the G-protein has a direct effect on the process (Jo et al. [2]) because if an isolated G-protein is bound with an insulin receptor, it may be internalized with the insulin receptor. Especially, binding G-protein with tubulin inhibits the formation of a microtubule [5], which means that a G-protein has multiple effects on hormone action.

In conclusion, pertussis toxin inhibits insulin binding and insulin receptor recycling, therefore, it is suggested that a pertussis toxin sensitive G-protein is closely associated with the insulin receptor and modulated on the multiple steps of insulin signaling.

References

1. Heyworth CM, Houslay MD. Insulin exerts action through a distinct species of guanine nucleotide regulatory protein: inhibition of adenylate cyclase. Biochem J 1983;214:547–552.
2. Jo HJ, Cha BY, Davis HW, Macdonald JM. Identification, partial purification and characterization of two guanosine triphosphate-binding proteins associated with insulin receptors. Endocrinology 1992;131:2855–2862.
3. Rodbell M. Metabolism of isolated fat cells. Effect of hormones on glucose metabolism and lipolysis. J Biol Chem 1964;239:375–380.
4. Ciaraldi TP, Maisel A. Role of guanine nucleotide regulatory proteins in insulin stimulation of glucose transport in rat adipocytes. Biochem 1989;264:389–396.
5. Wang N, Rasenik MM. Tubulin G-protein interactions involve microtubule polymerization domains. Biochem J 1991;30:10957–10965.

Recent Advances on the Pathogenesis and Management of Diabetes Mellitus.
S.H. Shinn, M. Shichiri and K.-W. Kim, editors.

Subcellular distribution and functional changes of GTP-binding proteins (G-proteins) in adipocytes of streptozotocin-induced insulin-dependent diabetic rats and changes in the amount and function of G-protein in adipocytes from type II diabetic patients

B.Y. Cha, S.D. Moon, S.A. Jang, Y.B. Ahn, K.H. Song, S.J. You, J.H. Han, J.M. Lee, H.S. Son, K.H. Yoon, M.I. Kang, K.W. Lee, H.Y. Son and S.K. Kang
Department of Internal Medicine, Catholic University Medical College, Seoul, Korea

Abstract. *Background.* It has been well known that GTP-binding proteins (G-proteins) are involved in insulin actions. Therefore, in order to evaluate whether the G-protein is involved in the pathogenesis of diabetes mellitus, we evaluated the subcellular distribution and functional changes of G-proteins in adipocytes from streptozotocin-induced diabetic rats and changes in amount and function of G-protein in adipocytes from patients with diabetes mellitus.

Methods. To induce the diabetes, 30 male rats were injected with streptozotocin (55 mg/kg, intravenously). After 7 days isolated adipocytes from epididymal fat pads of control and diabetic rats were fractionated into homogenate (HOM), plasma membrane (PM), high-density microsome (HDM), low-density microsome (LDM), mitochondria (MIT), crude nuclear fraction (CNF) and cytosol (CYT). For human studies, the isolated adipocytes obtained from lower abdominal subcutaneous adipose tissue of control and diabetic patients who underwent elective abdominal surgery, were fractionated into homogenate and postnuclear fraction. The Gi1α/Gi2α, Gi3α, Gsα and Gβ were quantitated on Western blots in fractions of rats. The Gi1α/Gi2α were quantitated on Western blots in fractions of control and diabetic patients. In order to evaluate the functional changes of G-proteins, pertussis toxin-catalyzed ADP-ribosylation and GTPγS binding activity of G-proteins were performed.

Results. In adipocytes from streptozotocin-induced diabetic rats, the Gi1α/Gi2α, Gi3α, Gsα and Gβ proteins were mainly located in plasma membrane. Specifically, Gi1α/Gi2α and Gi3α were enriched in plasma membrane of adipocytes from streptozotocin-induced diabetic rats. In contrast, pertussis toxin-catalyzed ADP-ribosylation of Gi-proteins in plasma membrane of adipocytes from streptozotocin-induced diabetic rats significantly decreased. The GTPγS binding activity of G-proteins in the plasma membrane of diabetic rats significantly decreased; it was restored to some extent by insulin treatment. However, there were no consistent changes in the amount of Gi1α/Gi2α, pertussis toxin-catalyzed ADP-ribosylation of Gi-protein was consistently decreased in adipocytes from patients with diabetes mellitus.

Conclusions. These results suggest that insulin-deficient diabetic state induces the quantitative and functional changes in Gi-proteins of adipocytes plasma membrane. Therefore, these changes in Gi-proteins may be an important compensatory reaction for the insulin resistance occurring in insulin-deficient state.

Keywords: diabetes mellitus, G-protein, GTP-binding protein, subcellular distribution.

Address for correspondence: Bong Yun Cha MD, Department of Internal Medicine, Catholic University Medical College, 505 Banpodong, Seochoku, Seoul 137-040, Korea.

Introduction

G-protein-coupled receptors not only have similar primary sequences but also have a common membrane-spanning configuration with seven transmembrane regions [1]. However, there is abundant evidence that receptors of several peptide ligands such as IGF-I [2], IGF-II [3], EGF [4], IL-1 [5] and insulin [6,7], which have a single transmembrane region, can also activate G-protein-mediated signal transduction pathways in intact cells and broken cell membranes.

There has been considerable evidence that G-proteins would be involved in insulin action [8]. In addition to a previous report about the identification and purification of G-proteins coupled with insulin receptors in human placental tissue [9,10], a recent report that a Gi2α-deficient transgenic mouse shows growth retardation and insulin resistance similar to the characteristics of patients with non-insulin-dependent diabetes, strongly suggests the involvement of Gi-proteins in insulin action [11].

Among the studies related to G-protein and insulin action, some studies suggest that the function and amount of Gi-proteins of hepatocyte and adipocyte could be changed in the diabetic state [12—14], but the results have been conflicting. Therefore, to further clarify the relationship between the function and expression of Gi-proteins and diabetic state, we examined the expression and the functional changes of Gi-protein in adipocytes from streptozotocin-induced diabetic rats and from type II diabetic patients.

Material and Methods

The antibodies (anti-Gi1α/Gi2α antibody (AS/7), anti-Gi3α antibody (EC/2), anti-Gsα antibody (RM/1) and anti-Gβ antibody (MS/1)) used were obtained from Calbiochem Co, La Jolla, CA, USA. The radioisotopes ([^{32}P]-NAD, [^{35}S]-GTPγS, [^{3}H]-5′-AMP) used were obtained from Amersham Co., Buckinghamshire, England. To induce the diabetes, 30 male Sprague-Dawley rats weighing 120—160 g were intravenously injected with 55 mg streptozotocin/kg body weight. Seven days after the induction of diabetes, animals were killed to isolate adipocytes from epididymal fat pads by the method of Rodbell [15]. They were then fractionated into homogenate (HOM), plasma membrane (PM), low-density microsome (LDM), high-density microsome (HDM), mitochondria (MIT), crude nuclear membrane (CNF) and cytosol (CYT) using the differential centrifugation method as described by Jarett [16].

For human study, adipose tissue was obtained from lower abdominal subcutaneous adipose tissue from control (four nondiabetics) and four type II diabetics who underwent elective abdominal surgery. From these, adipocytes were rapidly isolated and then fractionated into homogenate (HOM) and postnuclear fraction (PNF).

The Gi1α/Gi2α, Gi3α, Gsα and Gβ were quantitated on the Western blot in fractions of rat adipocytes. The Gi1α/Gi2α was quantitated on the Western blot

Table 1. Characteristics of rats 7 days after the induction of diabetes with streptozotocin in a group.

	Control (n = 30)	Diabetes (n = 30)
Blood glucose (nM)	7.58 ± 2.1	18.81 ± 9.34[a]
Weight gain (g)	28.0 ± 17.8	19.0 ± 17.7[a]

[a]$p < 0.05$ control vs. diabetes. Data expressed as mean ± SD.

in fractions of control and diabetic patients. In order to evaluate the functional changes of G-proteins, pertussis toxin (PTX)-catalyzed ADP-ribosylation and GTPγS binding activity of G-proteins were assessed.

To estimate the degree of contamination of the plasma membrane which is the main site of the G-protein action, 5′-nucleotidase activity was measured in each fraction. All of these studies were performed at least three times and the statistical significance of those experiments was analyzed by the Student's t test. The p value less than 0.05 was considered to be significant.

Results and Discussion

Results shown in Table 1 demonstrate that rats are hyperglycemic 7 days after streptozotocin treatment. The rate of weight gain was much lower in the diabetic group. When the densitometric values of Gi-proteins in each fraction were com-

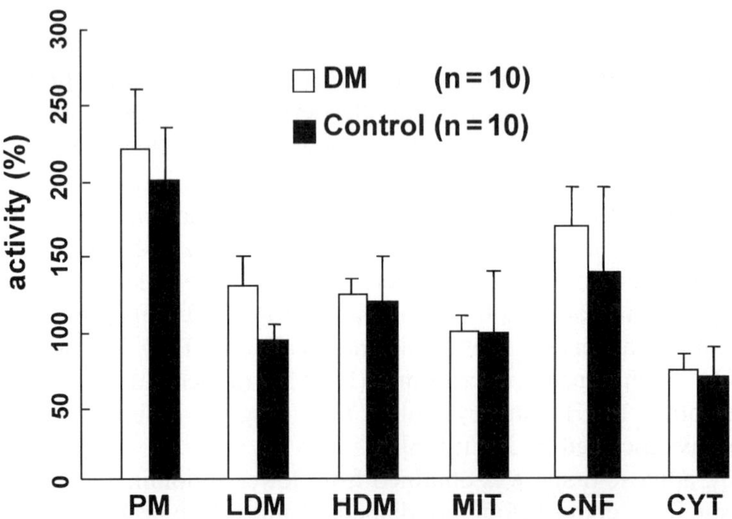

Fig. 1. Percent activities of 5′-nucleotidase in each subcellular fraction of streptozotocin-induced diabetic and control rats. Each value was expressed as mean ± SEM of three separate experiments. Activity (%) = cpm of each fraction/cpm of homogenate × 100. HOM: homogenate; PM: plasma membrane; HDM: high-density microsome; LDM: low-density microsome; MIT: mitochondria; CNF: crude nuclear fraction; CYT: cytosol.

Table 2. [^{35}S]-GTPγS binding activity in adipocyte plasma membranes from diabetic and control rats.

	[^{35}S]-GTPγS binding activity (% of total activity)	
	Without insulin	With insulin
Diabetic	40.8 ± 9.0[a]	45.6 ± 8.8
Control	49.9 ± 7.6	48.9 ± 9.2

Data shown are means ± SD for five preparations. [a]$p < 0.05$ compared with control. The insulin concentration used was 20 nM.

pared with the activity of 5′-nucleotidase activity, it was considerably enriched in PM fractions of both control and diabetic rats (Fig. 1). Therefore, our fractiona-

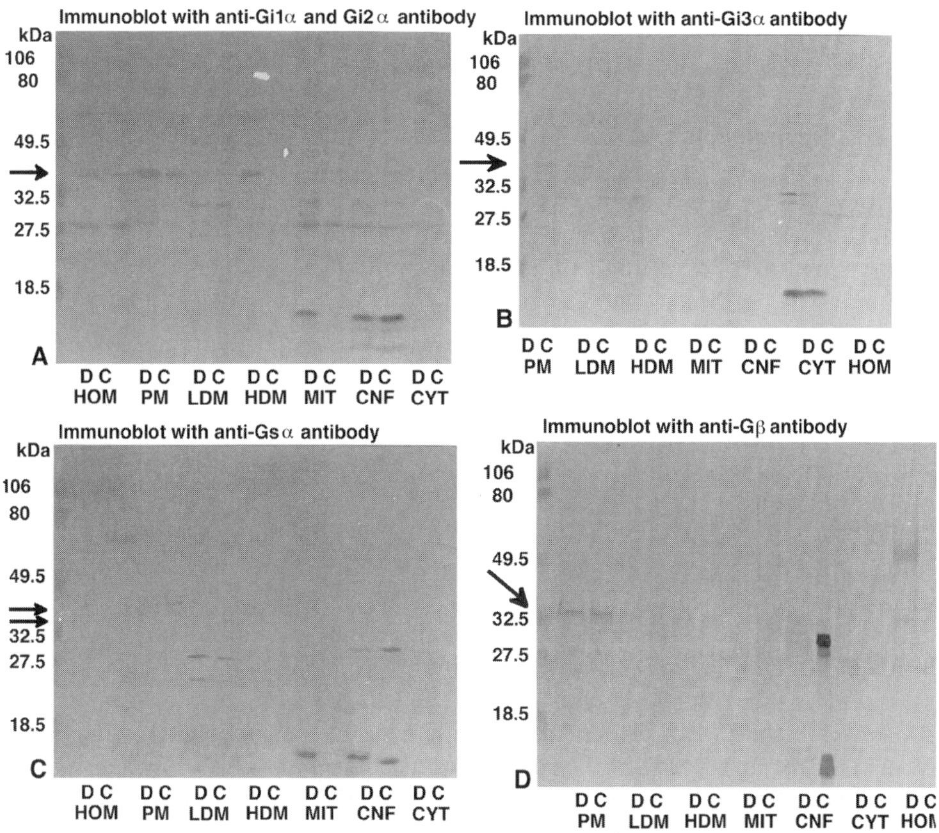

Fig. 2. Subcellular distribution of Gi1α and Gi2α, Gi3α, Gsα and Gβ (→) in rat adipocytes. Rat adipocytes from streptozotocin-induced diabetic rats (D) and control (C) were fractionated into homogenate (HOM), plasma membrane (PM), high-density microsome (HDM), low-density microsome (LDM), mitochondria (MIT), crude nuclear fraction (CNF) and cytosol (CYT). Cellular fractions were analyzed (10% resolving gel) after transferred to nitrocellulose. Immunoblottings were performed with antibodies for Gi1α and Gi2α **A**, Gi3α **B**, Gsα **C** and Gβ **D**.

Table 3. Characteristics of patients with NIDDM and control subjects.

	No.	Age	Sex	Diagnosis	DM duration (years)	Serum glucose		HbA1C (%)	Mode of therapy
						FBS (mM)	PP2h (mM)		
Controls									
	1	43	F	Myoma uteri					
	2	47	F	Myoma uteri					
	3	40	F	Myoma uteri					
	4	43	F	CIS in cervix					
Diabetes									
	5	34	F	Pregnancy	5 years	7.3	7.9	6.5	NPH 8U
	6	72	M	Rectal cancer	7 years	11.4	11.4	10.4	NPH 20U
	7	47	F	Adenomyosis	3 years	10.0	6.1	10.0	NPH 18U
	8	54	F	Endomyosis ca.	4 years	7.6	7.6	6.6	Diet

tion step is considered to be comparable to the originally reported Jarett's method [16].

In the immunoblots with anti-Gi1α/Gi2α antibodies, Gi1α/Gi2α were mainly distributed in the PM fraction, and a small amount in HDM and CNF. These were significantly expressed in PM of diabetic rats compared with that of control. In the immunoblots with anti-Gi3α antibodies, the expression of Gi3α was slightly higher in PM of diabetic rats (Fig. 2A,B). The immunoblots with anti-Gsα and Gβ antibodies showed that the two Gsα (44 and 48 kDa) proteins were mainly detected in PM and HDM fractions. Gβ was also detected mainly in PM and to some extent in HDM and CNF. There was no difference in the amounts of Gsα and Gβ in PM fractions between the two groups (Fig. 2C,D).

In the autoradiograph of PTX-catalyzed ADP-ribosylation, a 41-kDa Gi-protein was identified in PM and HDM fractions of control and diabetic rats. It was clearly decreased in PM and HDM of diabetic rats (Fig. 3A). In the Coomasie blue stain of gel after PTX-catalyzed ADP-ribosylation, each lane shows comparable density in each fraction (Fig. 3B). Therefore, it is clear that the remarkable difference in PTX-catalyzed ADP-ribosylation between the two groups was not due to the difference in the amount of loaded protein. In addition to the PTX-catalyzed ADP-ribosylation study, GTPγS-binding activity was also measured to see the functional changes of Gi-proteins. It was significantly decreased in the PM of diabetic rats compared with that of control. After treatment with insulin, it was increased somewhat, but without any statistical significance (Table 2). In view of the PTX-catalyzed ADP-ribosylation of inactive Gi-protein, the decreased PTX-catalyzed ADP-ribosylation in the diabetic state may reflect that most of the Gi-proteins are in an active state. This suggestion can be supported further by the evidence that GTPγS-binding activity was also significantly decreased in diabetic rats compared with that of control.

Table 3 shows the clinical characteristics of control and type II diabetic patients. The blood glucose of all the diabetic patients was controlled with insulin

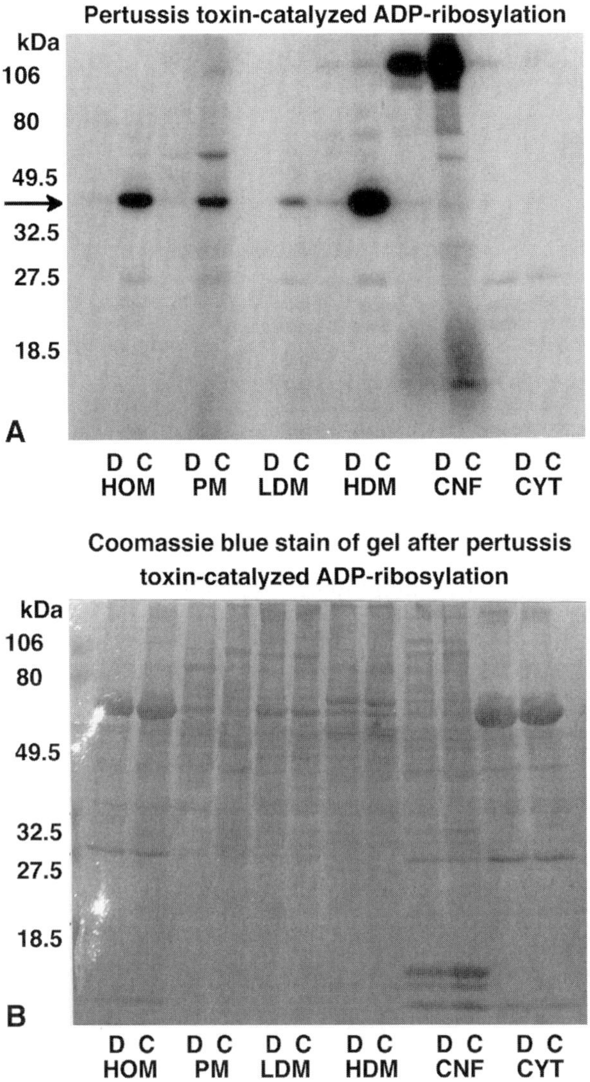

Fig. 3. Pertussis toxin-catalyzed ADP-ribosylation of Gi-protein (→) of fractions of adipocytes. **A:** Fractions of adipocytes from diabetic (D) and control (C) rats were incubated with activated pertussis toxin and [^{32}P] NAD, then analyzed by SDS/PAGE and autoradiography. **B:** Coomassie blue stained gel. Fractions from adipocytes from diabetic and control rats appeared very similar in the band shape of each other. Therefore, it suggests that the differences were not due to the gross differences in the amount of loaded protein.

and diet just before major surgery. In the immunoblots with anti-Gi1α/Gi2α antibody of postnuclear fraction of human adipocytes, there was no difference in the amount of protein between the two groups. However, the PTX-catalyzed ADP-ribosylation was clearly decreased in diabetic patients (Fig. 4).

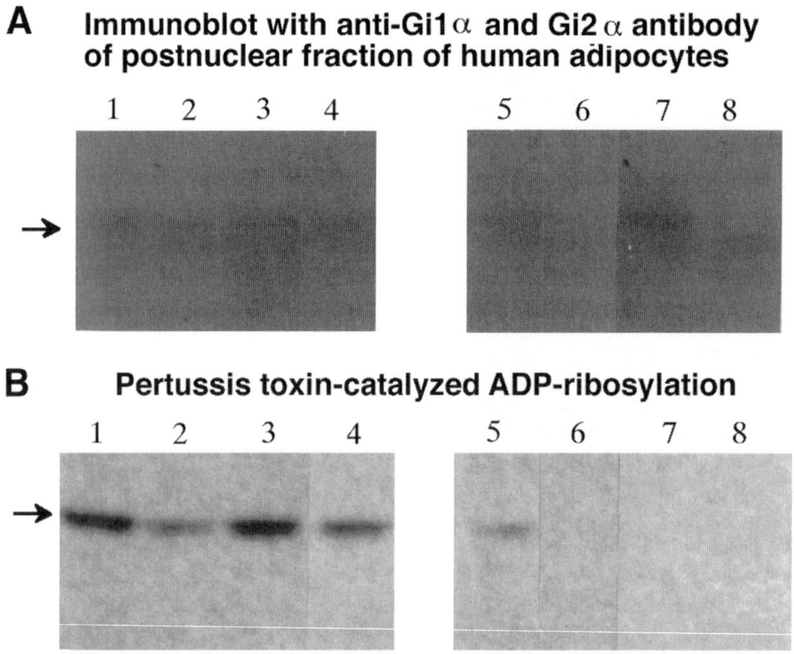

Fig. 4. Immunoblot of Gi1α and Gi2α (**A**) and pertussis toxin-catalyzed ADP ribosylation (→) (**B**) in the postnuclear membranes of abdominal adipocytes obtained from patients with diabetes mellitus (D) and control subjects (C).

Conclusion

These results suggest that insulin-deficient diabetic state induces the quantitative and functional changes in Gi-proteins of adipocytes plasma membrane. Therefore, these changes in Gi-proteins may be important compensatory reactions for the insulin resistance occurring in the insulin-deficient state.

References

1. Savarese TM, Fraser CM. In vitro mutagenesis and the search for structure-function relationships among G-protein-coupled receptors. Biochem J 1992;283:1—19.
2. Nishimoto I, Ogata E, Kojima I. Pertussis toxin inhibits the action of insulin-like growth factor-I. Biochem Biophys Res Commun 1987;148:403—411.
3. Nishimoto I, Ogata E, Ogata E, Kojima I. Insulin-like growth factor II stimulates calcium influx in competent BALB/c 3T3 cells primed with epidermal growth factor: Characteristics of calcium influx and involvement of GTP-binding protein. J Biol Chem 1987;262:12120—12126.
4. Church JF, Buick RN. G-protein-mediated epidermal growth factor signal transduction in a human breast cancer cell line. Evidence for two intracellular pathways distinguishable by pertussin toxin. J Biol Chem 1988;263:4242—4246.
5. Chedid M, Shirakawa F, Naylor P, Mizel SB. Signal transduction pathway for IL-1. Involvement of pertussis toxin-sensitive GTP-binding protein in the activation of adenylate cyclase. J Immunol 1989;142:4301—4306.

6. Goren HJ, Northup JK, Hollenber MD. Action of insulin modulated by pertussis toxin in rat adipocytes. Can J Physiol Pharmacol 1985;63:1017–1022.
7. Davis HW, McDonald JM. Insulin receptor function is inhibited by guanosine 5′-[r-thio]triphosphate (GTP-rs). Biochem J 1990;270:401–407.
8. Green A, Milligan G, Dobias SB. Gi down-regulation as a mechanism for heterologous desensitization in adipocytes. J Biol Chem 1992;267:3223–3229.
9. Jo H, Cha BY, Davis HW, McDonald JM. Identification, partial purification and characterization of two guanosine triphosphate-binding proteins associated with insulin receptors. Endocrinology 1992;131:2855–2861.
10. Jo H, Cha BY, McDonald JM. Characterization and purification of two unique GTP-binding proteins associated with the insulin receptor. Diabetes 1992;41(Suppl 1):8A.
11. Moxham CM, Malbon CC. Insulin action impaired by deficiency of the G-protein subunit Gia2. Nature 1996;379:840–844.
12. Allard WJ, Vicario PP, Saperstein R, Slater EE, Strout HV. The function but not the expression of rat liver inhibitory guanine nucleotide binding protein is altered in streptozotocin-induced diabetes. Endocrinology 1991;129:169–175.
13. Bushifield M, Griffiths SL, Murphy GJ, Pyne NJ, Knowler JT, Milligan G, Parker PJ, Mollner S, Houslay MD. Diabetes-induced alterations in the expression, functioning and phosphorylation state of the inhibitory guanine nucleotide regulatory protein Gi-2 hepatocytes. Biochem J 1990;271:365–372.
14. Strassheim D, Milligan G, Houslay MD. Diabetes abolishes the GTP-dependent, but not the receptor-dependent inhibitory function of the inhibitory guanine-nucleotide-binding. Biochem J 1990;266:521–526.
15. Rodbell M. Metabolism of isolated fat cells. I. Effects of hormones on glucose metabolism and lipocytes. Biol Chem 1964;239:375–380.
16. Jarett L. Subcellular fractionation of adipocytes. Meth Enzymol 1974;31:60–71.

Recent Advances on the Pathogenesis and Management of Diabetes Mellitus.
S.H. Shinn, M. Shichiri and K.-W. Kim, editors.

Fibroblast PC-1 mRNA content and insulin sensitivity in Korean NIDDM patients

H.-M. Kim, D.-B. Park, Y.-S. Chung and K.-W. Lee
Department of Endocrinology and Metabolism, Ajou University School of Medicine, Suwon, Korea

Abstract. *Background.* The clinical features of NIDDM in Korea seem to be quite different from those of western countries. It is reported that overexpression of PC-1 is related to insulin resistance in NIDDM patients. This study was performed to examine the significance of PC-1 mRNA in Korean NIDDM patients.

Methods. Eleven Korean NIDDM patients and 10 healthy controls were studied. C-peptide (pmol/l)/glucose (mmol/l) index (CGI) was calculated. Hyperinsulinemic euglycemic clamp tests were performed. Dermal fibroblasts were obtained from subjects by micropunched biopsy. Fibroblasts were grown to confluency, and then total RNA was isolated. PC-1 mRNA was measured by dot blot hybridization using 1.1 kb probe of full-length human PC-1 cDNA.

Results. NIDDM patients showed significantly lower CGI (13.8 ± 11.3 vs. 27.7 ± 14.6). Peripheral glucose utilization rate of NIDDM patients was significantly lower than that of controls (4.8 ± 2.6 vs. 8.0 ± 3.7 mg/kg/min). There was no significant correlation between BMI and glucose utilization rate or CGI. PC-1 mRNA contents were similar between NIDDM patients and controls, and there was significant correlation between BMI and PC-1 mRNA content (r = 0.485). However, there was no significant correlation between glucose utilization rate and PC-1 mRNA content in fibroblasts.

Conclusion. These results suggest that PC-1 in dermal fibroblasts is not related to insulin resistance in Koreans, and that NIDDM in Koreans is developed through insulin resistance superimposing relative insulinopenia.

Keywords: body mass index, C-peptide/glucose index, glucose utilization rate, PC-1.

Introduction

The most common form of diabetes mellitus in Korea is NIDDM. When compared with western patients, Korean NIDDM patients have different clinical characteristics, such as lower proportion of obesity [1] and lower insulin secretory capacity [2]. While the causes of NIDDM are unknown, a resistance to insulin and a defect in insulin synthesis or release seem to be equally significant in the development of NIDDM in Koreans.

The cellular mechanism causing insulin resistance is not fully understood. Recently, it was reported that overexpression of PC-1 was related to insulin resistance in NIDDM patients [3,4]. PC-1 is a type II transmembrane glycoprotein. In order to examine the significance of insulin resistance in the development of NIDDM in Koreans, we measured PC-1 mRNA content in dermal fibroblasts

Address for correspondence: Hyeon-Man Kim MD, Department of Endocrinology and Metabolism, Ajou University School of Medicine, 5 Woncheon-Dong, Paldal-Gu, Suwon 442-749, South Korea.

with insulin sensitivity by euglycemic hyperinsulinemic clamp test in 11 newly diagnosed NIDDM patients and 10 healthy control subjects. We also evaluated the relationships between PC-1 mRNA levels, insulin resistance of peripheral tissue and BMI.

Subjects and Methods

The study consisted of 11 Korean NIDDM patients and 10 healthy controls (Table 1). All NIDDM patients were newly diagnosed cases. C-peptide (pmol/l)/glucose (mmol/l) index (CGI) was calculated with the data of oral glucose tolerance tests. Hyperinsulinemic euglycemic clamp tests were performed by DeFronzo's method [5]. Dermal fibroblasts, which were obtained from subjects by micropunched biopsy, were cultured using modified Doyle's method [6]. Fibroblasts were grown to confluency and washed twice with ice-cold PBS, and then total RNA was isolated [7]. PC-1 mRNA was measured by dot blot hybridization using 1.1 kb probe of full-length human PC-1 cDNA (pSVT7B1HPC1; a gift from Dr Goding, Australia). The amount of PC-1 mRNA was measured by densitometer and was expressed as ADU (arbitrary densitometer unit). The results were expressed as mean ± SD. The statistical significance was evaluated by unpaired t test and Pearson's correlation coefficient.

Results

Mean age and body mass index (BMI) were similar in both groups. The range of BMI was 20.0–29.1. NIDDM patients showed significantly lower CGI than controls (13.8 ± 11.3 vs. 27.7 ± 14.6) (Table 1). Peripheral glucose utilization rate of NIDDM patients was significantly lower than that of controls (4.8 ± 2.6 vs. 8.0 ± 3.7 mg/kg/min, $p = 0.032$, Fig. 1). There was no significant correlation between BMI and glucose utilization rate or CGI. PC-1 mRNA content was similar between NIDDM patients and controls (2.1 ± 1.2 vs. 2.3 ± 1.5 ADU, $p = 0.776$, Fig. 2), and there was significant correlation between BMI and PC-1 mRNA content ($r = 0.485$, $p = 0.026$, Fig. 3). However, there was no significant

Table 1. Demographic features of subjects.

	NIDDM	Controls
Cases	11	10
Sex (M:F)	6:5	9:1
Age (years)	33.3 ± 4.0	29.1 ± 5.2
BMI	24.9 ± 2.3	22.7 ± 2.7
FBS (mmol/l)	8.1 ± 2.5[a]	5.2 ± 1.0
C-Parea (nmol/l)	3.31 ± 2.15	3.67 ± 1.69
CGI	13.8 ± 11.3[a]	27.7 ± 14.6

Notes: C-Parea: area under the curve of C-peptide during oral GTT. CGI: C-peptide/glucose index.
[a]$p < 0.05$.

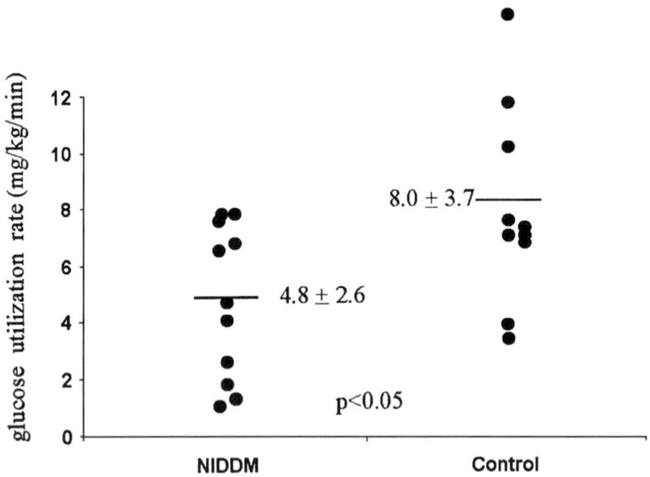

Fig. 1. Insulin sensitivity in NIDDM patients and controls.

correlation between glucose utilization rate and PC-1 mRNA content of fibroblasts (r = −0.156, p = 0.511, Fig. 4).

Discussion

Korean NIDDM patients showed a lower proportion of obesity [1] and lower insulin levels than those of western diabetics [2]. In the present study, newly diagnosed NIDDM patients showed significant defects in insulin synthesis or release as well as insulin resistance.

Maddux et al. [3] demonstrated that there was increased expression of PC-1 in muscle and fibroblasts of many patients with insulin resistance. However, PC-1

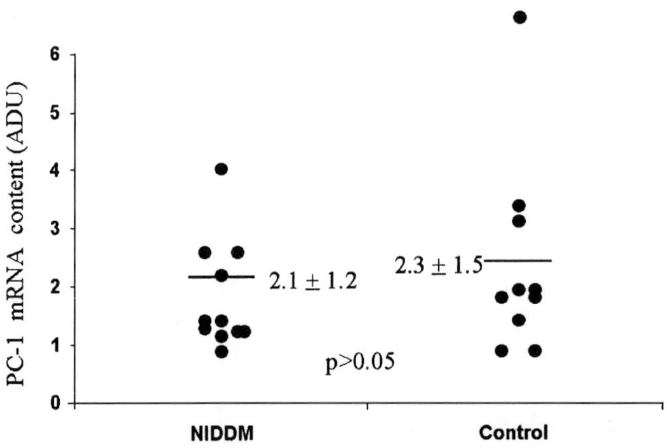

Fig. 2. PC-1mRNA content in dermal fibroblasts.

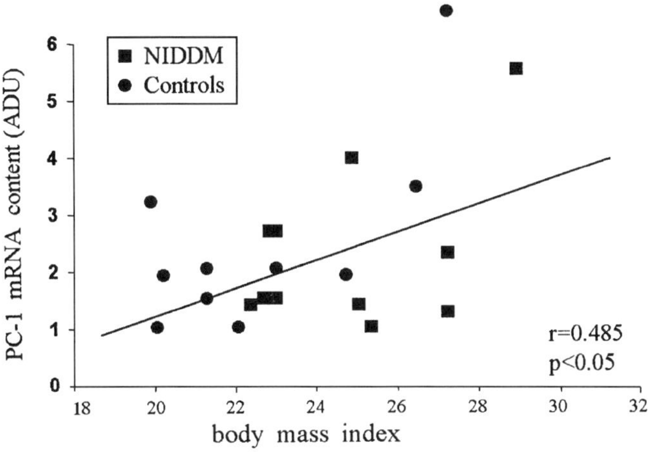

Fig. 3. Correlation between BMI and PC-1 mRNA content.

mRNA content in dermal fibroblasts was not increased in newly diagnosed Korean patients with NIDDM. Moreover, there was no significant correlation between glucose disposal rate and fibroblast PC-1 mRNA content.

These results suggest that PC-1 in dermal fibroblasts is not related to insulin resistance in Koreans, and that NIDDM in Koreans is developed through insulin resistance superimposing relative insulinopenia.

Acknowledgements

We wish to thank H.C. Lim, B.J. Lee, and Y.J. Kwak for their technical assis-

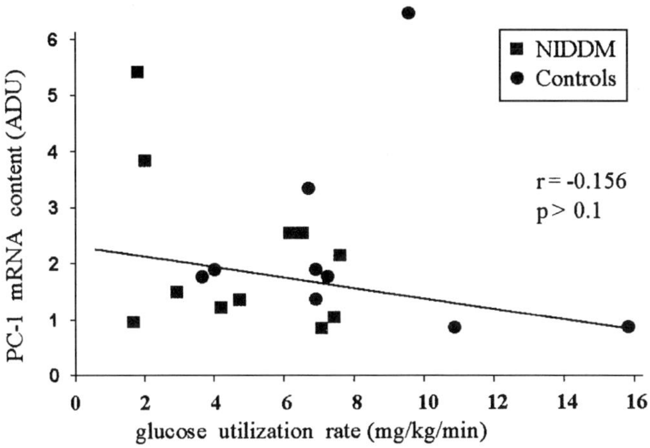

Fig. 4. Correlation between glucose utilization rate and PC-1 mRNA content in fibroblasts.

tance, and Heather Yu for editing the research paper. This study was supported by a grant (#HMP-96-M-2-0018) from the 1996 Good Health R&D Project, Ministry of Health & Welfare, ROK.

References

1. Lee TH. Prevalence of obesity in Korean non-insulin-dependent diabetic patients. Diabetes Res Clin Pract 1996;32:71–80.
2. Min HK. Non-insulin-dependent diabetes mellitus (NIDDM) in Korea. Diabetes Med 1996; 13(S6):S13–15.
3. Maddux BA, Sbraccia P, Kumakura S, Sasson S, Youngren J, Fisher A, Spencer S, Grupe A, Henzel W, Stewart TA, Reaven GM, Goldfine ID. Membrane glycoprotein PC-1 and insulin resistance in NIDDM. Nature 1995;373:448–451.
4. Youngren JF, Maddux BA, Sasson S, Sbraccia P, Tapscott EB, Swanson MS, Dohm GL, Goldfine ID. Skeletal muscle content of membrane glycoprotein PC-1 in obesity. Diabetes 1996; 45:1324–1328.
5. DeFronzo RA, Tobin JD, Andres R. Glucose clamp technique: A method for quantifying insulin secretion and resistance. Am J Physiol 1979;237:E214.
6. Doyle A, Griffiths JB, Newall DG. Rapid monolayer primary cell culture from tissue biopsy. In: Doyle A, Griffiths JB, Newall DG (eds) Cell and Tissue Culture. New York: John Wiley & Sons, 1993;3E:2.1–3E:2.7.
7. Chomczynski P, Sacchi N. Single-step method of RNA isolation by acid guanidium thiocyanate-phenol-chloroform extraction. Anal Biochem 1987;162:156–159.

Epidemiology

Recent Advances on the Pathogenesis and Management of Diabetes Mellitus.
S.H. Shinn, M. Shichiri and K.-W. Kim, editors.

Study on proinsulin levels in IGT and normal groups. Report 1: correlation between development of NIDDM and proinsulin levels

C. Ito and Y. Shibata
A-Bomb Casualty Council Health Management Center, Hiroshima, Japan

Abstract. This study was carried out to clarify whether proinsulin can be used as a predictor of diabetes mellitus. The subjects were 167 GTT examinees, composed of 55 normal cases and 112 IGT cases, tested from June–October 1996. The results are as follows: 1. Fasting IRI and proinsulin were higher in the IGT cases than in the normal group, but there was no difference in the proinsulin/IRI ratio. 2. In the IGT group, fasting IRI and proinsulin were higher in the obese patients than in the nonobese patients. However, the proinsulin/IRI ratio was lower in the obese patients. In the normal group, IRI was higher and the ratio was significantly lower in the obese patients than in the nonobese patients. 3. The IGT-2 (2 h PG $\geqslant$ 170 mg/dl) group tended towards higher fasting IRI and proinsulin levels, but no difference in the proinsulin/IRI ratio was seen.

These data suggested that the β-cell function of IGT and IGT-2 was normal based on the ratio of proinsulin to IRI. As it is not clear whether proinsulin levels or the proinsulin/IRI ratio can be used as predictors of diabetes mellitus, further investigation is needed.

Keywords: IGT, IGT-1, IGT-2, obese, proinsulin, proinsulin/IRI ratio.

Introduction

It has been reported that the ratio of proinsulin to insulin is high in diabetic patients, and that the ratio shows a pancreas β-cell function. IGT cases constitute the hyperglycemic group closest to diabetes mellitus, have a high development rate of diabetes mellitus and also may have β-cell dysfunction. If β-cell dysfunction is observed before the onset of diabetes mellitus, this would indicate that there may be many IGT cases with β-cell dysfunction. This study was undertaken to clarify whether proinsulin can be used as a predictor of diabetes mellitus.

Methods

The subjects of this study were GTT examinees from June to October 1996. The 50–59 year group was composed of 23 males and 18 females (41 cases in total); the 60–69 year group, 67 males and 54 females (121); and the 70–75 year groups; 2 males and 3 females (5); the total was 92 males and 75 females (167) cases. Mean age ± SD was 62.7 ± 5.9 years for the males and 62.4 ± 6.0 years

Address for correspondence: C. Ito, A-Bomb Casualty Council Health Management Center, 8–6, 3-chome Senda-machi Naka-ku, Hiroshima 730, Japan.

for the females. GTT results were analyzed using the WHO standard. IGT cases were divided into two groups using a 2-h plasma glucose level of 170 mg/dl at GTT. IGT-1 are cases with 2 h PG under 170 mg/dl and IGT-2 consists of cases with 170 mg/dl or more; there was no difference in the mean age of the two groups. Based on GTT results, there were 112 IGT (IGT-1, 57 cases, IGT-2, 55 cases) and 55 normal cases. Cases with diabetes mellitus under treatment, liver dysfunction and gastrectomy were excluded. Venous plasma glucose levels were measured by the glucose oxidase method. IRI and proinsulin were measured by double antibody and RIA methods, respectively. For the RIA method of proinsulin, Des 65,66 human proinsulin cross-reacted with this assay by 100%, and cross-reactivity to Des 32,33 human proinsulin was very weak; C-peptide and other pancreatic hormones were <0.01% [1]. Subjects were divided into two groups by BMI, an obese group in which BMI was 25 or more, and a nonobese group of BMI under 25.

Results

Comparison of mean plasma glucose levels and IRI levels by GTT results

Plasma glucose levels and IRI levels at GTT in both the normal and the IGT groups, including our IGT-1 and IGT-2, are shown in Table 1. In the IGT group, plasma glucose levels were higher than in the normal group at every point of GTT and peaked at 197.7 mg/dl 1 h after glucose challenge, but at 30 min in

Table 1. Plasma glucose levels, IRI levels and fasting proinsulin levels by GTT results (mean ± SD).

Items	Normal	IGT-1	IGT-2	IGT
Number of cases	55	57	55	112
Plasma glucose				
Fasting PG (mg/dl)	91.7 ± 6.6	102.4 ± 9.8	107.4 ± 11.6^a	104.8 ± 11.0^d
30 min PG (mg/dl)	145.2 ± 21.8	172.8 ± 23.6	183.2 ± 28.4^a	177.9 ± 26.6^d
1 h PG (mg/dl)	127.9 ± 21.1	182.5 ± 42.5	213.3 ± 38.2^b	197.7 ± 43.2^d
2 h PG (mg/dl)	100.0 ± 16.2	153.5 ± 9.0	181.4 ± 7.8^b	167.3 ± 16.3^d
3 h PG (mg/dl)	84.8 ± 21.0	109.7 ± 24.9	115.4 ± 31.4	112.5 ± 28.4^d
IRI levels				
Fasting IRI (pmol/l)	34 ± 12	42 ± 19	46 ± 23	44 ± 21^d
30 min IRI (pmol/l)	236 ± 133	197 ± 107	190 ± 127	194 ± 117^c
1 h IRI (pmol/l)	269 ± 169	249 ± 172	272 ± 164	260 ± 169
2 h IRI (pmol/l)	161 ± 94	283 ± 142	364 ± 213^a	323 ± 185^d
3 h IRI (pmol/l)	88 ± 10	172 ± 143	210 ± 174	191 ± 160^d
Fasting proinsulin (pmol/l)	2.8 ± 0.9	3.5 ± 1.3	46 ± 23	3.6 ± 1.4^d
Fasting proinsulin/IRI (%)	9.4 ± 4.6	9.4 ± 4.5	9.6 ± 4.4	9.5 ± 4.5

Significant difference between IGT-1 and IGT-2 groups: $^a p<0.05$; $^b p<0.001$. Significant difference between normal and IGT groups: $^c p<0.05$; $^d p<0.001$. IGT-1 are cases with 2-h plasma glucose levels at GTT under 170 mg/dl. IGT-2 are cases with 2 h plasma glucose levels at GTT 170 mg/dl or more.

the normal group, the level was 145.2 mg/dl. IRI levels were lower in the IGT group 30 min after glucose challenge, 194 pmol/l as opposed to 236 pmol/l in the normal; but IRI levels peaked at 2 h in the IGT and at 1 h in the normal. At 2 and 3 h fasting, IRI levels were significantly higher in the IGT. Thus IRI response at GTT in the IGT group showed a delayed hyperresponse. The IGT group was divided into two groups using 2 h plasma glucose levels. Comparing IGT-1 (2 h PG $<$ 170 mg/dl) and IGT-2 (2 h PG $\geqslant$ 170 mg/dl) groups, plasma glucose levels were higher in the latter than in the former at every point of GTT, and higher 2 h IRI levels were observed in IGT-2.

Fasting IRI, proinsulin and the ratio of proinsulin to IRI levels are compared in the IGT groups and the normal groups. Fasting IRI was 44 in the IGT and 34 pmol/l in the normal group; proinsulin was 3.6 and 2.8 pmol/l. Fasting IRI and proinsulin were significantly higher in the IGT group. The proinsulin/IRI ratio was 9.6% in the IGT and 9.4% in the normal, no difference being observed in the two groups. The fasting IRI, proinsulin and the proinsulin/IRI ratio were compared in the IGT-1 and IGT-2 groups. IRI and proinsulin levels were higher in IGT-1 and IGT-2 groups than in the normal group, and no difference in proinsulin levels was observed between the IGT-1 and the IGT-2. There was no difference in the proinsulin/IRI ratio among the normal, IGT-1 and IGT-2 groups.

Comparison of plasma glucose levels, IRI levels and proinsulin and the ratio of proinsulin to IRI between the obese and nonobese groups.

Subjects were divided into nonobese (BMI $<$ 25 kg/m^2) and obese (BMI $\geqslant$ 25 kg/m^2) groups. In the normal group, there were 45 nonobese cases and 10 obese cases, and in the IGT group, 81 and 31 cases, in the IGT-1, 39 and 18, in the IGT-2, 42 and 13 cases, respectively. Among the normal GTT subjects, fasting IRI in the obese group was 40, a value significantly higher than the 32 pmol/l in the nonobese. In both groups, fasting proinsulin was the same, 2.8 pmol/l. The ratio of proinsulin to IRI was 6.7% in the obese group, significantly lower than the 9.6% in the nonobese group. Nevertheless, there was no difference in plasma glucose levels at GTT between the two groups.

For the IGT group, fasting IRI in the obese patients was 58 and 39 pmol/l in the nonobese patients. Proinsulin levels were 4.3 and 3.3 pmol/l, respectively, both values being significantly higher in the obese group. Nevertheless, the proinsulin/IRI ratio was 8.2% in the obese group, a significantly lower rate than the 9.9% in the nonobese group.

In nonobese cases, fasting IRI levels were 32 pmol/l in the normal and 39 pmol/l in the IGT groups. Proinsulin was 2.8 and 3.3 pmol/l, respectively. The values were significantly higher in the IGT. No difference was observed in the proinsulin/IRI ratio between the two groups. In obese cases, fasting IRI was 58 pmol/l in the IGT group, a value significantly higher than the 40 pmol/l in the normal. Also, proinsulin levels were 4.3 and 2.8 pmol/l, respectively, significantly higher values being observed in the IGT. There was no difference between the two groups in the ratio of proinsulin to IRI.

No difference was observed in the fasting IRI, proinsulin and the proinsulin/IRI ratio between the IGT-1 and IGT-2 groups (Table 2).

Discussion

The prevalence of diabetes mellitus in Japan has increased rapidly, now reaching 10% in the population over 40 years old. Early detection of diabetes mellitus is very important to prevent diabetic complications. This study was made to clarify

Table 2. Comparison of plasma glucose levels, IRI levels and fasting proinsulin levels between obese and nonobese groups by GTT results (mean ± SD).

Items	Normal	IGT-1	IGT-2	IGT
Nonobese cases	45	39	42	81
Plasma glucose				
Fasting PG (mg/dl)	92.1± 6.8	101.7 ± 9.3	106.4 ± 11.5[d]	104.2 ± 10.8[c]
30 min PG (mg/dl)	145.0 ± 22.7	172.8 ± 23.2	182.0 ± 27.7	177.7 ± 26.1[c]
1 h PG (mg/dl)	127.7 ± 21.4	177.4 ± 43.8	212.0 ± 32.8[f]	195.8 ± 42.1[c]
2 h PG (mg/dl)	98.1 ± 17.0	152.8 ± 9.1	181.2 ± 7.2[f]	167.9 ± 16.4[c]
3 h PG (mg/dl)	84.9 ± 20.4	110.0 ± 25.4	117.7 ± 32.0	114.1 ± 29.3[c]
IRI levels				
Fasting IRI (pmol/l)	32 ± 12	37 ± 14	40 ± 18	39 ± 16[b]
30 min IRI (pmol/l)	230 ± 136	203 ± 113	169 ± 126	185 ± 121
1 h IRI (pmol/l)	255 ± 166	222 ± 148	234 ± 130	228 ± 139
2 h IRI (pmol/l)	146 ± 82	253 ± 102	318 ± 214	287 ± 174[c]
3 h IRI (pmol/l)	81 ± 62	151 ± 104	196 ± 175	175 ± 148[c]
Fasting proinsulin (pmol/l)	2.8 ± 0.9	3.2 ± 1.1	3.5 ± 1.1	3.3 ± 1.1[b]
Fasting proinsulin/IRI (%)	9.6 ± 3.9	9.6 ± 4.7	10.0 ± 4.8	9.9 ± 4.7
Obese cases	10	18	13	31
Plasma glucose				
Fasting PG (mg/dl)	90.2 ± 5.4	103.8 ± 10.9	110.5 ± 11.1	106.6 ± 11.4[c]
30 min PG (mg/dl)	145.8 ± 17.7	172.2 ± 25.0	187.1 ± 30.5	178.5 ± 28.4[c]
1 h PG (mg/dl)	128.8 ± 19.8	195.4 ± 36.9	217.3 ± 51.9	204.6 ± 45.1[c]
2 h PG (mg/dl)	108.3 ± 7.2	155.4 ± 8.6	181.5 ± 9.5[f]	166.4 ± 15.7[c]
3 h PG (mg/dl)	84.7 ± 23.5	107.7 ± 23.8	107.9 ± 28.0	107.8 ± 25.7[c]
IRI levels				
Fasting IRI (pmol/l)	40 ± 5[k]	52 ± 25[g]	67 ± 25[k]	58 ± 26[ck]
30 min IRI (pmol/l)	260 ± 117	175 ± 82	260 ± 105[h]	211 ± 102
1 h IRI (pmol/l)	328 ± 172	302 ± 208	399 ± 196[h]	343 ± 208[h]
2 h IRI (pmol/l)	224 ± 113[g]	346 ± 189[g]	518 ± 115[ek]	418 ± 183[ck]
3 h IRI (pmol/l)	117 ± 93	211 ± 195	256 ± 163	230 ± 184[b]
Fasting proinsulin (pmol/l)	2.8 ± 0.9	3.9 ± 1.5	4.8 ± 1.8[h]	4.3 ± 1.7[ch]
Fasting proinsulin/IRI (%)	6.7 ± 2.0[k]	8.6 ± 3.8	7.6 ± 2.3[h]	8.2 ± 3.3[g]

Significant difference between normal and IGT groups: [a]$p < 0.05$; [b]$p < 0.01$; [c]$p < 0.001$. Significant difference between IGT-1 and IGT-2 groups: [d]$p < 0.05$; [e]$p < 0.01$; [f]$p < 0.001$. Significant difference between nonobese and obese groups: [g]$p < 0.05$; [h]$p < 0.01$; [k]$p < 0.001$.

whether or not proinsulin can be used as a predictor of diabetes mellitus. The proinsulin/IRI ratio shows a pancreas β-cell function. IGT cases have a high development rate of diabetes mellitus, and because IGT constitutes the hyperglycemic group closest to diabetes mellitus, IGT cases possibly have β-cell dysfunction. However, although there are many papers on diabetic cases, few data are available on IGT cases. Since prevalence of IGT is more than 2—3 times higher than that of diabetes mellitus, it is very hard to follow all IGT cases. In the IGT group in this study, cases with 2-h plasma glucose levels of 170 mg/dl or more (IGT-2), have a 3 times higher rate of development of diabetes mellitus than those in the IGT-1 group in the short term. We reported at the 15th IDF in Kobe that the IGT-2 was a high-risk group for diabetes mellitus, for which more careful follow-up observations were needed. It is efficient to detect high-risk groups and intervene in the development of diabetes mellitus before onset. Therefore, this study was undertaken to determine whether proinsulin can be used as a predictor or not. A RIA method of proinsulin measurement cross-reacted with Des 65,66 human proinsulin, but Des 32,33 was very weak. Thus, these proinsulin levels were lower than with the use of other specific antibodies. As we mentioned before, cross-reactivity with other pancreatic hormones was very low. In fasting levels in the normal group, proinsulin and the conversion intermediate to IRI have each been estimated to account for some 10% of the total insulin-related material. This percentage coincides with our data, and no relationship among grades of glucose intolerance was observed. Kahn et al. reported that for the ratio of proinsulin to IRI, the ratio of cases who developed diabetes mellitus was higher than that of those who did not in the IGT group at initial test [2]. Nevertheless, differing results have also been reported [3,4]. Our data was from a cross-sectional study, but our subjects included many different grades of glucose intolerance. IGT-2 group was the hyperglycemic group closest to diabetes mellitus, but the proinsulin/IRI ratio was no different from the normal and the IGT-1 group. These differing results are attributable to different proinsulin RIA methods and subjects, therefore further investigation is needed with long follow-up observation of many cases.

As regards the difference between the nonobese and the obese cases, Shiraishi et al. reported that the proinsulin/IRI ratio depends only on the grade of glucose intolerance [5]. We found that in obese cases fasting proinsulin levels were higher than in nonobese cases, but the ratio was lower in the obese cases of the normal group and in the IGT group. Regardless of the fact that both IGT-1 and IGT-2 had a high development rate of diabetes mellitus, the proinsulin/IRI ratio was the same. These results were different from other papers, but as the number of obese subjects was small, further investigation with a large number of subjects is necessary. Our results underline the difficulty of using proinsulin as a predictor of development of diabetes mellitus. However, since no pancreas β-cell dysfunction was observed in either the IGT group or the IGT-2 group, it would be possible to decrease the pancreas β-cell load in the IGT-1 and the IGT-2 stages through effective lifestyle guidance.

Conclusions

1. Fasting IRI and proinsulin were higher in the IGT than in the normal group, but there was no difference in the proinsulin/IRI ratio.
2. In the IGT group, fasting IRI and proinsulin were higher in the obese patients than in the nonobese patients. But the ratio of proinsulin to IRI was lower in the obese patients. In the normal group, IRI was higher and the ratio was significantly lower in the obese patients than in the nonobese patients.
3. The IGT-2 group tended toward higher fasting IRI and proinsulin levels, but no difference in proinsulin/IRI ratio was seen.

These data suggested that β-cell function of IGT and IGT-2 were normal, based on the proinsulin/IRI ratio. As it is not clear whether proinsulin levels or proinsulin/IRI ratio can be used as predictors of diabetes mellitus, further investigation is needed.

References

1. Watanabe Y, Horie H, Hata K, Oono T, Tomono S, Kawazu T. Established RIA method of proinsulin and its clinical evaluation. Peptide Hormones in Pancreas 1993;13:69–73.
2. Kahn SE, Leonetti DL, Prigeon RL, Boyko EJ, Bergstrom RW, Fujimoto WY. Proinsulin as a marker for the development of NIDDM in Japanese-American men. Diabetes 1995;44: 173–179.
3. Haffner SM, Bowsher RR, Mykkanen L, Hazuda HP, Mitchell BD, Valdez RA, Gingerich R, Monterossa A, Stern MP. Proinsulin and specific insulin concentration in high- and low-risk populations for NIDDM. Diabetes 1994;43:1490–1493.
4. Saad MF, Kahn SE, Nelson RG, Pettitt DJ, Knowler WC, Schwarz MW, Kowalyk S, Bennett PH, Porte D Jr. Disproportionately elevated proinsulin in Pima Indians with non-insulin-dependent diabetes mellitus. J Clin Endocrinol Metab 1990;70:1247–1253.
5. Shiraishi I, Iwamoto Y, Kuzuya T, Matsuda A, Kumakura S. Hyperinsuliaemia in obesity is not accompanied by an increase in serum proinsulin/insulin ratio in groups of human subjects with and without glucose intolerance. Diabetologia 1991;34:737–741.

Diabetes education

Recent Advances on the Pathogenesis and Management of Diabetes Mellitus.
S.H. Shinn, M. Shichiri and K.-W. Kim, editors.

Self-assessment of the capability for patient education in diabetes clinics

Takayuki Asahina[1], Yoshihito Atsumi[1], Kazuhiro Hosokawa[1], Akira Shimada[1], Atsuko Mokubo[1] and Kempei Matsuoka[2]
[1]Saiseikai Central Hospital; and [2]Saiseikai Diabetes Center, Tokyo, Japan

Abstract. In order to elucidate an actual state of patient education and its infrastructure, or the influence of the number of outpatients, a survey with questionnaires at 508 clinics that contained a diabetic department was conducted in Japan. Most of the clinics assessed themselves to be adequate in the basic concept of diabetes education. However, in the long-term perspective, it looked obscure due to an increase in the number of beds. The higher the number of outpatients, the more necessary it is to hold clinical conferences including paramedical staff. The educators' activity itself is not properly assessed in general. Furthermore, the assignment of nurses does not seem to be satisfied by the doctors, and this is more significant in larger hospitals. The adequate existence of training staff is significantly correlated with the number of outpatients, however, it is not correlated with the size of the hospitals. The consolidated annual budget for training subspecialty staff tends to depend on the number of outpatients, however, it also tends to decrease according to the number of inpatients. The training of diabetes educators is preferably to be implemented in clinics which have a larger number of diabetic outpatients.

Keywords: diabetes educator, infrastructure, patient education.

Background

Patient education is essential for diabetic management, as strict metabolic control is recognized for preventing dreadful diabetic complications. Diabetes is a unique chronic disease which needs close alliance between patients and health professionals, who are well-trained in educational methods and psychology as well as in medical knowledge, in order to assess motivation for the best possible compliance for the treatment. Unfortunately, in Japan there are still lots of bottlenecks to overcome in order to provide appropriate patient education.

Methods

In order to elucidate an actual state of patient education and its infrastructure in Japan, a series of questionnaires consisting of 110 questions which concerned the factors surrounding diabetes primary care, was sent to 1,001 facilities which treated diabetics. 508 named responses among 543 responses in total were analyzed. Answers were given by the following five scores according to their self-

---

Address for correspondence: Takayuki Asahina, Saiseikai Central Hospital, 1-4-17 Mita, Minato-ku, Tokyo 108, Japan.

assessment: 5 means a very adequate existence or very active performance, 4: appropriate, 3: uncertain, 2: not appropriate, 1: no or none. The percentage of the hospitals and clinics responded as a very adequate existence or very active performance and "appropriate" as shown in the figures.

The clinics were classified into three groups according to the number of patients followed at outpatient clinics (1: under 500, 2: 501 ~ 1,000, 3: over 1,001) and four groups according to the number of the beds in the hospital (5: under 200, 6: 201 ~ 500, 7: over 501). Afterwards, we investigated the relationship between the answers and the number of the patients, followed by the number of the beds.

Results

Concerning the basic concept of diabetes education and its infrastructure, most clinics assessed themselves to have the basic concept of diabetes education, and there are no differences between groups (72 ~ 91%). However, in the the long-term perspective, clinics without inpatients were found to be the best, and it became obscured with the increasing number of beds (Fig. 1). They have a negative attitude toward charging the tuition fee for their educational program and educational admission, and for an outpatient diabetes course (2 ~ 20% and

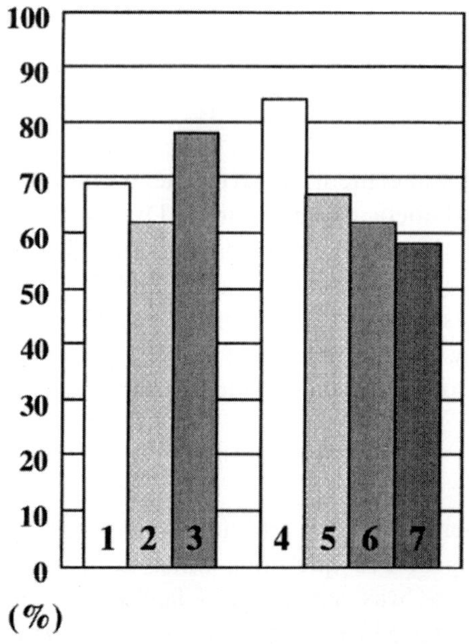

Fig. 1. Clinical conference with comedicals. The percentage of the hospitals and clinics responded as "a very adequate existence or a very active performance" and were "appropriate". The column numbers mean: 1—3 is a number of followed-up outpatients (1: under 500, 2: 501 ~ 1,000, 3: over 1,001), and 4—7 is the number of beds (4: none, 5: under 200, 6: 201 ~ 500, 7: over 501).

17 ~ 25%, respectively), and to expect economic bases from diabetes education (7 ~ 14%).

The percentage of a clinical conference, including paramedical staff, was rather low as shown in Fig. 2, and the result of education was poorly assessed for further strategy (30 ~ 63%, the proportion of each group resembles Fig. 2).

The educators' activity itself is not properly assessed in their personnel evaluation in general (10 ~ 16%, except 33% of group 4). The assignment of nurses does not seem to be satisfied by doctors (17 ~ 31%), and this is more significant among larger sized hospitals (31, 30, 24 and 17% of group 4, 5, 6 and 7, respectively).

Interest in the training of staff is significantly correlated with the number of outpatients (Fig. 3), however, it is interesting to see that it has nothing to do with the size of hospitals. The consolidated annual budget for training subspecialty staff slightly depends on the number of outpatients, however, it tends to decrease according to the number of inpatients (22, 21, 10 and 13% of group 4, 5, 6 and 7, respectively).

Discussion

As for the long-term perspective, clinics without inpatients were found to be the best, and it became obscured with the increasing number of beds. Furthermore, in large-scale general hospitals, they have difficulties in changing the system

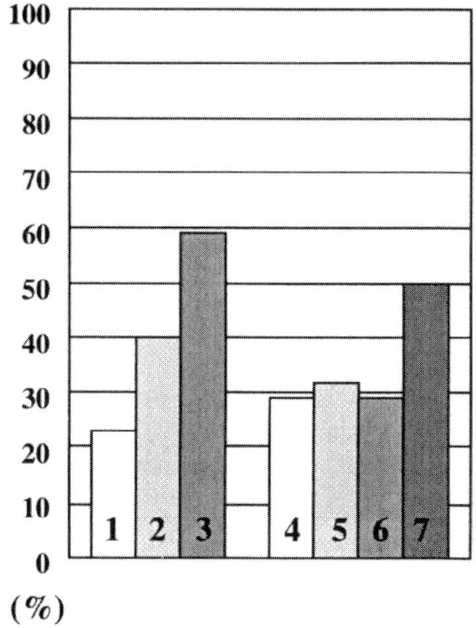

Fig. 2. Patient education in administrative scheme. For percentages and other data see Fig. 1.

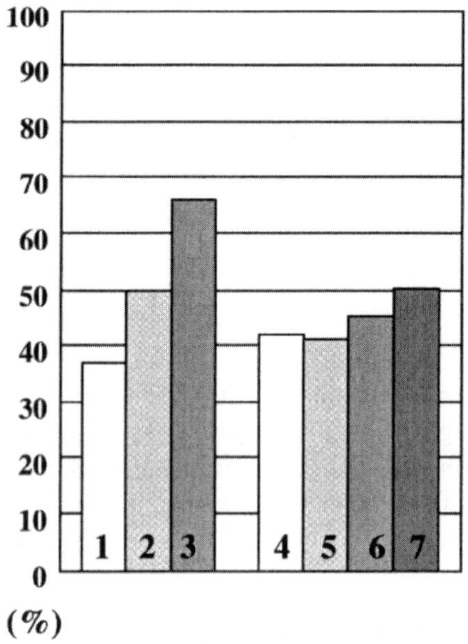

Fig. 3. Training for diabetic specialty. For percentages and other data see Fig. 1.

exclusively for a single section – a diabetes department. Moreover, educators' activity itself is not properly assessed, and the assignment of nurses does not seem to be satisfied by doctors, especially in larger sized hospitals. This is probably because of two reasons. Firstly, the request from one section cannot always be reflected in total administration. Secondly, in general they have the idea that nurses should have broad basic knowledge by rotation. To be a good nurse in Japan: this idea is the major substance in the way of educating specialists and causes inadequate positioning of potential nurses.

Concerning the quality of diabetes education and training educators, we found that the more outpatients there are, the more necessary it is to hold clinical conferences, and the larger sized hospitals (those with 500 beds or more) seem to have higher percentages because they may be licensed or certified educational hospitals, and have sufficient training systems not only in diabetes departments but also in other sections. However, these findings tell us that an infrastructure for training diabetes educators is not complete in larger sized hospitals.

In general, it is somehow believed by administrators that diabetes clinics are not a financially profitable division compared with other departments such as the cardiovascular or the oncology sections. It appears that they show a negative attitude toward expecting economic bases from diabetes education. However, without charge for education, they cannot plan to organize good educational teams to provide high-quality patient education, and they remain unchanged in empowerment. It appears to be a vicious circle. In Japan, the JDS (Japan Diabetic Society) and Ministry of Health and Welfare have recently emphasized the importance of primary care of diabetes in order to eliminate the total medical budget to spend an enormous amount of money for the treatment of complications. Although this idea is gradually accepted among administrations, it is not yet apparent in this survey. The cost performance of diabetes education must be further taken into consideration.

Conclusion

1. Understanding the importance of diabetes education is proportionately higher in hospitals or clinics which have a larger number of outpatients.
2. It is difficult to change the infrastructure by establishing the diabetes department as a single section in larger hospitals which hold many inpatients.
3. There are difficulties in alternating management for the sake of a single section (diabetes clinic) in hospitals holding a higher numbers of beds.
4. Although large hospitals have an excellent training system for paramedical staff, budget and training exclusively reserved for diabetes subspecialties remain incomplete.
5. From the above we can see that training of diabetes educators is preferably to be implemented in large-scale general hospitals, however, it is also desirable to choose clinics which have a large number of diabetic outpatients.

Recent Advances on the Pathogenesis and Management of Diabetes Mellitus.
S.H. Shinn, M. Shichiri and K.-W. Kim, editors.

Dietary habits in Korean type II diabetic patients

Sunmin Park[1], Eui Kwang Choi[1] and Soo Bong Choi[2]
[1]Department of Food and Nutrition, Hoseo University, Asan; and [2]Department of Internal Medicine, KunKok University, Chungjoo, Korea

Abstract. *Background.* Diet therapy is one of the most important methods of controlling blood glucose concentrations (BGC) in type II diabetic patients. A proper diet therapy should be reflected in dietary habits. The purpose of this study was to determine whether diabetic patients have a reasonable knowledge of diet therapy, and whether they have proper dietary intakes and dietary habits to maintain optimal BGC.

Methods. 150 type II diabetic patients with over 165 mg/dl of fasting BGC were interviewed prior to hospitalization. Questionnaires included recent weight change, income, education, diabetic duration, family history, lifestyles, diet therapy, folk therapy, and food consumption.

Results. Their diabetic history ranged from 3 months to 30 years (8.6 ± 5.8). Although the average of BMI was in the normal range, over 25% of the patients had a lower than normal BMI. Sixty-three percent of them were on the diet therapy, but only 25.3% of them performed it in the correct manner, even though they had received education about diet therapy. About 82% of the patients just tried to eat less foods and avoid sweets. However, they had snacks such as fruits, cookies and bread, at least once a day. Diet therapy showed a weak negative correlation to the prevalence of diabetic complications. According to dietary recall, the patients consumed daily 1,514 ± 573.5 kcal, composed of carbohydrates (68.6%), proteins (15.9%) and fats (15.4%). The caloric intake of almost all patients was below the RDA. Also, the quality and quantity of protein consumed was insufficient. This resulted from the consumption of less meals and more snacks.

Conclusion. Type II diabetic patients need better education of diet therapy to control BGC and to improve their health.

Keywords: diabetic complications, diet therapy, nutrient intakes, lifestyles.

Introduction

As the Korean economy has improved since the 1980s, the prevalence of type II diabetes has remarkably increased [1]. Type II diabetes mellitus is a serious and common chronic disease affecting an estimated 10% of the Korean population aged 25—75 years. The disease often leads to disability from vascular complications, including blindness, limb amputation, coronary artery disease and renal failure [2]. However, treatment is often unsuccessful in preventing these adverse outcomes. Prevention of type II diabetes may be achieved through modification of risk factors [3,4].

Most patients with type II diabetes mellitus have similar characteristics, including both insulin resistance and cell dysfunction [5]. These characteristics affect

Address for correspondence: Sunmin Park, 29-1 Sechulri Baebang-Myun Asan City, Chungnam-Do 336-795, South Korea.

glucose metabolism: the blood glucose concentration of the patients is much higher than the normal ranges. Thus, the treatment goal of type II diabetes is to achieve near normal or normal blood glucose levels. To maintain normal glucose levels, patients require comprehensive training in self-management modifying lifestyles. Self-management programs include the following components:

1) frequent self monitoring of blood glucose;
2) proper meal planning;
3) regular exercise;
3) insulin therapy; and
4) oral glucose lowering agent [6,7].

The patients should understand these self-management programs well, so that they can implement them in their life. Proper meal planning and regular exercise are important to assist the control of blood glucose levels. Most patients with type II diabetes had diet therapy (lifestyles) education, but simple diet education cannot fundamentally change dietary habits. Each patient modifies the diet therapy in their own way. The patient thinks that they follow the diet therapy correctly. However, this is not usually the case. Therefore, in the present study, we sought to:

1. Define the lifestyles and dietary habits of uncontrolled type II diabetes patients.
2. Ascertain whether dietary patterns and methods of diet therapy influence the prevalence of diabetic complications.
3. Determine the relations among diabetic conditions, lifestyles and dietary consumption patterns in type II diabetic patients.

Materials and Methods

Subjects

The subjects were 150 type II diabetic patients hospitalized in the Diabetic Center at KunKook University, Chungjoo. Prior to hospitalization, their fasting blood glucose levels were above 180 mg/dl, which means the blood glucose levels were not controlled, even though most of them were on treatments of insulin therapy, oral glucose lowering agent, diet therapy and exercise.

The survey period was from October 1996 to March 1997. The surveys were performed by well-trained interviewers. To determine how lifestyles and dietary habits would affect the control of blood glucose levels and the prevalence of diabetic complications, survey questionnaires were answered prior to hospitalization.

Measures

Risk factor assessment

Risk factor data for type II diabetes was collected prior to hospitalization. General characteristics which can influence controlling blood glucose levels were surveyed. These included weight, body mass index, recent weight change, income, education, duration of diabetes and family history. Medical doctors determined the diagnosis of diabetic complications. The survey was composed of questions about lifestyles, such as smoking, drinking, snacking, exercising, diet therapy, and folk therapy.

Assessment of nutrient intakes

A comprehensive dietary behavior assessment prior to hospitalization consisted of a 24-h recall, semiquantitative food frequency questionnaire, and food habit questionnaire. The 24-h recall was performed by a trained nutritionist. Food portion sizes were determined using a food model to help respondents report portions of foods consumed. The nutrient intakes were analyzed by data from 24-h recalls using the Food Processor II computer program. Daily nutrient intake was calculated based on the US Department of Agriculture nutrient database modified for Korean foods using food composition tables from the Department of Korean Agricultures. Food frequency data was collected from the questionnaires containing 30 food items. The questionnaires included a portion size of each food item and the number of the food items consumed.

Statistical analysis

Descriptive statistics, including means and percentage, were computed for age categories ($30 \leqslant$ age < 50, $50 \leqslant$ age < 70 and age $\geqslant 70$) diabetic complication (yes/no), and method of diet therapy (proper or improper method). Means in different categories were compared by multiple comparison by Tukey test using the SAS statistical package. Frequencies in different categories were compared by the χ^2 test. To determine the relationships among diabetic conditions, lifestyles and dietary consumption, Pearson's correlation coefficients were calculated. The significance level was set at $\alpha = 0.05$.

Results

Characteristics of lifestyles and food consumption relative to age categories

Table 1 presents the characteristics of subjects. The mean body mass index of patients was in the normal range. Most patients had lost weight since the diagnosis of type II diabetes. Huh et al. reported that these characteristics in Korean patients were different from those of type II diabetes in Western countries [8,9]. Type II diabetic patients in Korea radically lost weight at the onset of diabetes. About half of the patients aged less than 70 years had a family history of diabetes and/or other metabolic syndrome X. This syndrome included hypertension, coronary heart disease, obesity, and hypercholesterolemia. However, the patients over 70 years had a family history less than 10%. This may be due to early death of the patients with family history. Averaged duration of diabetes of the subjects was over 6 years. Patients over 50 years old had more diabetic complications.

Table 1. Characteristics of subjects.

	Age category		
	$30 \leqslant$ age < 50	$50 \leqslant$ age < 70	age $\geqslant 70$
Sample size	48	97	5
Weight (kg)	58.9 ± 11.0^a	58.6 ± 8.7	60.7 ± 4.3
Body mass index (kg/m^2)	22.0 ± 3.1	22.7 ± 3.5	23.0 ± 2.3
Income ($)	$1,700 \pm 780^b$	$1,500 \pm 820^{bc}$	$800 \pm 1,000^c$
Education (years)	11.3 ± 5.0	8.4 ± 4.5	7.2 ± 5.4
Diabetic history (years)	6.9 ± 4.8^d	9.3 ± 5.6^c	14.9 ± 8.2^b
Family history (%)^e	42.1	49.1	8.8
Weight change (kg)	-5.1 ± 5.7	-4.6 ± 7.8	-3.7 ± 3.8
Diabetic complications	19.4^f $(22.0)^g$	45.1 (71.9)	45.5 $(6.1)^h$

[a]Mean ± standard deviation; [b,c,d]alphabets with different superscripts are significantly different among the three age categories by Tukey tests; [e]percentage of patients with a family history of diabetes and/or other metabolic syndrome X in each age category; [f]percentage of patients in that age category that responded "yes"; [g]percentage of patients belonging to that age category from among all participants who responded "yes"; [h]the proportions of each variable are significantly different in three age categories at $\alpha = 0.01$. Without an asterisk they are not significantly different among three age categories at $\alpha = 0.05$.

This is related to the fact that diabetic complications were usually revealed after 6 years of diabetic history. Since the number of patients in the category of over 70 years was small compared to other age categories, it was low to the percentage of patients belonging to that age category from among all participants who responded "yes" in patients over 70 years old.

The characteristics of lifestyles relative to age categories are shown in Table 2. More than one-third of patients had had diabetic education more than once,

Table 2. Characteristics of lifestyles relative to age categories.

	Age category		
	$30 \leqslant$ age < 50	$50 \leqslant$ age < 70	age $\geqslant 70$
Diet education	44.0^a $(32.3)^b$	35.4 (63.9)	66.7 (3.9)
Diet therapy	54.4 (33.1)	52.8 (61.6)	77.8 $(5.2)^c$
Proper diet therapy	11.5 (31.0)	2.4 (62.4)	7.7 (6.6)
Folk therapy	46.7 (30.8)	32.5 (63.1)	33.3 (6.2)
Exercise	28.6 (33.8)	33.9 (59.9)	23.1 (6.3)
Smoke	15.9 (31.8)	24.0 (62.7)	33.3 (5.5)
Drink	14.3 (37.8)	32.5 (57.4)	40.0^d (4.9)
Snack	47.5 (35.9)	67.7 (58.2)	60.0 (5.9)

[a]Percentage of patients in that age category who responded "yes"; [b]percentage of patients belonging to that age category from among all participants who responded "yes"; [c]the proportions of each variable are significantly different in three age categories at $\alpha = 0.05$; [d]the proportions of each variable are significantly different in three age categories at $\alpha = 0.01$. Without an asterisk the proportions of each variable are not significantly different in three age categories at $\alpha = 0.05$.

and over half of them were on diet therapy. However, this is crucial since less than 10% of patients performed proper diet therapy in all age categories. Proper diet therapy is defined as a desirable caloric intake and a proper consumption of carbohydrates, protein and minerals using food exchange system. Most patients only follow whatever diet therapy they can easily apply into their everyday lives, such as the consumption of rice with other grains, small meals with snacks, and avoiding sweets. The diabetic patients believed that these were correct and effective methods. Nevertheless, they did not understand the diet therapy well; they did not consume candy since they avoided consuming sweets, but they ate cookies. More than one-third of the patients used folk therapy, such as consuming silk protein, but none received any beneficial effects from folk therapy. More than half of the patients ate snacks because they were instructed to consume smaller meals more frequently and having snacks between meals. Having snacks is not a bad idea for controlling blood glucose levels. However, snacks usually contain sugar and fats, which are harmful for diabetes. Thus, they needed a better education about diet therapy, and the education should be easily applicable to the patients' everyday lifestyles.

Table 3 shows the frequency of food consumption relative to age categories. There were no significant differences of various food groups among the three age categories. As the patients became older, their food consumption patterns seemed to improve; the elderly consumed more vegetables, fruits, and fish, and consumed less fatty foods, fried foods, meats, oils and fats, and ice cream. The patients' nutrient intakes were not significantly different among the three age categories.

Table 4 presents the relationship between the general characteristics of the patients' lifestyles and food consumption. Correlation data gave a similar explanation of the mean and frequency data. Age was positively correlated to the fre-

Table 3. Frequency of food consumption relative to age categories.[a,b]

	Age category		
	$30 \leqslant \text{age} < 50$	$50 \leqslant \text{age} < 70$	$\text{age} \geqslant 70$
Fast foods	6.9 ± 2.5^a	3.2 ± 3.7	0 ± 0^b
Fried foods	2.5 ± 3.7	1.8 ± 4.0	0 ± 0
Meats	13.4 ± 12.3	9.6 ± 12.8	6.0 ± 9.2
Fish	26.8 ± 18.5	22.6 ± 22.7	24.0 ± 23.1
Vegetable oil	23.5 ± 18.7	17.1 ± 12.9	18.0 ± 18.7
Animal fat	3.0 ± 1.0	4.0 ± 1.3	2.0 ± 3.0
Fruits	39.9 ± 22.2	47.0 ± 41.1	60.0 ± 33.7
Vegetables	25.5 ± 23.7	29.9 ± 25.7	42.0 ± 28.0
Ice cream	7.6 ± 13.8	3.0 ± 7.8	0.0 ± 0.0
Nuts	17.4 ± 9.1	15.4 ± 8.5	23.0 ± 7.9

[a]Mean ± standard deviation; [b]without an asterisk there are not significantly different among three age categories at $\alpha = 0.05$.

Table 4. Correlation among diabetic conditions, lifestyles and dietary consumption patterns.

	Smoke amount	Drink amount	# of snack	Protein intake	CHO[a] intake	# of exercise[b]	Activity[c]	Diet therapy[d]	Folk therapy[e]
Age	−0.05[f]	−0.01	0.15	0.41[g]	−0.34	0.27[g]	0.09	−0.15	0.15
Body mass index	0.04[g]	0.11	−0.11	−0.09	0.27	−0.01	0.01	0.06	0.03
Weight change	−0.09	−0.3[g]	0.05	0.09	−0.02	−0.09	−0.03	0.22[g]	−0.10
Diabetic complication	−0.01	0.27	0.03	0.08	0.03	−0.01	−0.15	0.12	0.03
Diabetic history	0.17	0.13	0.09	0.16	−0.04	0.01	0.04	−0.21	0.13

[a]Carbohydrate; [b]indicative variable: 1 = yes; 0 = no; [c]indicative variable: 1 = sedentary; 2 = light; 3 = moderate; 4 = hard; [d]indicative variable: 1 = proper way of diet therapy; 2 = improper way of diet therapy; [e]indicative variable: 1 = yes; 0 = no; [f]Pearson's correlation coefficient; [g]significantly correlated between two variables at $\alpha = 0.05$.

quency of exercise; the elderly patients exercised more than the young. The duration of diabetes was negatively correlated to the proper diet therapy. The patients with longer duration of diabetes performed diet therapy more improperly than those with a shorter duration. The diabetic complication was positively correlated to amount of drinking.

Characteristics of lifestyles and food consumption relative to diabetic complication

About 52% of subjects had more than one diabetic complication. The complications of diabetes are classified as microangiopathy such as retinopathy, nephropathy, neuropathy, and macroangiopathy, such as cardiovascular diseases. In our data, about 78% of patients with diabetic complications had microangiopathy, while the other 22% had macroangiopathy. Since some of the patients had more than one complication, it is difficult to calculate a separate percentage of patients with retinopathy, neuropathy, and nephropathy. About 17% of patients with diabetic complications had nephropathy. Most of the patients with diabetic complications had retinopathy and/or neuropathy.

We determined whether lifestyles and other characteristics of patients with diabetic complications were different from those without diabetic complications (Table 5). Patients with diabetic complications had a longer diabetic history than others. The prevalence of diabetic complications was influenced by improper diet therapy and the number of cigarettes smoked per day. Patients without complications performed diet therapy more properly, they smoked fewer cigarettes, and they ate no snacks. Although small meals and snacks between meals were recommended for the diabetic patients, patients who ate more snacks revealed diabetic complications. This phenomenon demonstrated that the problem was 2-

Table 5. Characteristics of lifestyles relative to diabetic complications.

	Diabetic complications	
	Yes	No
Sample size	78	72
Body mass index	22.7 ± 3.4[a]	22.5 ± 3.1
Diabetic history (years)	10.6 ± 3.8	6.9 ± 3.4[b]
Weight change (kg)	−4.6 ± 8.1	−5.2 ± 6.5
Proper diet therapy	8.3[c] (22.2)[d]	15.9 (77.8)[e]
Smoke (%)	21.6 (61.1)	61.1 (38.9)
Smoke amount (cigarette/day)	16 ± 3	13 ± 3[e*]
Drink (%)	30.4 (54.2)	35.4 (45.8)
Drink amount (cup)	9.6 ± 9.0	5.1 ± 5.9
Exercise (%)	29.3 (47.3)	70.7 (52.7)
Snack (%)	64.6 (54.8)	35.4 (45.2)[e*]

[a]Mean ± standard deviation; [b]significantly different between two groups at $\alpha = 0.05$. Without an asterisk there are not significantly different among diabetic complication categories at $\alpha = 0.05$; [c]percentage of patients in that diabetic complication categories that responded "yes"; [d]percentage of patients belonging to that diabetic complication categories from among all participants who responded "yes"; [e]the proportions of each variable are significantly different in two diabetic complication categories at $\alpha = 0.05$. Without an asterisk the proportions of each variable are not significantly different between diabetic complication categories at $\alpha = 0.05$.

fold: the education was not properly taught, nor was it fully understood. While patients learned to consume smaller meals more frequently and to have snacks, they did not understand the proper recommended types of snacks. They consumed ramien, cookies, and fried foods as snacks. Even though patients consumed smaller meals, the kinds and amounts of snacks consumed were counterproductive for controlling blood glucose levels.

From food frequency data, there were no significant differences of consumption of various foods between patients with and without complications (Table 6). Patients without complications tended to consume less meats, ice cream, and fast foods (such as pizza, hamburgers and ramien), compared to those with diabetic complications. However, patients without diabetic complications seemed to consume more oils and fats, and nuts. These differences were very minimal.

Patients with and without diabetic complications consumed daily similar amounts of each nutrient (Table 7). Most patients consumed lower caloric intakes than the Recommended Daily Allowances (RDA) by 200–300 kcal per day, which is recommended for obese diabetic patients to lose weight in Western countries [3]. However, in Korea the body weight of most patients ranged from normal to under normal, and they did not need to cut caloric intake. Concurrently, calorie and fat intakes tended to be a little less in patients with diabetic complications. The patients consumed 68.5 energy% (en%) of carbohydrates, 15.5 en% of protein and 16 en% of fat [6,7]. The proportion of carbohydrates was higher than the American Diabetes Association (ADA) recommendation, but this may

Table 6. Frequency of food consumption relative to diabetic complications. (Number of serving consumed per 1 week.)

	Diabetic complications	
	Yes	No
Fast foods	7.1 ± 10.2[a]	4.6 ± 8.9[b]
Fried foods	3.6 ± 9.0	3.5 ± 8.5
Meats	12.8 ± 13.6	9.5 ± 9.3
Fish	24.7 ± 13.6	23.1 ± 17.9
Vegetable oil	17.5 ± 17.8	20.1 ± 32.0
Animal fat	2.2 ± 6.9	4.8 ± 19.2
Fruits	35.7 ± 39.3	34.4 ± 37.8
Vegetables	27.9 ± 29.7	30.8 ± 33.6
Ice cream	10.3 ± 26.0	5.0 ± 17.7
Nuts	10.9 ± 22.1	14.0 ± 25.0

[a]Mean ± standard deviation; [b]without an asterisk they are not significantly different between diabetic complication categories at $\alpha = 0.05$.

be more reasonable for the Korean diet. The proportion of protein was within the recommended range. Nevertheless, Korean diabetic patients should consume more and better quality protein. This is especially true for patients with no nephropathy. Therefore, we need to reevaluate the ADA recommendations for Korean diabetic patients.

Patients with diabetic complications tended to consumed more antioxidants (vitamin E and C), however, this was not significant. Most patients consumed less vitamin A and calcium than RDA guidelines. The lifestyles and dietary habits were not significantly different among the various diabetic complications such

Table 7. Daily nutrient intake relative to diabetic complications.

	Diabetic complications	
	Yes	No
Calories (kcal)	1614.9 ± 878.4[a]	1407.7 ± 539.8[b]
Protein (%)	15.3 ± 3.8	15.7 ± 6.0
Fat (%)	16.0 ± 6.0	14.8 ± 5.2
Saturated fat (g)	6.8 ± 7.4	6.0 ± 4.4
Polyunsaturated fat (g)	6.2 ± 5.8	4.1 ± 3.5
Carbohydrates (%)	68.6 ± 8.1	69.2 ± 9.0
Vitamin C (mg)	87.5 ± 43.7	70.5 ± 50.3
Vitamin E (IU)	6.4 ± 8.4	4.9 ± 2.9
Vitamin A (RE)	356.6 ± 55.0	375.5 ± 55.2
Calcium (mg)	461.8 ± 235.9	444.0 ± 190.5

[a]Mean ± standard deviation; [b]without an asterisk they are not significantly different between diabetic complication categories at $\alpha = 0.05$.

as retinopathy, nephropathy, neuropathy, and cardiovascular diseases. Patients with neuropathy, however, were less concerned about changing their lifestyles and dietary consumption.

Characteristics of lifestyles and food consumption relative to methods of diet therapy

Table 8 shows general characteristics and lifestyles of patients performing a proper diet therapy and those who do not. Only about 20% of the patients with diabetic complications performed diet therapy properly. The patients who followed proper diet therapy tended to lose more weight than the others. Since most of type II diabetic patients were obese in Western countries, they needed to lose weight through diet therapy [9]. However, in Korea, type II diabetic patients had a normal weight [8]. They should not lose weight by proper diet therapy. Thus, the ADA recommendations should be reevaluated for Korean diabetic patients. The patients consuming foods improperly had a longer duration of diabetes, less diabetic education, smoked more, and exercised less. However, a proper diet therapy was not associated with drinking. As duration of diabetes became longer, patients increasingly did not pay attention to diet therapy, and they followed only the diet therapy which they could carry out easily. Therefore, diabetic patients should take diabetic education regularly and continuously. Diabetic education should include how to modify their diet and lifestyle such as drinking, smoking, and exercising.

Table 9 demonstrates the frequency of food consumption between patients performing proper and improper diet therapy. The patients performing diet therapy properly consumed less fried foods and ice cream, while they tended to consume

Table 8. Characteristics of lifestyles relative to methods of diet therapy.

	Methods of diet therapy	
	Proper method	Improper method
Sample size	34	116
Age (years)	49.8 ± 13.4[a]	54.6 ± 10.2[b]
Body mass index	22.2 ± 2.1	22.8 ± 3.4
Diabetic history (years)	5.6 ± 5.4	9.6 ± 6.2
Education (years)	11.7 ± 5.0	7.7 ± 4.7
Weight change (kg)	−8.1 ± 8.3	−4.1 ± 5.4
Diabetic education (%)	17.0[c] (69.2)[d]	5.9 (30.8)
Diabetic complication (%)	8.3 (22.2)	15.9 (77.8)
Smoke (%)	11.4 (22.1)	11.9 (77.9)
Drink (%)	25.1 (45.4)	12.8 (54.6)
Exercise (%)	16.7 (60.0)	6.0 (40.0)

[a]Mean ± standard deviation; [b]without an asterisk they are not significantly different between methods of diet therapy categories at $\alpha = 0.05$; [c]percentage of patients in that methods of diet therapy categories that responded "yes"; [d]percentage of patients belonging to that methods of diet therapy categories from among all participants who responded "yes".

Table 9. Frequency of food consumption relative to methods of diet therapy. (Number of servings consumed per 1 week.)

	Methods of diet therapy	
	Proper method	Improper method
Fast foods	4.5 ± 3.9[a]	53.8 ± 5.4[b]
Fried food	0.6 ± 1.1	3.1 ± 7.5[b]*
Meats	8.8 ± 11.2	12.7 ± 13.8
Fish	31.9 ± 23.6	25.9 ± 20.9
Vegetable oil	26.7 ± 58.4	18.3 ± 17.6
Animal fat	3.8 ± 10.6	4.1 ± 16.3
Fruits	56.4 ± 50.4	34.2 ± 38.9
Vegetables	29.9 ± 26.7	28.7 ± 25.6
Ice cream	0.4 ± 0.9	7.9 ± 21.9[b]*
Nuts	26.5 ± 39.7	13.3 ± 24.0

[a]Mean ± standard deviation; [b]*Significantly different between two groups at $\alpha = 0.05$. Without an asterisk they are not significantly different between methods of diet therapy categories at $\alpha = 0.05$.

more fish, vegetable oil, fruits, and nuts.

It is our finding that diabetic complications can only be reduced if patients perform proper diet therapy including consuming fewer snacks, smoking less cigarettes, and exercising moderately. Since diabetic complications are more prevalent in patients with longer diabetic histories, and family histories of diabetes and/or metabolic syndrome X, those people need to pay attention to other risk factors (related to lifestyles) for diabetic complication.

Discussions

The prevalence of type II diabetics in Korea was 0.2% in the 1960s, but it increased to 3–4% in the 1990s. Meanwhile from Park et al. it was reported that the prevalence was remarkably high (about 7%) in Yonchon county [11]. There was a sharp increase during these 30 years even though the collection of the prevalence data had some flaws. Very little data for diabetic complications was available. Some information included data on diabetes from the Ministry of Health and Welfare [1] and the Medical Insurance Management Association [12]. This data was based on information of known diabetic patients seen by doctors, and it gave much lower estimates of prevalence than research-based studies. There is a possibility of a further increase in Korea in the future. To prevent such an increase of the prevalence of diabetes and complications, continued efforts to collect accurate data in Korea is important. Further, the proper analysis of risk factors for the increasing prevalence of diabetes and complications should be undertaken.

In Western countries, most diabetic patients are overweight [10]. Type II diabetic patients need to lose weight and their diet therapy is usually geared to consuming less calories than their energy expenditure [13]. However, the Korean diabetic patients have different characteristics [8,9,14]. They are not usually obese, and still they lose weight after getting diabetes. They do not need to lose weight, yet they do so, because their diet therapy is similar to that prescribed for diabetics in Western (overweight) countries [6,7,15]. Thus, there is the need to reevaluate the caloric needs for Korean diabetic patients. Also, the proportion of carbohydrates, protein and lipids from total caloric intakes should be reevaluated. Since Koreans consume much more carbohydrates than the Western societies, and Koreans consume protein from grains not from animal meats, the proportion of carbohydrates, protein and lipids from total caloric intakes should be different from the Western countries [16,17]. Korea needs further study on the dietary requirements of Korean diabetic patients.

The goals of the nutrition therapy for diabetes are:

1) maintenance of normal or near-normal serum glucose concentration;
2) achievement of optimal serum lipid levels;
3) provision of adequate calories for maintaining or attaining reasonable weights for adults; and
4) improvement of overall health through optimal nutrition.

Achieving nutritional goals can reduce the prevalence of diabetic complications [18,19]. To achieve these goals, patients should adhere to meal planning principles, which must be learned by diabetic patients. These principles are related to diet requirements as well as lifestyle variables, such as exercise, smoking and drinking. Our data showed that diabetic complications were related to smoking, snacking, and exercise. Other studies reported that alcohol consumption had a harmful effect on the regulation of blood glucose levels. Also, moderate exercise can improve diabetic conditions and prevent the prevalence of diabetic complications, especially cardiovascular disease, without adverse effects such as hypoglycemia, ketosis, and hyperglycemia [20,21]. It is a prerequisite that patients themselves alter eating patterns and implement new eating behaviors. Also, patients can themselves evaluate the effectiveness of their nutritional therapy. Patients should receive the education about nutritional therapy to change their diet patterns and lifestyles [13]. The education should: 1) not be abstract; 2) integrate diet therapy, exercise, and the consumption of less alcohol and cigarettes; and 3) not just give knowledge but alter patients' attitudes and behaviors.

References

1. Korean Ministry of Health and Welfare. The National Annual Statistics of Health and Welfare, 1995.
2. The DCCT Research Group. Weight gain associated with intensive therapy in Diabetes Control and Complications trials. Diabetes Care 1988;11:567–573.
3. Franz MJ, Horton ES, Bantle JP, Beebe CA, Brunzell JD, Coulston AN, Henry RR, Hoogwerf BJ, Stackpoole PW. Nutrition principles for the management of diabetes and related complications. Diabetes Care 1994;17:490–518.

4. Kuzuya T. Prevalence of diabetes mellitus in Japan compiled from literature. Diabet Res Clin Practice 1994;24:S15–S21.
5. DeFronzo RA, Bonadonna RC, Ferrannini E. Pathogenesis of NIDDM. A balanced overview. Diabetes Care 1992;15:318–355.
6. American Diabetes Association. Nutrition recommendations and principles for people with diabetes mellitus. Diabetes Care 1995;18:16–19.
7. American Diabetes Association. Standards of medical care for patients with diabetes mellitus. Diabetes Care 1995;18:8–15.
8. Huh KB. The characteristics of Korean diabetes mellitus. Kor J Diabetes 1995;19:1–4.
9. Min H. Clinical characteristics of Korean diabetes mellitus. Kor J Diabetes 1992;16:163–174.
10. Knowler WC, McCance DR, Nagi DK, Pettitt DJ. Epidemiologic studies of the causes of non-insulin-dependent diabetes mellitus. In: Leslies RDG (ed) Causes of Diabetes. Sussex, UK: Churchill Livingston, 1993;187–218.
11. Park Y, Lee H, Koh CS, Min H, Yoo K, Kim Y, Shin Y. Prevalence of diabetes and IGT in Yonchon County, South Korea. Diabetes Care 1995;18:545–549.
12. Medical Insurance Management Association. 1994 Medical Diagnosis, 1995.
13. Wing RR, Shoemarker M, Marcus MD, McDermott M, Gooding W. Variables associated with weight loss and improvements in glycemic control in type II diabetic patients in behavioral weight control programs. Int J Obes 1990;14:495–503.
14. Huh KB, Kim HM, Lim SK. Non-traditional diabetes mellitus in Korea. Kor J Int Med 1987; 33:762–770.
15. Korean Diabetes Association, Korean Dietetic Association, and Korean Nutrition Society. Diet Therapy Guidelines for Diabetes. Medical Publication, 1995.
16. US Department of Agriculture. Nationwide Food Consumption Survey of Food Intakes of Individuals 1985. Hyattsville, MD, Nutrition Monitoring Division, Human Nutrition Information Service, 1987 (Report no. 85-3).
17. Korean Ministry of Health and Welfare. '93 National Nutrition Survey Report. 1995.
18. Friedman EA. Diabetic nephropathy: strategies in prevention and management. Kidney Int 1990;38:136–144.
19. Stamler J, Vaccaro, O, Neaton JD, Wentworth D. Diabetes, other risk factors, and 12-yr cardiovascular mortality for men screened in multiple risk factor intervention trial. Diabetes Care 1993;16:434–444.
20. Bjorntorp P, de Jounge K, Sjostrom L, Sullivan L. Physical training in human obesity. II. Effects of plasma insulin in glucose-intolerant subjects without marked hyperinsulinemia. Scand J Clin Lab Invest 1973;32:41–45.
22. Eriksson K-F, Lindgarde F. Prevention of type 2 diabetes mellitus by diet and physical exercise: the 6-year Malmo feasibility study. Diabetologia 1991;34:891–898.

Recent Advances on the Pathogenesis and Management of Diabetes Mellitus.
S.H. Shinn, M. Shichiri and K.-W. Kim, editors.

Medical optical memory card system to construct a medical information network for diabetic patients

M. Nomura, M. Ohashi, Y. Yamada, T. Kamada and H. Abe
Center for Diabetes Mellitus, Osaka Rosai Hospital, Sakai, Osaka, Japan

Abstract. To treat diabetic complications properly and to improve clinical care of diabetic patients at any place they may move to, it is necessary to construct a medical information managing network among medical centers for the smooth exchange of medical information. In order to construct a medical information network, we have tried to develop and evaluate the medical optical memory card system.

Materials and Methods. The medical optical memory card system was constructed with: 1) an optical memory card (size: 54 × 85.5 mm), 2) a card reader/writer (LC-304, Conlux, Japan), 3) a personal computer, 4) a color image scanner, and 5) a printer.

In this optical memory card system, various medical records including laboratory data and imaging data (X-ray, CT, MRI, RI) can be recorded.

Results and Conclusions. The optical memory card system is useful for diabetic patient's medical information managing because of tight security of recorded data, large capacity of memory size, and high-speed reading and recording capacity. Although further studies may be necessary to improve handling of imaging data, we could construct the medical information network by this medical optical memory card system.

Keywords: medical information network, optical memory card, security.

Introduction

To improve the clinical care of diabetic patients at any place they may move to, it is necessary to develop a new device to transfer personal clinical data, and to construct a medical information network for the smooth communication between medical centers. For this purpose, we have tried to evaluate and develop the medical optical memory card (optical card) system for diabetic patients.

Method and Material

To develop a new device to transfer various clinical data, we have compared three card systems:
1) the magnetic card,
2) the IC-card, and
3) the optical card system [1].

In this study we have further evaluated the optical card system. The size of the

Address for correspondence: Makoto Nomura MD, PhD, Center for Diabetes Mellitus, Osaka Rosai Hospital, 1179-3, Nagasone-cho, Sakai, Osaka 591, Japan. E-mail: m.nomura@orh.go.jp

optical card is the same as that of a credit card. In this optical card, a recording layer is covered by several protective layers. About 2,500 memory tracks were lined precisely with a 12-μm pitch. Data were recorded as quite a small pit made by the laser beam. When reading out the data, the change in the reflection rate of the scanning laser beam focused on memory track is detected by the specific sensor. By the highly advanced autofocusing and autotracking technique, mechanical errors in recording and reading the data are almost negligible (Fig. 1). The total optical card system consists of:

1) an optical card,
2) a card reader/writer (LC-304, Conlux, Japan),
3) a personal computer system,
4) a color image scanner, and
5) a printer (Fig. 2) [2].

Results and Discussion

The optical card is easy to carry everywhere by the patient himself and it has a larger memory capacity than other card systems. Total memory capacity is 4.11 Mbits and the user memory capacity is 2.8 Mbits. As a result, in a single optical card, about 3 million characters or imaging data such as chest X-ray, CT, MRI and fundoscopy that usually require a large memory size are able to be recorded.

When recording data, both in the magnetic and IC-card, it is easy to modify the original data. On the contrary, in the optical card, it is impossible to modify the original data – only addition of new data are possible. Therefore, the security

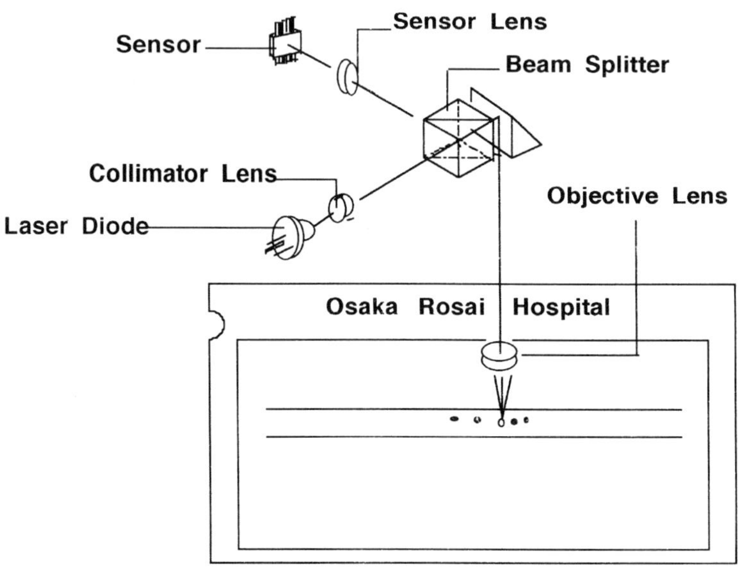

Fig. 1. Recording and reading mechanism of the medical optical memory card system.

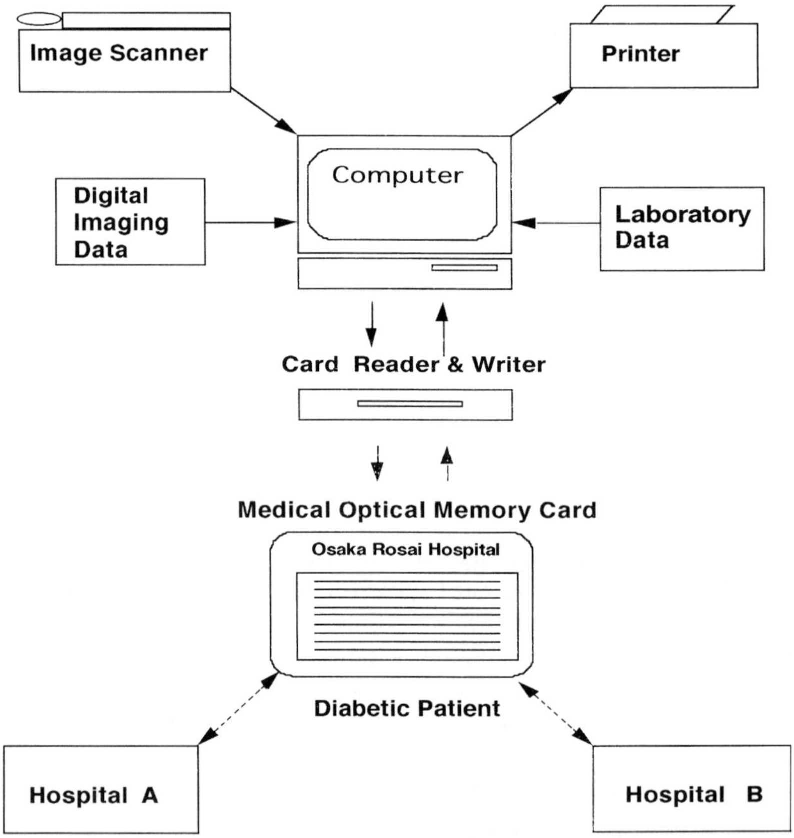

Fig. 2. Medical information network with the medical optical memory card system.

of the recorded data is greater in the optical card than that of other systems. Reading speed of recorded data is faster in the optical card. In summary, the

Table 1. Comparison of three memory card systems.

	Magnetic card	IC-card	Optical card
Recording capacity (user memory)	72 bits 72 characters	8 Kbits 8,000 characters	2.8 Mbits 2,800,000 characters
Recording method	Rewrite previous data	Possible to rewrite previous data	Addition of new data to previous recorded data
Security	Low security	Moderate security	High security
Speed for reading	2.4 Kbits/s	9.6 Kbits/s	160 Kbits/s
Cause of crash down	Magnet physical damage	Static electricity physical damage radiation, magnet	Physical damage

(M: $\times 10^6$, K: $\times 10^3$).

optical card is quite suitable for the memory device of personal medical information (Table 1).

To obtain easy operability, the basic operating software adapted for the optical card system is Microsoft Windows®. Moreover, the program is able to choose either Japanese or English as a language. For security reasons, a specific operating number is needed as the identification is necessary to read out stored data and to add new data with the reader and writer system.

As for the basic personal information, it will be able to record:

1) identification of the patient (such as name, blood type, birth date, sex, nationality, home address and telephone number);
2) name of working company and address;
3) social insurance number and medical insurance number; and
4) information of the hospital or clinic (such as name, address, telephone or fax number, and the doctor's name).

Clinical laboratory and physical examination data (such as blood pressure, results of electrocardiography) are able to be recorded according to the time sequence. In addition, imaging data such as chest X-ray, MRI, CT and color fundoscopy can be stored using the scanner system. By using this optical card system, it is quite easy to construct a medical information network among medical centers (Fig. 2).

In summary, the optical card system is useful for the management of diabetic patient's medical information, because of:

1) tight security of the recorded data,
2) a large capacity of memory size, and
3) a high-speed reading and recording capacity.

Although further studies may be necessary to improve the handling of imaging data, we could construct the medical information network by this medical optical card system.

Acknowledgements

Part of this research was supported by the Labor Welfare Corporation and West Japan KSD Research Foundation.

References

1. Smart MN. Cards in health care: A solution in search of a problem. Proc Med Inform 1989; 1151–1155.
2. Nomura M, Ohashi M, Abe H. Medical information net work system using optical medical card. Jpn J Traumatol Occupat Med 1996;44:469–472.

Recent Advances on the Pathogenesis and Management of Diabetes Mellitus.
S.H. Shinn, M. Shichiri and K.-W. Kim, editors.

Nutrition knowledge and dietary management of Korean diabetics living in the Suwon area

H.R. Park[1], K.H. Lee[1], K.S. Lee[1], H.M. Kim[2], A.H. Ha[2] and S.J. Choi[2]
[1]*Myongji University, Department of Food and Nutrition; and* [2]*Ajou University, School of Medicine, Kyonggi-do, Korea*

Abstract. *Background.* Diabetes mellitus is one of the most representative diseases requiring dietary care for treatment. This study was designed to evaluate the association of nutrition knowledge and adhering to dietary care for Korean diabetics living in the Suwon area.

Methods. In Korea, 143 diabetic patients who attended the Diabetes Walking Festival participated in the study. Data were obtained from a survey which was conducted by dietitians and students who majored in nutrition. The questionnaire included questions about nutrition knowledge related to DM and about the degree of adherence to dietary care. Fasting blood glucose was also measured.

Results. It was found that 70% of the subjects had previously had nutrition education at hospitals. The average nutrition knowledge score was relatively high (52.6/60), but the score of adhering to dietary care was very low (2.7/7). Formal education level, age and sex variables were not related to nutrition knowledge, nor to adhering to dietary care. No differences were found in the nutrition knowledge score or in the adhering to dietary care score between the subjects who had experienced nutrition education and those who had not.

Conclusion. The results showed that nutrition education was not effective for these subjects and that it is important to target and tailor nutrition education programs for diabetics of different conditions.

Keywords: dietary care adherence, nutrition education.

Introduction

Diabetes mellitus is one of the major diseases that causes a considerable increase in morbidity or mortality due to diabetic complications [1]. This complication can be reduced by early diagnosis and treatment, including nutrition [2—4]. It has generally been accepted that assessment of the individual patient's nutrition knowledge of diabetes and its management is critical before effective educational programs are implemented [4—6,8]. However, only a few studies which measured nutrition knowledge and dietary practice existed in Korea [1,7,9]. This study was designed to evaluate the relationship between the nutrition knowledge and dietary management of Korean diabetics.

Address for correspondence: Haeryun Park PhD, Department of Food and Nutrition, Myongji University, San 38-2, Nam-dong, Yongin-city, Kyonggi-do 449-728 Korea.

Subjects and Methods

In October 1996, 143 diabetic patients who attended the Diabetes Walking Festival in Korea participated in this study. The survey was conducted by dietitians and students who majored in nutrition. The questionnaire included 15 questions on nutrition knowledge related to DM, which consisted of three for etiology, four for DM symptoms, seven for dietary care and one for exercise effect which scored 1–4 points depending on their conviction for the correct answer. Another seven questions were also included to estimate the degree of adhering to dietary care, scoring one point for each case of practicing dietary care. Fasting blood glucose was also measured.

Results

Among the subjects, 47.4% were male and 52.6% were female. The average age was 53 years and the average duration of suffering from DM was less than 10 years. More than 70% had the experience of nutrition counseling at hospital. In answer to the questions about the treatment method, 66.7% were employing both insulin and diet, 49.3% using exercise, and 4% using the traditional type. The difference between males and females in using management methods is shown in Table 1. In general, the nutrition knowledge score was relatively high (52 out of 60). The rate of correct answers for questions related to dietary care such as the C:F:P ratio, fiber or sodium intake, carbohydrate metabolism, and food exchange was relatively low (24.8, 47.4, 58.3, 37.1 and 52.6%, respectively) compared to those of diabetic symptoms (72.6%). The nutrition knowledge score distribution is reported in Table 2. The subjects showed poor adherence to dietary care except for meal regularity, of which the score was 2.7 out of 7. However,

Table 1. Employed therapy for DM management according to sex.

Kind of therapy	Male	Female	p-value
Insulin	1.51 ± 0.5[a]	1.56 ± 0.5	0.404
Diet	1.6 ± 0.49	1.76 ± 0.43	0.000[c]
Exercise	1.7 ± 0.46	1.6 ± 0.49	0.027[b]
Traditional type	1.97 ± 0.16	1.98 ± 0.13	0.328

[a]Mean ± SD, 1 for not employing the therapy, 2 for employing the therapy; [b]$p < 0.05$; [c]$p < 0.001$.

Table 2. Nutrition knowledge score distribution.

Nutrition knowledge score[a]	No.	Percentage (%)
Under 40	1	0.1
40–50	40	27.8
Over 50	102	71.1

[a]4 points for giving the correct answer, 1 point for giving the incorrect answer.

Table 3. Correlation coefficients among variables.

	1	2	3	4
1. Duration of suffering DM				
2. Nutrition knowledge score	NS			
3. Adhering to dietary care score	NS	0.3001[b]		
4. Number of employed therapies	0.1882[a]	NS	0.3778[b]	
5. Formal education level	NS	NS	NS	NS

[a]$p < 0.05$; [b]$p < 0.01$.

the worst area was the counting of energy intake, estimating nutrient compositions and having someone for diet planning (28.3, 30.4 and 18.8%, respectively).

There was no difference in the nutrition knowledge scores between male and female subjects ($p > 0.05$), although male subjects had a higher level of education than females ($p < 0.05$). However, female subjects more frequently attended DM nutrition education class ($p < 0.05$) and employed dietary therapy as their major treatment ($p < 0.0001$) while male subjects employed more exercise therapy ($p < 0.05$). The highly educated subjects tended to know their DM types compared to less educated subjects ($p < 0.05$).

The duration of DM was not related to nutrition knowledge, nor to dietary adherence score while it was related to fasting blood glucose level or to the number of treatments employed. Nutrition knowledge was not related to the number of management methods employed, nor to the formal education level, but was positively related to the dietary adherence score (Table 3). A most interesting finding was that the nutrition education and counseling was not very effective for improving nutrition knowledge or for dietary adherence (Table 4). However, the dietary adherence score was high among those employing dietary management and those with a high nutrition knowledge score.

Discussion

The study showed that formal education level or nutrition education experience was not related to nutrition knowledge nor to the nutrition care adherence score, while the subjects who had a higher nutrition knowledge score showed better dietary adherence. These results suggested that diet counseling was not very use-

Table 4. Differences in nutrition knowledge and adhering dietary care according to experience of nutrition education.

Nutrition education experience	Nutrition knowledge score[a]	Adhering to dietary care score[b]
Yes	52.9 ± 4.9	3.12 ± 2.06
No	51.7 ± 4.6	2.0 ± 2.21
p-value	0.74 (NS)	0.67 (NS)

[a]Same scoring system as Table 2; [b]1 for practicing, 0 for not practicing for each question.

ful for improving DM-related knowledge and dietary care adherence for these subjects. Therefore, more targeted and tailored nutrition counseling and education programs for the subjects of different conditions have to be designed.

References

1. Kim YS, Seung JJ, Kim DM, Kim SB, You HJ. A study on the evaluation of nutrition education for diabetic patients. Diabetes 1986;10(2):191–204 (in Korean).
2. Franz MJ, Monk A, Barry B, Weaver T, Cooper N, Bergenstal PU, Mazze RS. Effectiveness of medical nutrition therapy provided by dietitians in the management of non-insulin-dependent diabetes mellitus: a randomized, controlled clinical trial. J Am Diet Assoc 1995; 95:1009–1017.
3. Dunn SM, Bryson JM, Hoskins PL, Alford JB, Handelsman DJ, Turtle JR. Development of the diabetes knowledge (DKN) scales: forms DKNA, DKNB and DKNC. Diabetes Care 1984; 7(1):36–41.
4. Franz MJ, Splett PL, Monk A, Barry B, McClain K, Weaver T, Bergenstal PU, Mazze RS. Cost-effectiveness of medical nutrition therapy provided by dietitians for persons with non-insulin-dependent diabetes mellitus. J Am Diet Assoc 1995;95:1018–1024.
5. Monk A, Barry B, McClain K, Weaver T, Cooper N, Franz MJ. Practice guidelines for medical nutrition therapy provided by dietitians for persons with non-insulin-dependent diabetes mellitus. J Am Diet Assoc 1995;95:999–1006.
6. Carey M. Diabetes guidelines, outcomes, and cost-effectiveness study. A protocol, prototype, and paradigm. J Am Diet Assoc 1995;95(9):976–978.
7. Oh HO, Kim BG. Diet counseling and its effect for diabetic patients. Korean Dietetic Assoc Ann Meeting Proceeding 1990:94–100 (in Korean).
8. Connell JE, Thomas-Dobersen D. Nutritional management of children and adolescents with insulin-dependent diabetes mellitus: a review by the Diabetes Care and Education Dietetic Practice Group. J Am Diet Assoc 1991;91:1556–1564.
9. Park CO, Paik HY, Lee HG, Min HK. The effect of nutrition knowledge and practice on management of diabetes mellitus. Diabetes 1988;12(1):79–88 (in Korean).

Recent Advances on the Pathogenesis and Management of Diabetes Mellitus.
S.H. Shinn, M. Shichiri and K.-W. Kim, editors.

Implementation of a practice guideline to diabetes management

Kenichi Nakata[1], Taiji Yonei[1], Tatsuya Itoshima[1] and Kempei Matsuoka[2]
[1]Okayama Saiseikai General Hospital, Okayama; and [2]Saiseikai Diabetes Center and Saiseikai Central Hospital, Tokyo, Japan

Abstract. For better clinical decision-making, a management program is helpful for general practitioners and healthcare providers. Staged Diabetes Management (SDM™) is a guideline with a flowchart, edited by the International Diabetes Center, Minneapolis, MN. In order to assess the feasibility of SDM in Japanese patients, the original SDM was modified to fit the background of our hospital and we conducted a trial in 30 patients. By using a practice guideline, improvement and assurance of the quality of management with a consensus among the healthcare team were expected. After the trial, it was found that firstly, physicians and healthcare professionals were well-motivated to manage the patients from the same standpoint, and secondly, an informed consent was fairly easily obtained on showing the management plan. On the other hand, several disadvantages were noted. There was a difficulty in controlling certain patients using the guidelines and the decision path had to be revised. Also, for some patients the descriptions of guidelines were difficult to understand and a translation by staff was necessary. In conclusion, the practice guideline was beneficial, however, the physicians effort is necessary to support the program.

Keywords: decision path, flow chart, informed consent, management plan, Staged Diabetes Management.

Introduction

In managing diabetic patients, general practitioners and healthcare providers can make a clinical decision easily with a guideline [1]. At the International Diabetes Center in Minneapolis, they edited an excellent guideline with a flowchart named "Staged Diabetes Management (SDM)" [2,3].

In our hospital, we intend to improve the quality of management by using a guideline. Moreover, we expect to obtain consensus among the healthcare team. For that purpose, we modified the original SDM to fit the background of our hospital and conducted a trial with 30 patients to assess the feasibility in Japanese patients.

Practice guideline

The management plan of our practice guideline is shown in the figures. The inclusive plan is depicted in Fig. 1. When a patient comes to the hospital with a diagnosis, he is examined for diabetes and complications. After evaluating the

Address for correspondence: Kenichi Nakata, Okayama Saiseikai General Hospital, 1-17-18 Ifukucyo, Okayama 700, Japan.

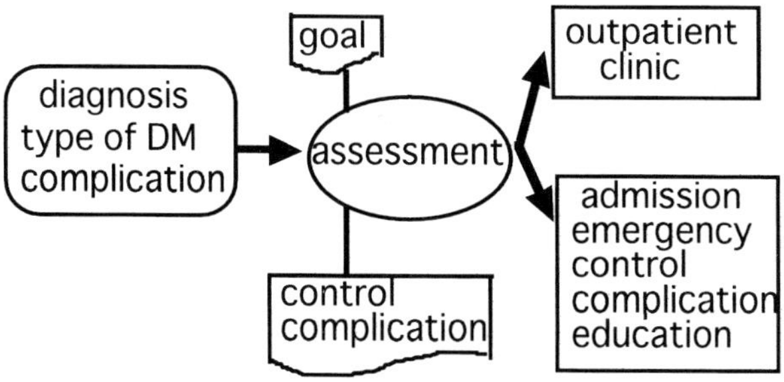

Fig. 1. Inclusive plan.

diabetic control and complications, a goal is set for each patient. This is important because an improper goal will cause many problems. After that, clinical decision making is along the pathway to outpatient clinics or to admission. The purpose of admission is divided into emergency, diabetic control, treatment of complication and education.

The guideline of dietary management is illustrated in Fig. 2. If the fasting blood glucose level is less than 140 mg/dl or random blood glucose level is less than 200 mg/dl, diet therapy is started. After the assessment of the patient for his eating habits, amount of energy intake, alcohol drinking, exercise and lifestyle, his diet plan is made. Every 4 weeks the patient is examined for blood glucose, hemoglobin A1c (HbA1c), body mass index (BMI) and serum cholesterol. If he reaches the goal, dietary management is continued. However, if he cannot achieve his goal, oral agents or insulin will be started.

The guideline with oral antidiabetic agents is shown in Fig. 3. If the fasting blood glucose level is greater than 140 mg/dl, random blood glucose level is more than 200 mg/dl, or if HbA1c remains much greater than 7.0% for 2 or 3 months with dietary management, oral antidiabetic agents will be started after the evaluation of serum immunoreactive insulin (IRI) and BMI. If the serum IRI level is low, sulfonylurea will be administered. If the IRI level is 5 μU/ml or more and BMI is more than 24.0 kg/m^2, troglitazone will be used. Especially

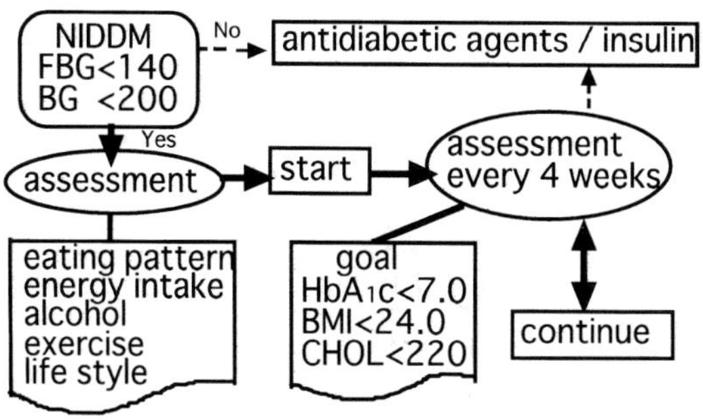

Fig. 2. Guideline of dietary management.

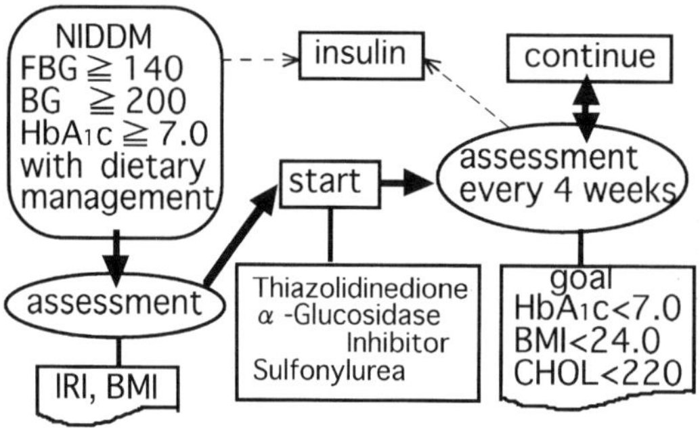

Fig. 3. Guideline with oral antidiabetic agents.

when the postprandial blood glucose is high, α-glucosidase inhibitor will be chosen. Every 4 weeks we evaluate HbA1c, MI and serum cholesterol. If they are within the goal, oral agents will be continued. If they do not reach the goal, insulin therapy is to be considered.

The guideline of insulin therapy on emergency is shown in Fig. 4. When a patient comes to hospital due to diabetic ketoacidosis, hyperosmolar nonketotic coma and for other sicknesses, insulin therapy needs to be started after an emergency workup. In case of a diabetic coma, drip infusion of low-dose insulin is initiated. After the recovery from a coma, and in case of other sicknesses or operations, a baseline plan of four divided injections of insulin is started. According to the algorithm, doses of insulin are adjusted retrospectively. We can then confirm the patient arriving at the goal, and evaluate the insulin therapy to be continued or to be changed to oral agents.

The guideline of insulin therapy in an ordinary condition is illustrated in Fig. 5. After the recovery from a diabetic coma or in case of failure of oral antidiabetic agents and diet, insulin therapy is undertaken after the estimation of serum C-peptide level, condition of diet and exercise. Intensive insulin therapy is chosen, however, conventional insulin therapy is also selected if a patient does not meet the educational plan or a social factor does not allow them. Insulin doses

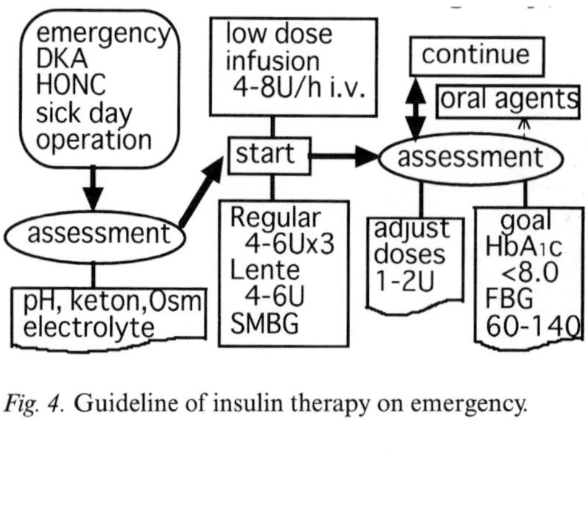

Fig. 4. Guideline of insulin therapy on emergency.

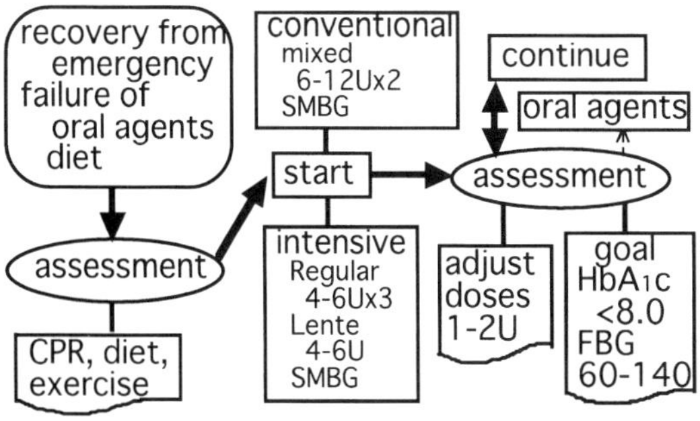

Fig. 5. Guideline of insulin therapy in ordinary condition.

are gradually adjusted to obtain the goal. After that, we can decide to continue insulin therapy or change to oral antidiabetic agents.

Trial in patients

A trial was conducted using the practice guideline in 30 patients. Four of the six patients with dietary management, four of the six with oral antidiabetic agents and 13 of 18 with insulin therapy were managed well with this practice guideline.

However, some patients failed to be managed along this guideline. Two patients with dietary management could not reach the goal; as we could not confirm whether the patients were adhering to the prescribed diet. It was also difficult to initiate the treatment with oral agents. Two patients with oral antidiabetic agents failed to reach the goal, because again they apparently did not keep to the diet. Without keeping the diet regimen, oral agents will have little effect.

As for insulin therapy, consent to insulin injection was easily obtained from patients. However, one patient could not inject insulin in the correct manner. She proved to have a mental disorder and her goal had to be changed from strict blood glucose control to avoid diabetic emergencies. The doses of insulin could not be adjusted in four patients due to failure in dietary management.

Results

As regards the benefits of a practice guideline, two items could be pointed out. Firstly, physicians and healthcare professionals could manage the patients from the same standpoint. Secondly, informed consent went fairly well and was easily obtained. On the other hand, two disadvantages could be found. Firstly, it was difficult to use the guideline in some patients. Secondly, it was difficult for some patients to understand the descriptions.

According to the results, conclusions were as follows:

1) practice guidelines are beneficial;
2) the physician's effort is necessary to support the program, e.g., the decision

path and guideline are to be customized according to the conditions of a patient; and
3) the guideline has to be revised continuously.

References

1. Mazze RS, Etzwiler D, Stock E et al. Staged Diabetes Management, toward an integrated model of diabetes care. Diabet Care 1994;17(Suppl 1):56–66.
2. Mazze RS, Strock E, Etzwiler D. Staged Diabetes Management. Minneapolis: International Diabetes Center, 1989.
3. Mazze RS, Strock E, Etzwiler D. Staged Diabetes Management, Decision Paths. Minneapolis: International Diabetes Center, 1995.

Recent Advances on the Pathogenesis and Management of Diabetes Mellitus.
S.H. Shinn, M. Shichiri and K.-W. Kim, editors.

The relationship between plasma glucose and insulin secretion on 75-g OGTT

Sekiya Masashi, Hoshi Mituru, Yoshiuchi Kazutoimi, Sanada Mituru, Takimoto Tadashi and Hatanaka Ikuo
Department of Medicine, Osaka Kousei-Nenkin Hospital, Osaka, Japan

Abstract. The Japan Diabetes Society recommends the classification of glucose tolerance after 75-g oral glucose load and does not consider insulin secretion for diagnosis. We therefore evaluated insulin secretion against the plasma glucose level (PG) as a basal insulin by fasting the serum insulin level, the first phase after glucose loading by ΔIRI/ΔPG, and the total insulin level after glucose loading by ΣIRI. 626 outpatients of our diabetic clinic were eligible for analysis from 1992 to 1997. They were administered 75-g OGTT and measured with both plasma glucose and serum insulin concentration before and at 30, 60 and 120 min after glucose loading. The fasting insulin level had no correlation with fasting plasma glucose, and the basal level was prevented from increasing fasting plasma glucose levels from 70 to 300 mg/dl. ΔIRI/ΔPG seemed to decrease at around 140 mg/dl of the fasting glucose level. ΣIRI seemed to decrease at around 200 mg/dl of the 2-h plasma glucose level in OGTT. In conclusion, the Japan Diabetes Society's recommendation of the plasma glucose level was supported by the dynamic insulin secretion on OGTT.

Keywords: classification of diabetes mellitus, insulin secretion, oral glucose loading.

Introduction

As the diagnostic standard of diabetes mellitus we utilized, by the Japan Diabetes Society's classification, glucose tolerance after 75-g oral glucose load (75-g OGTT). However, since there have recently been many new findings on the causation of diabetes mellitus, the classification of diabetes mellitus demands many other factors. The Japan Diabetes Society's recommendation for the classification of glucose tolerance after 75-g OGTT is not considering insulin secretion for diagnosis. We therefore evaluated insulin secretion against the plasma glucose level (PC).

Methods

626 outpatients from our diabetic clinic from 1992 to 1997 were eligible for analysis. They were administered 75-g OGTT and measured with both plasma glucose

Address for correspondence: Sekiya Masashi, Department of Medicine, Osaka Kousei-Nenkin Hospital, Fukushima 4-2-78, Osaka, Japan. Tel.: +81-06-441-5451. Fax: +81-06-445-8900.

Table 1. The Japan Diabetes Society's classification of glucose tolerance after 75-g oral glucose load.

	Glucose level		
	Plasma glucose	Capillary whole blood	Whole blood
Diabetes mellitus			
fasting	≥140 mg/dl (≥8.0 mmol/l)	≥120 mg/dl (≥7.0 mmol/l)	≥120 mg/dl (≥7.0 mmol/l)
2 h	≥200 mg/dl (≥11.0 mmol/l)	≥200 mg/dl (≥11.0 mmol/l)	≥180 mg/dl (≥10.0 mmol/l)
Normal			
fasting	<110 mg/dl (<6.5 mmol/l)	<110 mg/dl (<6.5 mmol/l)	<110 mg/dl (<6.5 mmol/l)
1 h	<160 mg/dl (<9.0 mmol/l)	<160 mg/dl (<9.0 mmol/l)	<140 mg/dl (<8.0 mmol/l)
2 h	<120 mg/dl (<7.0 mmol/l)	<120 mg/dl (<7.0 mmol/l)	<110 mg/dl (<6.5 mmol/l)

Borderline: belong to neither DM nor normal.

and serum insulin concentration before and at 30, 60 and 120 min after glucose loading. Moreover, we judged them using the Japan Diabetes Society's classification of 75-g OGTT.

We evaluated insulin secretion against the plasma glucose level, such as basal insulin, by fasting the serum insulin level – the first phase after glucose loading by insulinogenic index that was calculated by $\Delta IRI/\Delta PC$, and the total insulin level after glucose loading by ΣIRI.

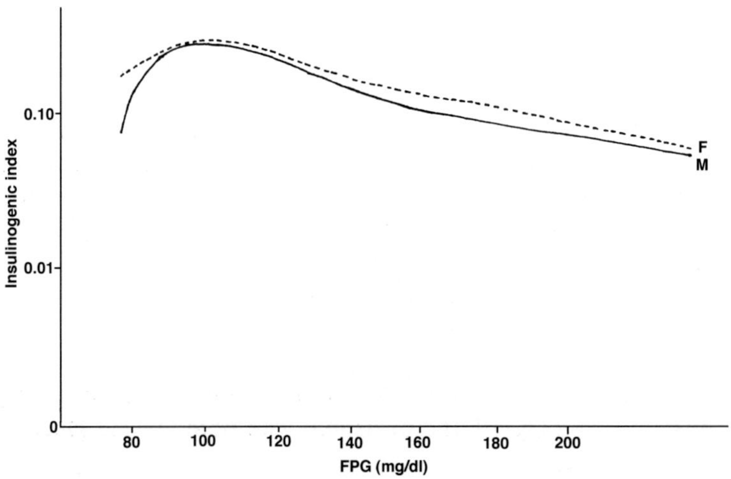

Fig. 1. The relationship between insulinogenic index and fasting plasma glucose.

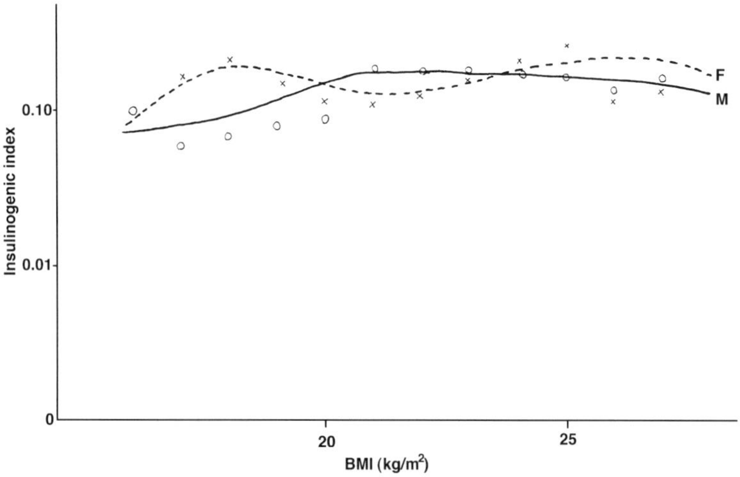

Fig. 2. The relationship between insulinogenic index and body mass index.

Results

573 patients showed a diabetic pattern, 10 patients showed a normal pattern, and 53 patients showed a borderline pattern (Table 1).

The relationship between insulinogenic index and fasting plasma glucose level

The first phase of insulin secretion seemed to decrease at around 140 mg/dl of

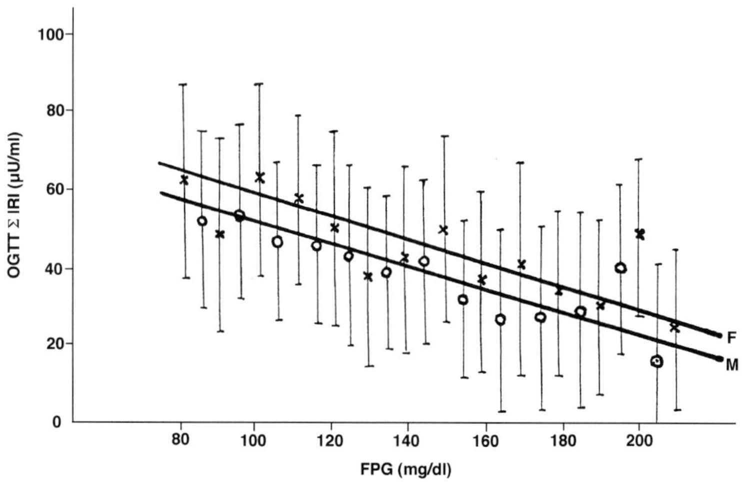

Fig. 3. The relationship between ΣIRI and fasting plasma glucose.

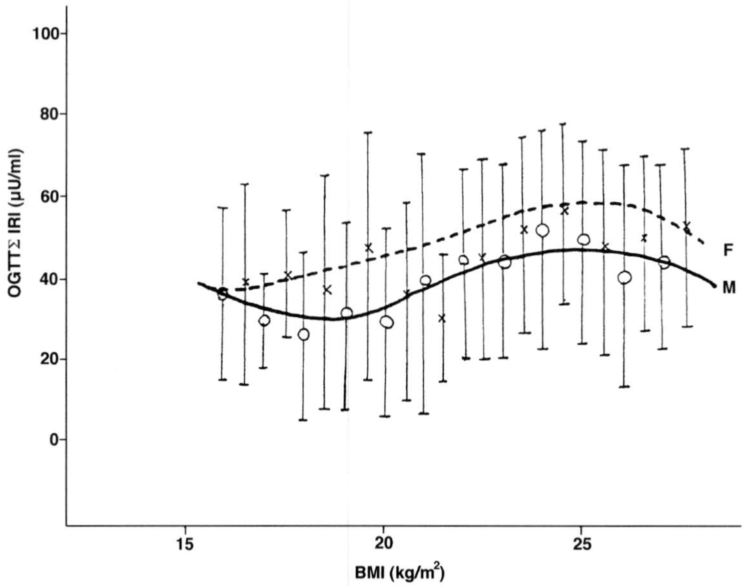

Fig. 4. The relationship between ΣIRI and body mass index.

fasting plasma glucose, and the maximum insulin secretion was at around 100 mg/dl. However, the first phase of insulin secretion had no correlation with sex, body mass, index and age (Figs. 1 and 2).

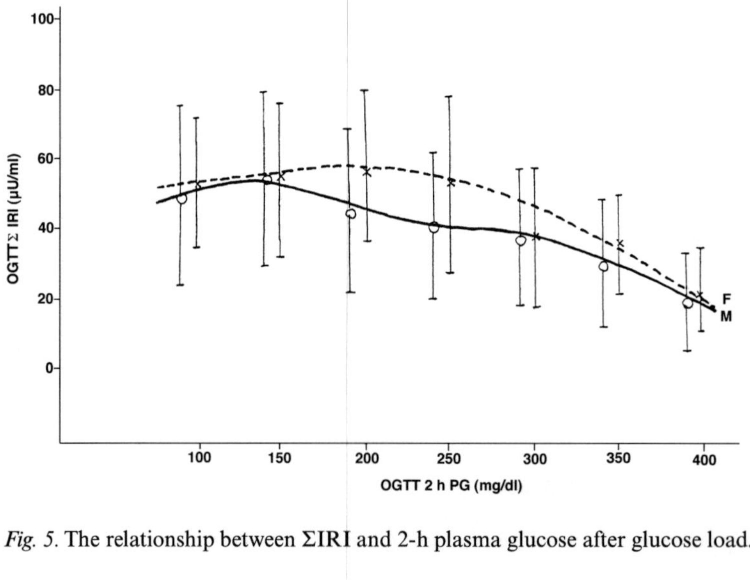

Fig. 5. The relationship between ΣIRI and 2-h plasma glucose after glucose load.

The relationship between ΣIRI and the fasting plasma glucose level (Fig. 3)

In increasing fasting plasma glucose, the total insulin secretion decreased. However, the basel insulin level was kept against increasing fasting plasma glucose from 70 to 300 mg/dl.

The relationship between ΣIRI and body mass index

ΣIRI seemed to decrease over 25 kg/m^2 (Fig. 4). Also, the relationship between ΣIRI and the 2-h plasma glucose level after glucose loading was that total insulin secretion seemed to decrease at around 200 mg/dl (Fig. 5).

Conclusion

Glucose which was absorbed from gastrointestinal tract affects insulin secretion. Therefore, insulin secretion was variable on glucose loading. However, the patient with low insulin response on glucose loading would become diabetic in the future [1]. Moreover, the diabetic group who had over 140 mg/dl of fasting plasma glucose and over 200 mg/dl of 2-h plasma glucose after glucose loading showed a decrease in insulinogenic index and ΣIRI. Therefore, the Japan Diabetes Society's recommendation of the plasma glucose level was supported by the dynamic insulin secretion on oral glucose tolerance.

Reference

1. Kosaka K et al. Insulin secretory response of diabetics during the period of improvement of glucose tolerance to normal range. Diabetologia 1974;10:775.

Complications

Recent Advances on the Pathogenesis and Management of Diabetes Mellitus.
S.H. Shinn, M. Shichiri and K.-W. Kim, editors.

Ultrastructure of neuromuscular junction in Vacor-induced diabetic rats

Tai Hee Lee[1], Jae Su Ahn[1] and Min Chul Lee[2]
Departments of [1]Internal Medicine and [2]Pathology, Chonnam National University Medical School, Kwangju, Korea

Abstract. *Background.* Rodenticide Vacor causes a severe peripheral neuropathy in humans. Electrophysiologic studies on a peripheral motor-nerve skeletal system of Vacor-treated rat showed decreased amplitude of muscle action potential without conduction velocity abnormalities. The ultrastructural studies of the neuromuscular junction were performed to clarify the anatomic site of the Vacor-induced peripheral neuropathy in male Wistar rats.

Methods. After oral administration of a single dose of Vacor, 80 mg/kg of body weight, to the experimental animals, neuromuscular junctions within the interosseous muscles of the hind foot were observed following time.

Results. No axon terminal change was noted until 24 h after the administration of Vacor. Remarkable loss of presynaptic vesicles and swollen endoplasmic reticulum in the axon terminal were developed at 3 days after Vacor treatment. Progressive degenerative changes consisting of marked loss of presynaptic vesicles, focal disruption of the membrane in the axon terminal with the disappearance of the number of the damaged axon terminal appeared, and flattening of postsynaptic folds was also seen.

Conclusion. These results suggest that degenerative changes in axon terminal at the neuromuscular junction may contribute to the peripheral neuropathy developed in the early phase of Vacor poisoning.

Keywords: axonal degeneration, peripheral neuropathy, Vacor poisoning.

Introduction

Vacor (N-3-pyridylmethyl-N′-p-nitrophenylurea)-poisoned patients had complained of various neurological symptoms such as urinary retention, a burning sensation of the foot, areflexia, and orthostatic hypotension [1–4]. Various neurotoxicities of Vacor were reported in the acute toxic phase, however, the cause of neurotoxicity is not well known [5].

In the electrophysiologic studies of the peripheral nerve, Vacor did not affect the conduction velocity, however, the decrease of action-potential amplitudes was developed on the sciatic-tibial nerve of Vacor-treated rat [6]. The decrement of action-potential amplitude indicates that axonal or muscular dysfunction might be induced by Vacor.

In order to define these electrophysiologic abnormalities in the Vacor-induced

Address for correspondence: Tai Hee Lee MD, Department of Internal Medicine, Chonnam University Medical School, Hakdong 8, Dongku, Kwangju 501-757, Korea.

peripheral neuropathy, an ultrastructural study was carried out on the neuromuscular junction in the interosseous muscle of Vacor-treated rat.

Material and Methods

Male Wistar rats (n = 30), weighing 200—250 g, were used in this study. A single dose of Vacor (N-3-pyridylmethyl-N′-p-nitrophenylurea, MW 272), 80 mg/kg of body weight, was administrated by orogastric canule, while distilled water was given in controls. The experimental animals were sacrificed at 1, 3, 7 and 14 days after administration of Vacor. The animals were perfused through the jugular vein with 5% glutaraldehyde in 0.1 M sodium phosphate buffer.

In order to examine the morphological changes of the neuromuscular junction, tissues were taken from interosseous muscles of the hind foot. The tissue fragments were divided into small blocks, 2 × 2 × 1 mm each, and subsequently immersed in 2.5% glutaraldehyde for 12 h at 10°C. They were postfixed in 2% osmium tetroxide for 4 h at room temperature. After dehydration in graded ethanol, they were embedded in epon mixture for 3 days at 50°C. Thick sections, 1 μm in thickness and stained with toluidine blue, were prepared for light microscopy. Thin sections, 80 nm in thickness, were obtained from the representative areas, and stained with uranyl acetate and lead citrate. The sections were examined with a Zeol 100 CXII electron microscope.

Results

In control rats, myelinated axons and axon terminals at neuromuscular junctions of the hind foot interosseous muscle maintained their structural integrity well.

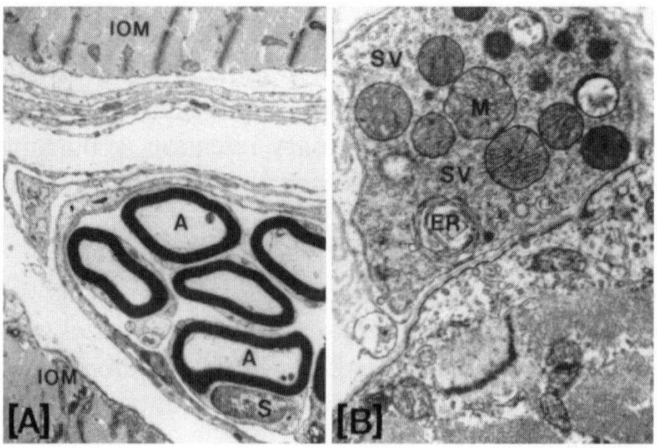

Fig. 1. **A**: Normal posterior tibial nerve. Note intact myelinated axons (A) and Schwann cell (S) between the interosseous muscle (IOM) of the hind foot (× 11,200). **B**: Normal neuromuscular junction. Note the axon terminal filled with many presynaptic vesicles (SV), mitochondria (M), and lamellated endoplasmic reticulum (ER) (× 32,000).

No degenerative changes were seen in myelinated nerve fibers (Fig. 1A). The axon terminal contained mitochondria, concentrically lamellated endoplasmic reticulum and numerous small round presynaptic vesicles (Fig. 1B), and was in close contact with the sarcoplasmic membrane of myocyte.

Morphological change of the axon terminals at neuromuscular junctions was not evident within 1 day after Vacor administration (Fig. 2). The synaptic cleft between the axon terminal and postsynaptic folds of sarcoplasm was not widened. At 3 days after Vacor administration, there was remarkable loss of presynaptic vesicles and swollen ER in the axon terminal (Fig. 3). The papillary postsynaptic folds were partially flattened. A progressively decreasing number of presynaptic vesicles, and disruption of membrane of the axon terminal with myeloid body formation were seen at 7 days after Vacor administration (Fig. 4). The synaptic cleft was widened. The axon terminals significantly reduced in number at 14 days after Vacor administration. A few presynaptic vesicles were engulfed in irregular Schwann cell processes identified by a delicate lining of their basal lamina (Fig. 5). Some axon terminals had only a few synaptic vesicles, and postsynaptic folds were markedly flattened and simplified (Fig. 6).

Discussion

Degenerative changes and segmental demyelinations were developed in diabetic neuropathy with long duration. In the acute phase of experimental diabetes induced by streptozotocin, pathologic changes of the nervous system were not found and it required many more days or weeks to develop.

The diabetes induced by Vacor has various neurological complications such as urinary retention, burning sensation of the foot, areflexia, and orthostatic hypotension, etc. [1–4,7,8]. Lee et al. [5] had reported that rats given Vacor show vari-

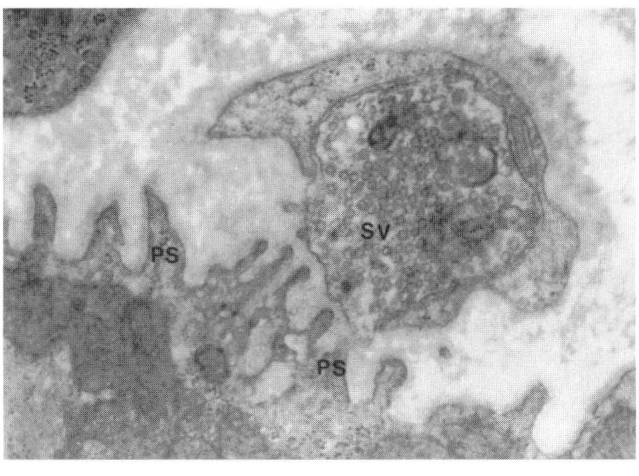

Fig. 2. Neuromuscular junction 1 day after Vacor administration (80 mg/kg). No degenerative change is seen. Note intact axon terminal containing many presynaptic vesicles (SV), synaptic cleft and delicate papillary postsynaptic folds (PS) of sarcoplasm (× 88,000).

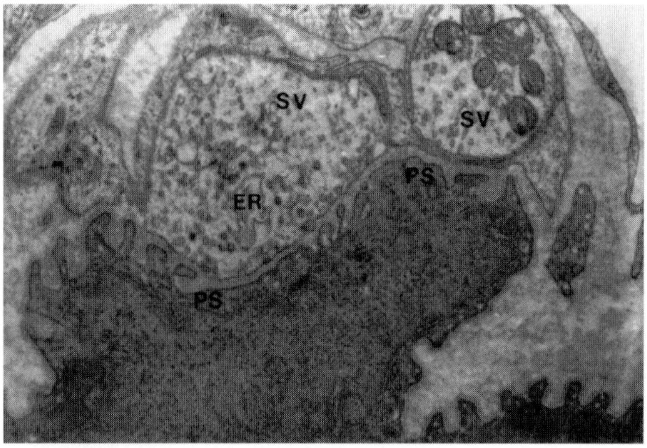

Fig. 3. Neuromuscular junction 3 days after Vacor administration. Note mild degenerative changes considering of significantly reduced number of presynaptic vesicles (SV) and dilatation of endoplasmic reticulum (ER) in the axon terminal, and flattening of postsynaptic folds (PS) (× 52,000).

ous morphological changes such as necrosis of axon, myelin sheaths and glial cells in the spinal cord with unchanged organelles of the peripheral nerves, but its correct mechanism is not clear.

Park et al. [6] reported that the amplitude of the compound muscle action potential decreased but the conduction velocity of the sciatic-tibial nerve of Vacor treated rat was unchanged. Na^+, K^+-ATPase activity and inositol content of sciatic nerve were unchanged, which was different from those of streptozotocin diabetes. However, neurotoxicity was reported in the acute toxic phase of Vacor poisoning. Lewitt [9] reported the active breakdown of myelin sheath in

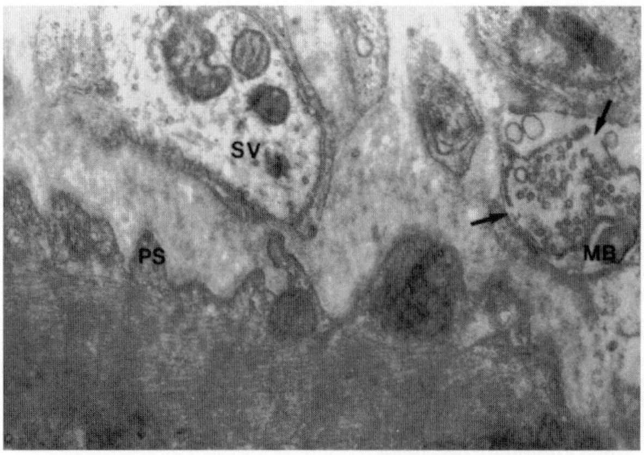

Fig. 4. Neuromuscular junction 7 days after Vacor administration. Note progressive degenerative changes consisting of marked loss of presynaptic vesicles (SV) and focal disruption of membrane (arrow) in the axon terminal with myeloid body (MB) formation and flattened postsynaptic folds (PS) (× 52,000).

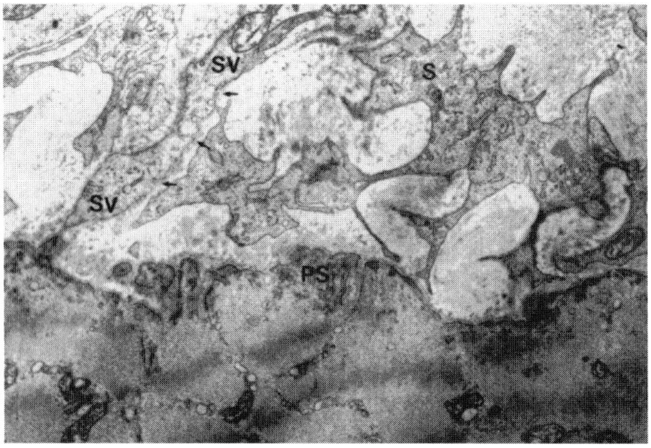

Fig. 5. Neuromuscular junction 14 days after Vacor administration. Some presynaptic vesicles disappeared, and the lesion is replaced by irregularly elongated processes of Schwann cell (S) which engulfed a few presynaptic vesicles (SV). Note thin delicate basal lamina along the processes (arrow). Postsynaptic folds (PS) were simplified (× 22,400).

streptozotocin diabetic animal.

In this study morphological changes of axon terminals at neuromuscular junction were not evident within 1 day after Vacor treatment, however, loss of presynaptic vesicles in axon terminal and swollen endoplasmic reticulum were developed at 3 days after Vacor administrations. These abnormalities of axon terminal progressed at 7 and 14 days after Vacor treatment.

These findings may give us the evidence that decreased amplitude of compound muscle action potential was through axonal degeneration.

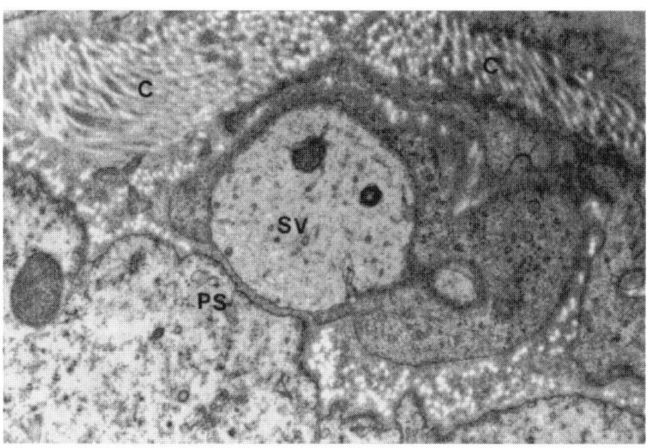

Fig. 6. Neuromuscular junction 14 days after Vacor administration. Note markedly decreased number of presynaptic vesicles (SV) in the axon terminal surrounded by collagenous fibers (C) and flattened postsynaptic folds (PS) of sarcoplasm of myocyte (× 40,000).

Acknowledgements

The authors thank Jae Hong Park for his valuable assistance in this project.

References

1. Lee TH. Diabetes mellitus by rodenticide, RH-787 poisoning. Kor J Int Med 1976;19:618–624.
2. Lee TH, Kang JC, Kim JS, Rho JW, Chung MY, Choi BJ. Clinical observation of rodenticide, RH-787 poisoning. J Kor Diab Assoc 1977;4:43–51.
3. Prosser PR, Karam JH. Diabetes mellitus following rodenticide ingestion in man. JAMA 1978;239:1148–1150.
4. Karam JH, Lewitt PA, Young CW, Nowlain RE, Frankel BJ, Fujiya H, Freedman ZR, Grodsky GM. Insulinopenic diabetes after rodenticide (Vacor) ingestion. Diabetes 1980;29:971–978.
5. Lee TH, Doi K, Yoshida M, Baba S. Morphological study of nervous system in Vacor-induced diabetic rats. Diabet Res Clin Pract 1988;4:275–279.
6. Park CJ, Ryu HJ, Chung MY, Lee TH. Functional study on peripheral neuropathy in Vacor-treated rat (Abstract). Kor J Int Med 1995;47(Suppl 1):63.
7. Felig P. Disorders of carbohydrate metabolism. In: Bondy PK, Rosenberg LE (eds) Duncan's Metabolic Control and Disease, 8th edn. Philadelphia: Saunders, 1980;348–350.
8. Sharma AK, Thomas PK. Peripheral nerve structure and function in experimental diabetes. J Neurol Sci 1974;23:1–15.
9. Lewitt PA. The neurotoxicity of the rat poison Vacor. N Engl J Med 1980;302:73–77.

Recent Advances on the Pathogenesis and Management of Diabetes Mellitus.
S.H. Shinn, M. Shichiri and K.-W. Kim, editors.

Significance of the sympathetic skin response (SSR) and F wave in IDDM with neuropathy

Shinichiro Takayama, Yoshiatsu Takahashi, Takeshi Ito, Yasuko Uchigata, Yasue Omori and Yasuhiko Iwamoto
Diabetes Center, Tokyo Women's Medical College, Tokyo, Japan

Abstract. To detect the early dysfunction of the autonomic nervous system and peripheral nerve in IDDM, we examined sympathetic skin response (SSR) and F wave in IDDM with (n = 22) or without (n = 23) diabetic complications and healthy controls (n = 23). In IDDM without complications, the amplitude and latency of SSR were significantly lower than those of controls. The latency and nerve conduction velocity of the F wave were significantly lower in IDDM than in healthy controls. In IDDM, there was a linear correlation between the mean HbA1c for the previous 5 years and the amplitude of SSR, the latency and amplitude of the F wave. These results suggest that SSR and the F wave may be useful for the early detection of diabetic autonomic and peripheral neuropathy in IDDM.

Keywords: diabetes, diabetic autonomic neuropathy, human.

Introduction

Diabetic autonomic neuropathy may manifest as a dysfunction of several different organs [1]. The symptoms are important in individual patients but difficult to evaluate quantitatively. Several objective measurements of autonomic function have been developed. These tests measure end-organ responses to activation of neural reflex arcs. They can be influenced by end-organ failure, intercurrent illness, drugs and age. Clinically, various tests have been used to diagnose autonomic and peripheral neuropathy. The aim of this study was to detect the early dysfunction of the autonomic nervous system and the peripheral nerve in IDDM by the sympathetic skin response (SSR) and the F wave.

Subjects and Methods

The subjects consisted of 45 IDDM patients who were consecutively referred to our hospital. Twenty-three nondiabetic healthy controls were matched for sex and age with IDDM patients. The IDDM patients were divided into two groups, i.e., group 1 (IDDM without diabetic complications) and group 2 (with diabetic complications), which were defined by patella tendon reflex or Achilles tendon reflex, retinopathy and microalbuminuria (Table 1). The patients with heart, renal

Address for correspondence: S. Takayama, Diabetes Center, Tokyo Women's Medical College, Kawada-cho 8-1, Shinjuku-ku, Tokyo 162, Japan.

Table 1. Clinical features of healthy controls and IDDM patients [8].

	Control	IDDM	
		Group 1 Retinopathy (−) Nephropathy (−) PTR or ATR (+)	Group 2 Retinopathy or Nephropathy (+) PTR or ATR (−)
n	23	23	22
Sex (M/F)	12/11	12/11	12/10
Onset age (years)		15.6 ± 6.7	13.8 ± 7
Age (years)	26 ± 3	25 ± 4	27 ± 5
Duration of DM (years)		9.1 ± 5.5[a]	13.2 ± 6.7
HbA1c (%)		7.4 ± 1.6[b]	8.2 ± 1.6

Mean ± SD, [a]p = 0.0336, [b]p= 0.0194 vs. group 2.

or hepatic failure were excluded from the subjects. SSR was elicited with electrical stimuli, rectangular pulses of 0.2 ms and 20 mA by using Neuropack-2. The reference electrode was placed at the right hand and foot. The stimulating electrode consisted of a pair of felt pads mounted on a plate, attached to the frontal head or the volar surface of the forearm just above the wrist so as to stimulate the median nerve. The SSR parameters measured included latency and peak-to-peak amplitude. The F wave was recorded from medial and tibial nerves using the same electrode. The F wave was elicited with electrical stimuli, rectangular pulses of 0.2 ms and 20 mA. The minimal F latency was determined for each series of 16 or 20 F waves. Data are expressed as mean ± SD, unless stated. Statistical analyses were done using the Student's t test and Mann-Whitney's U test. The significance was defined as $p < 0.05$.

Results

SSR

In group 1 (IDDM without complications), the amplitude of SSR was significantly lower than that in healthy controls. In group 2 (IDDM with complications), the amplitude of SSR was significantly lower than that in group 1 (Fig. 1). We had the same results in the latency of SSR.

F wave

In group 1 (IDDM without complications), the F wave conduction velocity was significantly lower than that of healthy controls. In group 2 (IDDM with complications), the F wave conduction velocity was significantly lower than that of group 1 (Fig. 2). We had the same results in the median nerve.

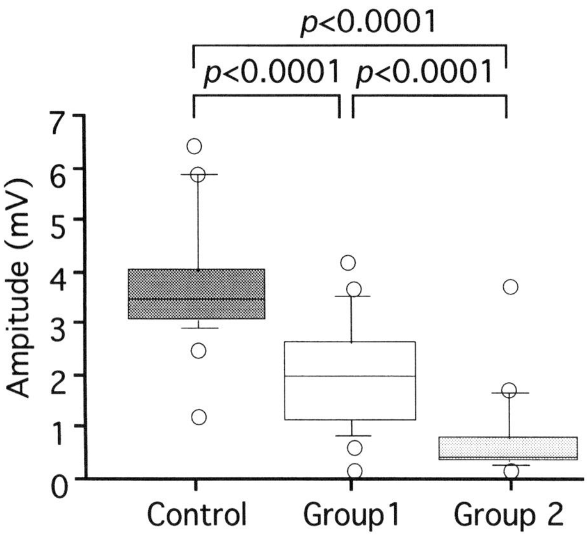

Fig. 1. The amplitude of SSR at foot by head stimulation [8].

Correlation between SSR, F wave and glycaemia control in IDDM

In IDDM, there was a significantly linear correlation between the mean HbA1c for the previous 5 years and the amplitude of SSR (Fig. 3). We also found a linear correlation between the latency of SSR, F wave and glycaemia control.

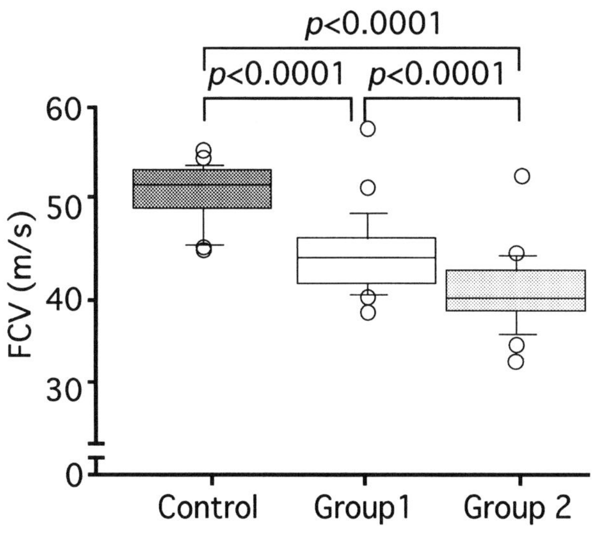

Fig. 2. The nerve conduction velocity of the F wave at the tibial nerve [8].

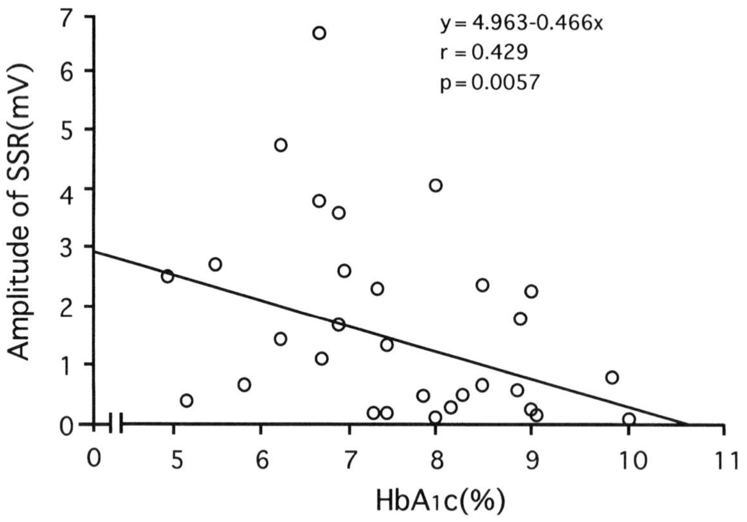

Fig. 3. Correlation between the mean HbA1c for the previous 5 years and SSR; stimulating median nerve and recording at foot [8].

Discussion

SSR is an established electrophysiological phenomenon reflecting activity in a part of the sympathetic nervous system, and has been shown to be independent of the vasoconstrictor reflex [2]. The method for the recording of SSR is well-established and has been standardized for clinical use. In some reports, microneurography can directly measure the peripheral autonomic nerve activity [3,4]. However, this technique is very difficult and needs a long time for measurement. In this study, the latency and amplitude of SSR were decreased in IDDM without complications. These results suggested that SSR may be useful for the early detection of diabetic autonomic neuropathy in IDDM.

The abnormalities of the F wave are present in a large variety of peripheral neurons, the central nervous system and the spinal cord [5]. In diabetic neuropathy, the motor conduction abnormalities are diffuse over the total length of the nerve [6]. In this study, the latency and amplitude of the F wave were decreased in IDDM without complications. These results suggested that the F wave may be useful for the early detection of diabetic peripheral neuropathy in IDDM, and that diabetic neuropathy may affect not only the peripheral nerve system but also the central nervous system and the spinal cord.

Previous metabolic control is a major determinant of nerve damage, and lowering of blood glucose levels may have some beneficial effects on the neural function [7]. In this study, there was a significant correlation between SSR, F wave and previous metabolic control. We assume that abnormalities of SSR and the F wave may be present before the appearance of overt complications and these abnormalities seem to be correlated with previous metabolic control status.

We conclude that the measurements of SSR and F wave could produce better clinical care and an early diagnosis of neurological complications of diabetic autonomic and peripheral neuropathy even in IDDM patients without any neurological symptoms [8].

References

1. Ewing DJ, Clarke BF. Diabetic autonomic neuropathy: Present insights and future prospects. Diabet Care 1986;9:648–665.
2. Bini G, Hagbarth KE. Thermoregulatory and rhythm-generating mechanism governing the sudomotor and vasoconstrictor outflow in human cutaneous nerves. J Physiol 1980;306: 537–552.
3. Takayama S, Nakajima Y. Increased muscle sympathetic nerve activity after glucagon administration in man. J Auton Nerve Syst 1995;54:171–175.
4. Mano T. Sympathetic nerve mechanisms of human adaptation to environment-findings obtained by recent microneurographic studies. Env Med 1990;34:1–35.
5. Lachman T. Late responses as aids to diagnosis in peripheral neuropathy. J Neurol Neurosurg Psychiat 1980;43:156–162.
6. Fierro B, Modica A. Analysis of F-wave in metabolic neuropathies: A comparative study in uremic and diabetic patients. Acta Neurol Scand 1987;75:179–185.
7. Duck SC, Wei F. Role of height and glycosylated hemoglobin in abnormal nerve conduction in pediatric patients with type 1 diabetes mellitus after 4–9 yr of disease. Diabet Care 1991;14: 386–392.
8. Takayama S. Significance of the F wave and sympathetic skin response (SSR) in IDDM patients with neuropathy. Tokyo Joshi Ikadaigaku Zasshi 1996;66:422–428.

Recent Advances on the Pathogenesis and Management of Diabetes Mellitus.
S.H. Shinn, M. Shichiri and K.-W. Kim, editors.

Analysis of diabetic neuropathy symptoms and pathophysiology

Kiyoshi Takekawa, Eiji Yamato and Takeshi Hata
Higashiosaka Municipal Central Hospital, Higashiosaka, Japan

Abstract. In order to determine the relevance of pathophysiological examination of neuropathy to the patients' symptoms, we originally designed an interview-based test for neuropathy. We scored the subjective data for neurological symptoms, measured sensory nerve conduction velocity (SCV), motor nerve conduction velocity (MCV), coefficient of variation of R-R intervals (CV-RR) and vibration perception threshold (VPT).

The subjects were 33 diabetic patients admitted to our hospital. VPT was elevated in all patients studied and significantly elevated in the patients with long duration of diabetes. High total scores for subjective symptomatic test (SST) for diabetic neuropathy was significantly associated with deterioration of vibration sense and tended to be associated with deterioration of SCV and CV-RR. High scores for vascular factor in SST for diabetic neuropathy tended to be associated with deterioration of vibration sense and SCV. These results suggested that vibration sense was a most sensitive index for diabetic neuropathy and SST for diabetic neuropathy was suggested to be useful for the detection of diabetic neuropathy, especially for deterioration of vibration sense.

Keywords: coefficient of variation of R-R intervals, diabetic neuropathy, motor nerve conduction velocity, sensory nerve conduction velocity, subjective symptomatic test, vibratory perception threshold.

Introduction

Neuropathy is an uncomfortable complication and injures a person's QOL. It is also known to increase risk of mortality [1], and occasionally is a major cause of sudden death in diabetic patients. It is also difficult to diagnose and to heal it. The underlying mechanism of development of diabetic neuropathy has not been fully clarified, although metabolic disturbance and/or vascular disorder have been suggested [2].

According to lack of objectivity about the patients' symptoms of diabetic neuropathy and lack of specificity to inspections of diabetic neuropathy, the diagnostic criteria and the treatment of diabetic neuropathy have not yet been established. The aim of this study is to establish and quantify the subjective symptoms of diabetic neuropathy and to determine the relevance of pathophysiological examinations of neuropathy to the patients' symptoms.

Address for correspondence: Kiyoshi Takekawa MD, PhD, Higashiosaka Municipal Central Hospital, 2-3-1 Mikuriaminami, Higashiosaka, Osaka 577, Japan.

Subjects and Methods

The subjects were 33 diabetic patients admitted to our hospital (male/female: 15/18, NIDDM/IDDM: 28/5, diet/OHA/insulin: 1/11/21). Subjects with chronic alcoholism and neurological disease were excluded. For objective neurological examination, sensory nerve conduction velocity (SCV), motor nerve conduction velocity (MCV), and coefficient of variation of R-R intervals (CV-RR) have been measured. SCV was measured at the palm segment of the left median nerve, using antidromic technique. MCV was measured at the left median nerve, by NRS-1100 (Aster, Japan). CV-RR was measured in 100 counts of heart stroke at rest. The vibratory perception threshold (VPT) was also measured at bilateral radial tubercle by SMV-5 (Technoloag, Japan) [3]. The standard values of SCV, MCV, CV-RR and VPT were instituted by preliminary study.

In order to obtain the subjective data for neurological symptoms, we originally designed an interview-based, subjective symptomatic test (SST) for diabetic neu-

Table 1. Subjective symptomatic test for diabetic neuropathy (SST).

	Score			
	0	1	2	3
Neurogenic				
1) Smart sense in fingers	none	sometimes	slight	severe
2) Smart sense in distal foot	none	sometimes	slight	severe
3) Dysesthesia in fingers	none	sometimes	slight	severe
4) Dysesthesia in distal foot	none	sometimes	slight	severe
5) Numbness in distal limbs	none	sometimes	slight	severe
6) Hypesthesia	none	sometimes	slight	severe
7) Paresthesia of soles	none	sometimes	slight	severe
8) Muscle cramp in leg	none	sometimes	slight	severe
9) Muscle weakness in limbs	none	sometimes	slight	severe
10) Leg pain at resting	none	sometimes	slight	severe
11) Unaware injury in limbs	none	sometimes	slight	severe
12) Burn by hot-water bottle	none	sometimes	slight	severe
Vascular				
13) Sense of cold limbs	none	sometimes	slight	severe
14) Sense of hot limbs	none	sometimes	slight	severe
15) Sense of swollen limbs	none	sometimes	slight	severe
16) Intermittent claudication	none	sometimes	slight	severe
Autonomic				
17) Postural hypertension	none	sometimes	slight	severe
18) Dizziness	none	sometimes	slight	severe
19) Constipation	none	sometimes	slight	severe
20) Diarrhoea	none	sometimes	slight	severe
21) Abnormal sweating	none	sometimes	slight	severe
22) Troubles in urination	none	sometimes	slight	severe
23) Impotence	none	sometimes	slight	severe

Table 2. Duration of DM and diabetic neuropathy.

	Short duration	Long duration
MCV	45.9 ± 2.3	45.9 ± 1.6
SCV	39.3 ± 2.2	38.9 ± 1.4
Vibration sense	14.1 ± 2.0	27.7 ± 6.2[a]
CV-RR	2.7 ± 0.6	2.1 ± 0.4
Total scores for neuropathy	9.4 ± 2.2	9.8 ± 2.6

MCV, SCV (m/s). CV-RR (%). [a]p = 0.017: vs. short duration.

ropathy (Table 1). There were 23 questionnaires divided into three categories, neurogenic, vascular and autonomic. Each questionnaire was scored by 0, 1, 2 and 3 points, and was added in each group and in total. A score of 0 means that a patient claims no symptoms, 1 indicates that the patient sometimes suffers from the symptoms, 2 signals that a patient suffers slightly from the symptoms, and 3 denotes that a patient suffers severely from the symptoms.

Statistical analysis was performed by unpaired t test.

Results

In order to elucidate the effect of duration of diabetes on diabetic neuropathy, duration was divided into two groups over or under the mean number, i.e., 12 years (Table 2). There were no differences in MCV, CV-RR and total scores of SST between the two groups for duration of diabetes. However, SCV was disturbed regardless of duration and VPT was elevated in patients with short duration of diabetes and was significantly elevated in the patients with long duration of diabetes.

To demonstrate the effect of previous control of blood sugar on diabetic neuropathy, patients were divided into three groups, NDR, SDR and PDR (Table 3). In the patients with SDR, MCV was slightly but significantly disturbed compared with NDR. In the patients with PDR, CV-RR was significant, SCV and VPT tended to be disturbed compared with NDR.

Patients were divided into two groups, by low and high score according to the mean of 9.5 points of SST (Table 4). There were no significant differences in

Table 3. Retinopathy and neuropathy.

	NDR	SDR	PDR
MCV	48.9 ± 1.8	41.1 ± 0.3[a]	45.5 ± 2.8
SCV	42.3 ± 2.6	40.6 ± 1.8	36.6 ± 2.1
Vibration sense	13.7 ± 3.1	10.6 ± 2.4	25.5 ± 4.8
CV-RR	3.9 ± 0.9	1.5 ± 0.4	1.9 ± 0.3[b]
Total scores for neuropathy	6.6 ± 2.5	14.3 ± 5.8	10.2 ± 2.2

MCV, SCV (m/s). CV-RR (%). [a]p = 0.009: vs. NDR; [b]p = 0.03: vs. NDR.

Table 4. Subjective symptomatic test for diabetic neuropathy and neuropathy.

	Low score	High score
MCV	49.3 ± 2.1	46.9 ± 2.5
SCV	49.7 ± 2.0	39.2 ± 2.5
Vibration sense	11.3 ± 1.5	25.7 ± 5.9[a]
CV-RR	3.3 ± 0.7	2.3 ± 0.4

MCV, SCV (m/s). CV-RR (%). [a]p = 0.013: vs. low score.

MCV or CV-RR between low and high score. In contrast, VPT was significantly elevated in the high-score group compared with that in the low-score group. SCV tended to be disturbed in high score, compared with low score.

Moreover, to determine which factors of SST contribute to the progression of neuropathy, we have divided SST into three categories as mentioned above, neurogenic, vascular and autonomic (Table 5). There were no significant differences in MCV and CV-RR among each category. However, in high scores of the vascular factor group, SCV and VPT tended to be disturbed compared with the low scores of the vascular factor group.

Discussion

Although diagnosis of diabetic neuropathy depends upon patients' symptoms, physical examinations and neurological examinations, it is difficult to evaluate the objective and quantitative state of diabetic neuropathy. Furthermore, the discrepancy between subjective symptoms and objective data is an important problem in the diagnosis of diabetic neuropathy. In order to solve these problems, the first step was establishing and quantifying the subjective symptoms of diabetic neuropathy and trying to determine the relevance of pathophysiological examination of neuropathy to the patients' symptoms. Among neurological examinations, VPT is known to be a highly sensitive method in diabetic neuropathy [4] and that was also observed in this study. High total scores for the subjective symptomatic test (SST) for diabetic neuropathy were significantly associated

Table 5. Subjective symptomatic test for diabetic neuropathy and neuropathy [2].

	Neurogenic		Vascular		Autonomic	
	Low	High	Low	High	Low	High
MCV	48.8 ± 2.0	45.9 ± 2.5	48.0 ± 1.7	47.3 ± 2.6	49.9 ± 2.2	45.6 ± 2.5
SCV	40.4 ± 1.9	39.1 ± 2.4	42.7 ± 2.3	37.3 ± 1.9[a]	40.2 ± 2.2	39.9 ± 2.5
Vibration sense	18.1 ± 4.2	20.4 ± 5.7	11.1 ± 1.9	23.4 ± 5.3[b]	22.1 ± 5.5	17.1 ± 4.1
CV-RR	3.0 ± 0.7	2.7 ± 0.4	2.7 ± 0.6	3.0 ± 0.7	2.4 ± 0.5	3.1 ± 0.8

MCV, SCV (m/s). RR-CV (%). [a]p = 0.07: vs. low. [b]p = 0.07: vs. low.

with deterioration of vibration sense and tended to be associated with deterioration of SCV and CV-RR. From the result that vascular factor of SST tended to be associated with deterioration of VPT and SCV, vascular factor of SST was suggested to contribute to the progression of neuropathy. These results suggested that SST for diabetic neuropathy was useful for detection of diabetic neuropathy, especially for deterioration of vibration sense.

This study will lead to a pathophysiological approach to diabetic neuropathy and to an accurate choice for therapy of diabetic neuropathy.

References

1. Ziegler D, Cicmir I, Mayer K, Gries FA. The natural course of peripheral and autonomic neural function during the first 2 years after diagnosis of type I diabetes. Klin Wochenschr 1988; 1085–1092.
2. Green DA, Lattimer SA, Sima AAF. New Engl J Med 1987;316:599–606.
3. Matsuoka K, Suzuki Y, Atsumi Y, Hosokawa K. Detection and symptomatic treatment of diabetic neuropathy. In: Goto Y, Lee TH, Kaneko T, Shiga Y (eds) Prevention and Treatment of NIDDM. London: Smith-Gordon, 1992;367–371.
4. Tchen PH, Chiu HC, Fu CC. Vibratory perception threshold in diabetic neuropathy. Taiwan I Hsueh Hui Tsa Chih 1990;89:23–29.

Recent Advances on the Pathogenesis and Management of Diabetes Mellitus.
S.H. Shinn, M. Shichiri and K.-W. Kim, editors.

Cognition disorder in elderly diabetic patients is related to glycemic control

Yoshikazu Goriya[1], Satoshi Takizawa[2], Eiji Miyauchi[2], Yoshiaki Tsukio[2] and Mikihiro Takasaki[2]
Departments of [1]General Medicine and [2]Gerontology, Kanazawa Medical University, Ishikawa, Japan

Abstract. The recent increase in elderly diabetic patients causes another complication of cognition disorder, i.e., senile dementia, which brings complicated problems and a poor prognosis. In this regard, we studied the mode of the onset of dementia and its relation to the glycemic control. Subjects consisted of 15 newly developed demented diabetics, and 69 nondemented elderly diabetics served as a contrast group. The age of demented patients was significantly higher than that of the nondemented patients, and were exclusively over the age of 75 years. Prevalence rates of demented patients treated by insulin and oral agents were higher than in the diet therapy. It was also revealed that dementia was more frequent in the well-controlled and the poorly controlled diabetics from an analysis of the frequency distribution of fasting blood glucose and HbA1c. The type of dementia based on brain CT examination was mostly nonvascular in the former and vascular in the latter. From these results it was suggested that chronic hyperglycemia could be a risk factor of vascular dementia, a sequela of diabetic macroangiopathy and also chronic asymptomatic hypoglycemia could be a risk factor of hypoglycemic dementia especially in elderly diabetic patients treated by insulin or oral hypoglycemic agents.

Keywords: dementia, elderly diabetics, hyperglycemia, hypoglycemia.

Introduction

As the number of elderly diabetic patients increases, the number of diabetic patients with cognition disorders increases proportionately. This other complication, senile dementia, brings about many complicated problems for the management of diabetes mellitus and a very poor prognosis. Therefore, it is very important to know the situation of dementia in the elderly diabetics and to prevent its occurrence from the viewpoints of the maintenance of better quality of life in the elderly patients. In this regard, we studied the mode of the onset of dementia and its relation to the glycemic control in elderly diabetics.

Subjects and Methods

Subjects consisted of 15 newly developed demented elderly diabetics who were diagnosed as being demented by means of the revised Hasegawa's dementia

Address for correspondence: Dr Yoshikazu Goriya, Department of General Medicine, Kanazawa Medical University, 1-1-50 Daigaku, Uchinada, Kahoku-gun, Ishikawa 920-02, Japan.

scale. Moreover, 69 nondemented elderly diabetics served as a contrast group. Firstly, prevalence rates of dementia according to age and diabetic treatment were investigated among these elderly diabetics. Secondly, frequency distribution of HbA1c in every 1% step in elderly diabetics of each treatment was studied in order to see the relationship of the development of dementia and the glycemic control. Thirdly, HbA1c in those elderly diabetics were investigated retrospectively for 2 years from the onset of dementia just to see the effects of preceding glycemic control, who this time were divided into the following three groups according to the degree of their glycemic control:

1) well-controlled demented group whose HbA1c at onset was below 8% (n = 7),
2) poorly controlled demented group whose HbA1c at onset was above 8% (n = 6), and
3) nondemented group (n = 69).

Fourthly, in order to see the relationship of glycemic control and the type of dementia, i.e., vascular or nonvascular in origin designated by brain CT examination, a plotting of fasting blood glucose (FBG) and HbA1c of each case was drawn according to the type of dementia.

Results

Prevalence rates (PR) of dementia

PR of dementia in the elderly diabetics in every 5-year step revealed that dementia appeared much more frequently after the age of 75 years ($p<0.05$). PR of dementia in elderly diabetics according to the diabetic treatment revealed that PR in insulin treatment (46.2%) was significantly higher than those in oral hypoglycemic agents (OHA: 14.6%, $p<0.05$) and diet (8.7%, $p<0.01$) treatments.

Frequency distribution of HbA1c according to treatments

HbA1c of diet therapy distributed symmetrically with a peak level of 6%. Moreover, HbA1c of OHA also distributed symmetrically with peak levels of 7—8%. In contrast to these, frequency distribution of HbA1c in insulin therapy was quite different and was divided into two groups. The first group was HbA1c with a 6% level (well-controlled group) and the other was HbA1c with more than 8% (poorly controlled group). Moreover, it was noted that dementia appeared in every case with HbA1c with a 6% level and in a quarter of the cases with HbA1c with a level of more than 11%.

Retrospective analysis of HbA1c

Although there were no changes in the level of HbA1c among the three groups 24 months before the onset of dementia, HbA1c in the well-controlled group became significantly lower than both the poorly controlled group and the nondemented contrast group 6 months before ($p<0.05$) and also at the onset of dementia ($p<0.001$).

A plot of FBG and HbA1c in elderly diabetics treated by insulin or OHA (Fig. 1)

Vascular dementia spread in the area of HbA1c over 7%, however, it was not specific as there was also high nondementia in the same area. In contrast, nonvascular dementia presented restrictively in the area of both FBG below 150 mg/dl and HbA1c below 7%.

Discussion

Since the recent report of DCCT [1], strict glycemic control has been approved for the treatment of diabetes mellitus. Although this strict glycemic control is worth it for the prevention of diabetic microangiopathy, it sometimes causes hypoglycemia. This hypoglycemia can be somewhat tolerated by ordinary patients but not by the elderly patients. It is rather dangerous for the elderly diabetics in that hypoglycemia used to be a trigger of myocardial infarction and cerebral infarction. Moreover, it may cause a cognition disorder [2]. As there were some reports of cognition disorder in young diabetics who had experienced frequent hypoglycemia [3—4], the elderly have a higher chance of having dementia. Accordingly, we studied the occurrence of dementia in the elderly diabetics. We investigated PR of dementia in the elderly diabetics and several important obser-

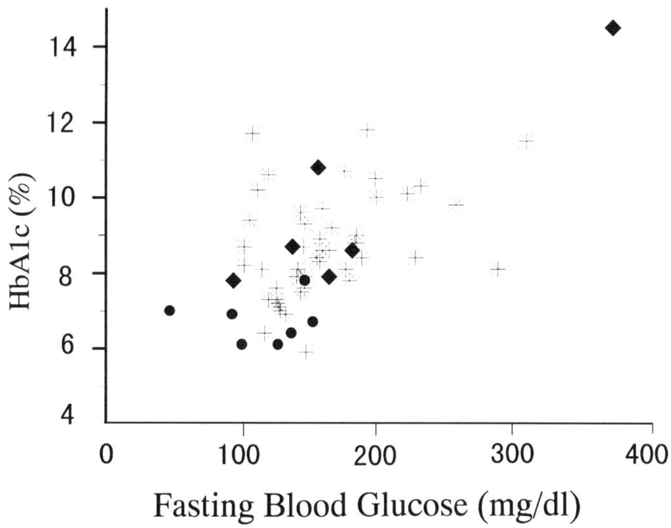

Fig. 1. A plot of fasting blood glucose and HbA1c in elderly diabetics treated by insulin or by an oral hypoglycemic agent. ●: Nonvascular dementia (n = 7), ◆: vascular dementia (n = 6), *: nondementia (n = 69).

vations were noted. The first one is that PR of dementia in the patients over 75 years of age was significantly higher than those below 74 years of age. However, this is not a specific phenomenon to the elderly diabetics but a common phenomenon to the elderly in general. The second one is that PR of dementia in insulin treatment was significantly higher than those in diet or OHA treatments. In order to see the effects of glycemic control on dementia if this was due to the severity of diabetes (hyperglycemia) or due to the adverse effects of insulin (hypoglycemia), the frequency distribution of HbA1c in elderly diabetics and PR of dementia in each HbA1c level was studied and it was revealed that dementia happened more frequently both in those well-controlled and poorly controlled elderly diabetic patients treated by insulin. Then in order to see whether these glycemic effects were acute or chronic, HbA1c in demented patients was studied retrospectively for the preceding 2 years and it was revealed that HbA1c in the well-controlled demented group had been significantly lower than the other two groups since 6 months earlier. This implies that a long-time depression of blood glucose concentration in the well-controlled group could affect the development of dementia. In addition to the relation of dementia and the glycemic control, the type of dementia is also important to be identified. In other words, which type of dementia, namely vascular or nonvascular dementia, tends to occur in those well-controlled or poorly controlled patients? For this purpose, demented patients were divided into vascular or nonvascular dementia groups by means of a brain CT examination and their FBG and HbA1c were plotted. This plot revealed that vascular dementia spread over the area of HbA1c more than 7% and nonvascular dementia located restrictively in the area of both FBG below 150 mg/dl and HbA1c below 7%. This demonstrated that vascular dementia seen in poorly controlled diabetics derived from diabetic macroangiopathy due to the long-standing hyperglycemia and aging, but it was not so specific as many nondemented patients also showed such a degree of glycemic control. Nonvascular dementia which was exclusively found in well-controlled patients can be the result of long-standing hypoglycemia, i.e., hypoglycemic dementia. With all these results, we can point out the characteristics of dementia in elderly diabetics as follows:

1) they were found in almost all of those over 75 years old; and
2) they were found in cases that were either well-controlled or poorly controlled, suggesting the former to be hypoglycemic dementia due to chronic asymptomatic hypoglycemia and the latter to be vascular dementia, a sequela of diabetic macroangiopathy.

Moreover, the characteristics of hypoglycemic dementia can be pointed out further as follows:

1) they were found in almost all of those over 75 years old,
2) they were found more frequently in drug-treated patients, especially insulin-treated ones, and
3) their glycemic control was strict enough to keep the fasting blood glucose below 150 mg/dl and also HbA1c below 7% for at least more than 6 months.

In other words, we should keep the following in our mind that in the treatment of elderly diabetics over 75 years old, by way of insulin or oral hypoglycemic agents, such a strict glycemic control could be a risk factor for the hypoglycemic dementia, a factor considerably deteriorating the quality of life in the elderly diabetic patients.

References

1. The Diabetes Control and Complication Trial Research Group. The effect of intensive treatment of diabetes on development and progression of long-term complications in insulin-dependent diabetes mellitus. N Engl J Med 1993;329:977–986.
2. Goriya Y et al. Dementia in the elderly diabetic patients – effects of glycemic control. J Jpn Diabet Soc 1995;38:267–273.
3. Langan SJ, Deary IJ, Hepburn DA, Frier BM. Cumulative cognitive impairment following recurrent severe hypoglycemia in adult patients with insulin-treated diabetes mellitus. Diabetologia 1991;34:337–344.
4. Ryan CM, Williams TM, Finegold DM, Orchard TJ. Cognitive dysfunction in adults with Type 1 (insulin-dependent) diabetes mellitus of long duration: Effects of recurrent hypoglycemia and other chronic complications. Diabetologia 1993;36:329–334.

Recent Advances on the Pathogenesis and Management of Diabetes Mellitus.
S.H. Shinn, M. Shichiri and K.-W. Kim, editors.

Power spectral analysis of heart rate in microalbuminuric diabetic patients

Jinbae Kim[1], Yongsoo Park[1], Youhern Ahn[1], Taewha Kim[1], Mokhyun Kim[1], Youngju Lee[2] and Myunggul Yum[3]

Departments of [1]Internal Medicine, [2]Neurology and [3]Pediatrics, Hanyang University College of Medicine, Seoul, Korea

Abstract. *Background.* Autonomic dysfunction in diabetic patients is related to an increased incidence of arrhythmic deaths. The prognostic importance of subclinical cardiac autonomic neuropathy emphasizes the need for a diagnosis of alterations of cardiac autonomic modulation at the earliest possible stage.

Methods. We performed autoregressive power spectral analysis of fluctuation of RR interval duration in the electrocardiogram in 37 NIDDM patients and 42 healthy controls. Patients were divided according to urinary albumin excretion as normo- (<20 μg/min, n = 18), micro- (>20 and <200 μg/min, n = 12) and macroalbuminuria (>200 μg/min, n = 7). Forty-three matched healthy subjects served as controls.

Results. NIDDM patients had reduced amplitude of the lower frequency power (LFP) and the total power (TP) (LFP: 248 ± 45 m^2, TP: 1,154,252 m^2) compared with the control group (LFP: 30,741 m^2, TP: 1,365 ± 215 m^2, p = 0.07). The high-frequency power (HFP) in NIDDM patients (476 ± 196 m^2) increased more than that of the control group (178 ± 20 m^2, p = 0.09). Microalbuminuric NIDDM patients had a decreased amplitude of the LFP and TP (LFP: 172 ± 158 m^2, TP: 733 ± 454 m^2) compared with the normoalbuminuric NIDDM patients (LFP: 246 ± 336 m^2, TP: 897 ± 1,164 m^2). The HFP in microalbuminuric NIDDM patients (132 ± 114 m^2) decreased more than that of the normoalbuminuric NIDDM patients (168 ± 201 m^2, p = 0.09). In contrast, macroalbuminuric NIDDM patients had increased amplitude of all three powers (LFP: 363 ± 538 m^2, TP: 1,503 ± 2,069 m^2, HFP: 597 ± 924 m^2). However, they did not significantly differ from neither the normoalbuminuric nor the microalbuminuric NIDDM patients.

Conclusions. NIDDM patients with microalbuminuria had reduced amplitude of the low-frequency and high-frequency oscillations. Microalbuminuric diabetic patients had significantly impaired vagal function and abnormal sympathovagal interaction. However, the tendency was not further deranged in macroalbuminuric NIDDM patients. We believe that this unexpected discrepancy is due to the relatively small numbers of study subjects and the heterogeneity of macroalbuminuric NIDDM subjects.

Keywords: autonomic neuropathy, heart-rate variability, microalbuminuria.

Introduction

Autonomic dysfunction in ischemic heart disease is related to an increased incidence of arrhythmic death, and symptomatic autonomic neuropathy carries a

---

Address for correspondence: Yongsoo Park MD, Department of Internal Medicine, Hanyang University Hospital, 249-1 Kyomun-dong, Kuri, Kyunggi-do, Seoul 471-020, Japan.

worse prognosis than any other complication of diabetes [1]. The subclinical diabetic autonomic neuropathy, in the form of cardiac autonomic neuropathy, evolves early in the course of diabetes, even in the absence of other microvascular complications [2]. The prognostic importance of subclinical cardiac autonomic neuropathy emphasizes the need for a diagnosis of alterations of cardiac autonomic modulation at the earliest possible stage. The hallmark and earliest indicator of cardiac autonomic neuropathy is a reduced heart-rate variability (HRV) [3]. Cardiac autonomic neuropathy is diagnosed by using a battery of cardiac autonomic function tests that evaluate changes in HRV. Recently, power spectral analysis of HRV has proved a useful tool in evaluating cardiovascular autonomic activity [4].

Microalbuminuria predicts proteinuria and cardiovascular mortality in NIDDM [5] and IDDM patients [6]. A previous report indicated that IDDM patients had impaired autonomic balance even at the microalbuminuric stage [7]. The aim of the present study was to evaluate sympathovagal balance in relation to microalbuminuria in NIDDM patients.

Materials and Methods

Forty-three healthy subjects and 79 NIDDM patients were studied. Forty-two of the 79 NIDDM patients were divided into groups according to their urinary albumin excretion as normoalbuminuria group (<20 μg/min, $n = 18$), microalbuminuria group (>20 and <200 μg/min, $n = 14$), and proteinuria group (>200 μg/min, $n = 10$). We assessed autonomic system activity by power spectrum analysis of HRV in 37 NIDDM patients and compared the results with those of a 43 age-matched control group.

Study subjects were invited to a metabolic ward at 9.00 am. When the subject had rested for about 10 min in a calm and dark room, an electrocardiogram (ECG) was recorded for 15 min. The ECG signal was immediately digitalized and sampled at 500 Hz. Data were transferred and stored on a hard-disk memory of a personal computer. In a three-step spectral estimation technique, an autoregressive algorithm was used to detect the QRS complex, compute the statistical evaluation of the RR intervals, and analyze the power spectral density of the time series. The R wave was detected automatically by the classic adaptive/threshold algorithm. Statistical data on the RR intervals, including the mean RR duration and variance and the normalized RR series (after subtracting the mean), were then computed and stored on hard-disk. The software program executed the autoregressive model in a repeated process – it applied the autocorrelation functions to the complete RR series and used the Levinson-Durbin algorithm to compute the coefficients of the Yule-Walker matrix (the autocorrelation matrix). Anderson's test was used to check the validity of the assumed model, and Aikake's Information Criterion was used to choose the order of the model. Spectral power was then calculated and the spectral series memorized on hard-disk. In this study we examined a high-frequency (HF) spectral component

(0.15 Hz <) reflecting parasympathetic activity, and a low-frequency component (LF) (0.03 ~ 0.15 Hz) corresponding to sympathetic activity.

Results

Comparison of the HRV at each frequency component between NIDDM patients and control group

NIDDM patients had reduced amplitude of the lower frequency power (LFP) and the total power (TP) (LFP: 248 ± 45 m^2, TP: 1,154 ± 252 m^2) compared with the control group (LFP: 307 ± 41 m^2, TP: 1,365 ± 215 m^2), but these did not reach statistical significance ($p = 0.07$). The high-frequency power (HFP) in NIDDM patients (476 ± 196 m^2) increased more than that of the control group (178 ± 20 m^2), but this did not reach statistical significance ($p = 0.09$).

Heart rate variability in the NIDDM patient in relation to the grade of albuminuria

Microalbuminuric NIDDM patients had decreased amplitude of the LFP and TP (LFP: 172 ± 158 m^2, TP: 733 ± 454 m^2) compared with the normoalbuminuric NIDDM patients (LFP: 246 ± 336 m^2, TP: 897 ± 1,164 m^2), but these did not reach statistical significance ($p = 0.09$). The HFP in microalbuminuric NIDDM patients (132 ± 114 m^2) decreased more than that of the normoalbuminuric NIDDM patients (168 ± 201 m^2), but this did not reach statistical significance. In contrast, macroalbuminuric NIDDM patients had increased amplitude of all three powers (LFP: 363 ± 538 m^2, TP: 1,503 ± 2,069 m^2, HFP: 597 ± 924 m^2). However, they did not significantly differ from neither those of normoalbuminuric NIDDM patients nor from those of microalbuminuric NIDDM patients.

Discussion

The subclinical diabetic autonomic neuropathy in the form of cardiac autonomic neuropathy evolves early in the course of diabetes, even in the absence of other microvascular complications [2]. The prognostic importance of subclinical cardiac autonomic neuropathy emphasizes the need for a diagnosis of alterations of cardiac autonomic modulation at the earliest possible stage. The hallmark and earliest indicator of cardiac autonomic neuropathy is a reduced HRV [3]. HRV is the amount of heart rate fluctuations around the mean heart rate, and is a valuable tool to investigate the sympathetic and parasympathetic function of the autonomic nervous system. Cardiac autonomic neuropathy is diagnosed by using a battery of cardiac autonomic function tests that evaluate changes in HRV. The diagnosis of cardiac autonomic neuropathy is usually established by cardiovascular autonomic function tests like the Valsalva maneuver, deep breathing test, and isometric hand-grip test [8]. Recently, power spectral analysis of HRV has proved a useful tool in evaluating cardiovascular autonomic activity [4]. This method allows a reliable quantification of the low-frequency (LF) and high-frequency (HF) components of the heart rate power spectral density; these are considered to be under mainly sympathetic and pure parasympathetic control, respectively.

It has been stated that parasympathetic damage occurs more commonly than sympathetic damage [9]. The clinical significance of early and reliable detection of diabetic cardiac autonomic neuropathy, as possible with heart rate spectral analysis, is obvious because the 5-year mortality rate in diabetic patients with neuropathy is increased 4–5 times compared with diabetic patients without neuropathy [1,10]. It was established that in diabetic patients, without abnormal cardiac autonomic function tests, parasympathetic tone was lowered [11,12]. It was concluded that cardiac (parasympathetic) autonomic activity might be diminished in diabetic patients before clinical symptoms of neuropathy became evident.

Recently it has been suggested that microalbuminuria predicts proteinuria and cardiovascular mortality in diabetes [5–7], and early autonomic dysfunction in IDDM patients [7]. From this study, NIDDM patients with microalbuminuria had reduced amplitude of the LF and HF oscillations. Microalbuminuric diabetic patients had significantly impaired vagal function and abnormal sympathovagal interaction. However, the tendency was not further deranged in macroalbuminuric NIDDM patients. We expected to see the lowest level of all three powers in the proteinuria group, however, the results showed us a disturbing increase in all three powers instead. We believe that this unexpected discrepancy was due to the relatively small numbers of study subjects and the heterogenecity of macroalbuminuric NIDDM subjects, which deserves further examination on this matter.

References

1. Ewing DJ, Campbell IW, Clarke BF. The natural history of diabetic autonomic neuropathy. Q J Med 1980;49:95–108.
2. Ewing DJ, Neilson JM, Shapiro CM, Stewart JA, Reid W. Twenty four hour heart rate variability: Effects of posture, sleep, and time of day in healthy controls and comparison with bedside tests of autonomic function in diabetic patients. Br Heart J 1991;65:239–244.
3. Ewing DJ, Campbell IW, Clarke BF. Assessment of cardiovascular effects in diabetic autonomic neuropathy and prognosis implications. Ann Intern Med 1980;92:308–311.
4. Mancia G, Paleari F, Parati G. Early diagnosis of diabetic autonomic neuropathy: Present and future approaches. Diabetologia 1997;40:482–484.
5. Mogensen CE. Microalbuminuria predicts clinical proteinuria and early mortality in maturity-onset diabetes. N Engl J Med 1984;310:356–360.
6. Mogensen CE, Christensen CK. Predicting diabetic nephropathy in insulin-dependent patients. N Engl J Med 1984;311:89–93.
7. Molgaard H, Christensen PD, Hermansen K, Sorensen KE, Christensen CK, Mogensen CE. Early recognition of autonomic dysfunction in microalbuminuria: Significance for cardiovascular mortality in diabetes mellitus? Diabetologia 1994;37:788–796.
8. Ewing DJ, Clarke BF. Autonomic neuropathy: Its diagnosis and prognosis. Clin Endoclinol Metab 1986;15:855–888.
9. Bellavere F, Bosello G, Cardone C, Girardello L, Ferri M, Fedele D. Evidence of early impairement of parasympathetic reflexes in insulin-dependent diabetics without autonomic symptoms. Diabet Metab 1985;11:152–156.

10. O'Brien IA, McFadden JP, Corrall RJ. The influence of autonomic neuropathy on mortality in insulin-dependent diabetes. Q J Med 1991;79:495–502.
11. Pfeifer MA, Cook D, Brodsky J, Tice D, Reenan A, Swedine S. Quantitative evaluation of cardiac parasympathetic activity in normal and diabetic man. Diabetes 1982;31:339–345.
12. Malpas SC, Maling TJ. Heart-rate variability and cardiac autonomic function in diabetes. Diabetes 1990;39:1177–1181.

Recent Advances on the Pathogenesis and Management of Diabetes Mellitus.
S.H. Shinn, M. Shichiri and K.-W. Kim, editors.

Glycemic threshold for lowering urinary albumin excretion

Kazuko Iwashima[1], Rieko Anaguchi[1], Yasuhisa Yamamoto[1], Takashi Ohoshi[1] and Kishio Nanjo[2]
[1]Third Department of Medicine, Osaka-Minami National Hospital, Osaka; and [2]First Department of Medicine, Wakayama University of Medical Science, Wakayama, Japan

Abstract. The extent of glycemic control necessary for lowering urinary albumin excretion was evaluated in diabetic patients without overt proteinuria. Urinary albumin excretion was measured in at least three random urine samples obtained 6 months before admission to our hospital. The median value of the ratios of albumin to creatinine (m-Alb) was compared with the 24-h urinary albumin excretion rate (AER) for each patient on admission ($\ln y = \ln 2.9 + 0.51 \ln x$, n = 27, r = 0.48). The mean value of glycated hemoglobins (m-HbA1c) 6 months after discharge correlated with the change in m-Alb between preadmission and postdischarge ($y = -2.71 + 0.3x$, n = 34, r = 0.4). Then, from the level of m-HbA1c after discharge, three patient groups were selected (A: $<7\%$, n = 7, B: $7\leqslant\ <8$, n = 9, C: $8\leqslant$, n = 18). Body mass index, blood pressure or serum lipids did not change between preadmission and postdischarge in any group, however, m-Alb decreased in group A only ($p<0.05$ from Wilcoxon's test). "m-Alb" is a clinically available marker for screening and follow-up of early-stage nephropathy, and the target level of glycated hemoglobin would be lower than 7% for lowering urinary albumin excretion.

Keywords: early-stage nephropathy, glycemic control, ratio of albumin to creatinine in random urine.

Background

In the diabetic patients without overt proteinuria, we aimed to answer the following two questions;

1. Is it possible to use urinary albumin excretion in random urine samples as the substitute for a 24-h urinary albumin excretion rate which is a clinically established marker for early-stage nephropathy [1]?
2. What extent of glycemic control is necessary for lowering urinary albumin excretion?

Methods

1. Urinary albumin excretion was measured in at least three random urine samples obtained 6 months prior to admission to our hospital. The median value of the ratios of albumin to creatinine (m-Alb) was compared with the 24-h urinary albumin excretion rate (AER; µg/min) on admission in each patient.

Address for correspondence: Kazuko Iwashima, Third Department of Medicine, Osaka-Minami National Hospital, 2-1, Kido-higashi machi Kawachinagano-shi, Osaka 586, Japan.

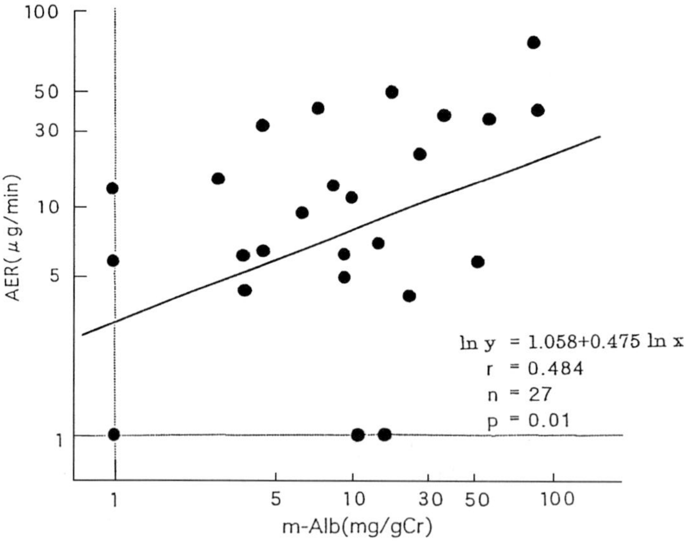

Fig. 1. Relationship between m-Alb and 24-h urinary albumin excretion rate (ER) on admission.

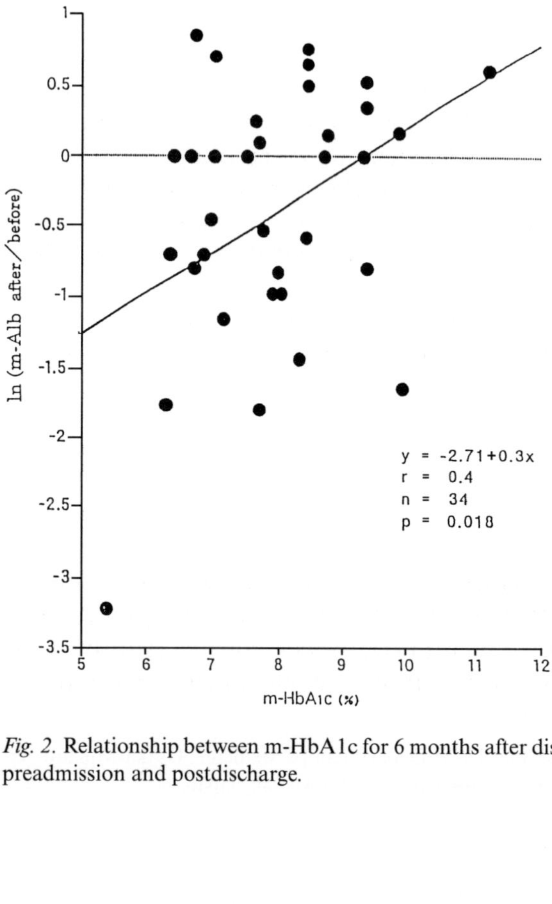

Fig. 2. Relationship between m-HbA1c for 6 months after discharge and the change in m-Alb between preadmission and postdischarge.

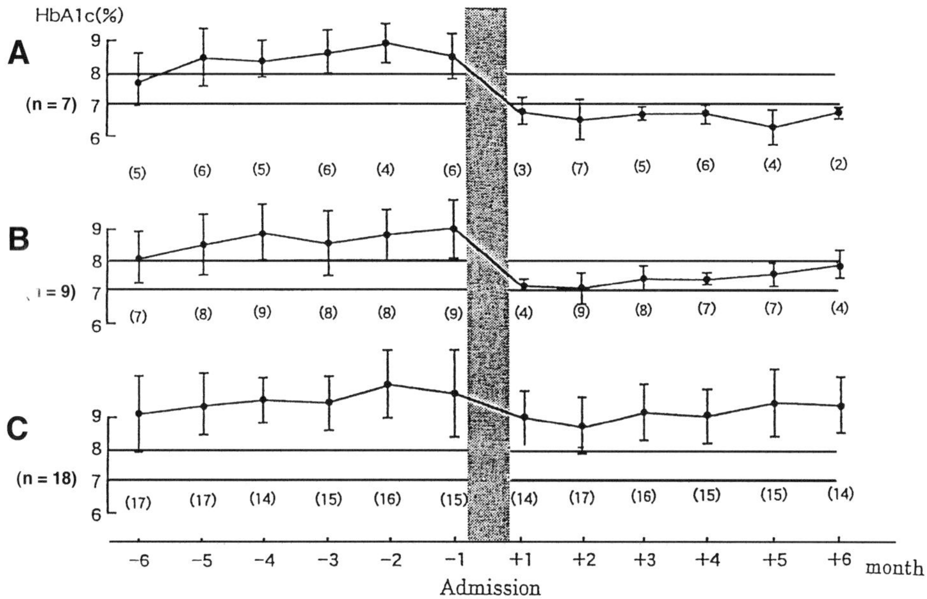

Fig. 3. Selection of three patient groups (**A, B and** C) from the level of HbA1c after discharge.

2. The mean value of glycated hemoglobins (m-HbA1c) 6 months after discharge was compared with the change in m-Alb from preadmission to postdischarge.
3. Urinary albumin was measured by turbidimetric immunoassay.
4. For the regression analysis, logarithms of m-Albs and AERs were used and the changes in m-Albs from preadmission to postdischarge were expressed as ln (x_1/x_2) where x_1 and x_2 were determined postdischarge and preadmission, respectively. χ^2 test and F tests were used for comparison between the three subgroups of patients; unpaired t test for comparison between each two subgroups; and a paired t test and Wilcoxon's test for a comparison of changes between preadmission and postdischarge.

Results

1. m-Alb correlated with AER (Fig. 1).
2. m-HbA1c correlated with the change in m-Alb from preadmission to postdischarge (Fig. 2). Although BMI, serum lipids and blood pressure did not change in any of the three patient groups (A,B and C) selected from the level of HbA1c after discharge (Fig. 3), m-Alb decreased from preadmission to postdischarge only in group A (Table 1).

Table 1. Comparison of clinical profiles between three groups (mean ± SD).

	A (n = 7)	B (n = 9)	C (n = 18)
Sex (male:female)	3:4	3:6	8:10 NS
Age (years)	69 ± 10	68 ± 10	60 ± 13 NS
Duration of DM (years)	17 ± 6	16 ± 8	14 ± 9 NS
SCr (mg/dl)	0.7 ± 0.1	0.8 ± 0.3	0.8 ± 0.2 NS
Ccr (ml/min)	73.4 ± 17.5	75.3 ± 29.3	73.3 ± 26.1 NS
BMI (kg/m^2)			
Before	21.8 ± 3.3	22.7 ± 3.5	24.6 ± 3.1
After	21.5 ± 2.7	22.4 ± 3.4	24.3 ± 3.2
T-chol (mg/dl)[a]			
Before	156 ± 47	196 ± 41	198 ± 38
After	172 ± 24	201 ± 61	208 ± 32
TG (mg/dl)[a]			
Before	72 ± 21	112 ± 43	137 ± 76
After	74 ± 28	104 ± 41	130 ± 89
HDL-chol (mg/dl)[a]			
Before	59 ± 6	55 ± 19	43 ± 9
After	69 ± 12	64 ± 18	57 ± 16[b]
m-SBP (mmHg)			
Before	148 ± 11	154 ± 16	140 ± 18
After	145 ± 14	155 ± 16	141 ± 17
m-DBP (mmHg)			
Before	79 ± 5	82 ± 9	78 ± 8
After	79 ± 8	84 ± 6	78 ± 7
m-HbA1c (%)			
Before	8.4 ± 0.5[c]	8.6 ± 0.7[d]	9.5 ± 0.8
After	6.5 ± 0.5[b]	7.4 ± 0.3[b]	9.0 ± 0.8
m-Alb (mg/gCr)			
Before	13.3 (−20.3 ~ 97.3)	22.0 (10.5 ~ 61.7)	18.0 (9.0 ~ 60.8)
After	5.6 (−12.6 ~ 50.2)[f]	19.0 (9.2 ~ 60.2)	14.5 (8.2 ~ 65.8)

[a]A, n = 5; B, n = 6; C, n = 14; [b]$p < 0.01$; [c]$p < 0.01$; [d]$p < 0.02$ (vs. C); [e]median value (95% confidence limits); [f]$p < 0.05$ (vs. before).

Conclusions

1. "m-Alb" is a clinically available marker for screening and follow-up of early-stage nephropathy.
2. The target level of glycated hemoglobin would be lower than 7% for lowering urinary albumin excretion.

Reference

1. Woolerton J, Jury DR, Dunn PJ, Speed JF. Urine albumin creatinine ratio and clinical correlates in a diabetic population. NZ Med J 1987:100:130–134.

Recent Advances on the Pathogenesis and Management of Diabetes Mellitus.
S.H. Shinn, M. Shichiri and K.-W. Kim, editors.

Intrarenal resistive index (RI) and the extracellular matrix in NIDDM patients with nephropathy

Hosojima Hiroyuki[1], Uchida Kenzo[1] and Yamamoto Itaru[2]
[1]Division of Endocrinology, Department of Internal Medicine; and [2]Department of Radiology, Kanazawa Medical University, Uchinada, Ishikawa, Japan

Abstract. Since biochemical and structural changes of the extracellular matrix (ECM) in the basement membrane are responsible for the progression of diabetic complications, we investigated the relationship between the components of ECM: type IV collagen, laminin, fibronectin or sialic acid, and the intrarenal resistive index (RI), which is obtained from duplex Doppler sonography of the kidney and a marker of the renal vascular resistance, in 137 NIDDM subjects with nephropathy. Serum creatinine and urinary albumin excretion values correlated with levels of ECM or RI, and urinary albumin excretion values correlated with levels of ECM or RI, and the RI also had significant correlations with type IV collagen, laminin or sialic acid. The RI, serum levels of type IV collagen and laminin, and plasma fibronectin increased in parallel with the severity of diabetic nephropathy in these subjects. Thus, it is suggested that the deterioration or proliferation of ECM in the capillary and glomerular basement membrane may contribute to the progression of intrarenal arterial resistance.

Keywords: diabetic nephropathy, fibronectin, laminin, NIDDM, RI, sialic acid, type IV collagen.

Introduction

It is suggested that the widening or proliferation of the capillary basement membrane must be responsible for the onset and development in diabetic microangiopathy [1,2]. The type IV collagen laminin, sialic acid, fibronectin or heparin-sulfate proteoglycan, which are high molecule glycoproteins, constitute the extracellar matrix (ECM) in the basement membrane of the capillary wall and glomerulus. The chronic hyperglycemia affects the protein constitution by enhanced nonenzymatic glucosylation, and produces the advanced glycated end-products (AGEs) in diabetic patients consequently [3]. Therefore, the glycated biochemical deterioration of the ECM is supposed to lead the progression of diabetic microangiopathy [4]. On the other hand, the intrarenal resistive index (RI), which is obtained from the duplex Doppler sonography of the kidney, is related to the severity of diabetic nephropathy and the RI is thought to be a marker of renal vascular resistance [5,6]. In the present study, we investigated the relationships between the renal RI and changes of ECM in NIDDM subjects with nephropathy.

Address for correspondence: Hosojima Hiroyuki, 1-1 Daigaku Uchinada, Ishikawa 920-02, Japan.

Materials and Methods

137 NIDDM subjects with nephropathy (64 men and 73 women, mean age: 62.9 ± 1.0, mean ± SE) and 12 nondiabetic subjects with normotension (six men and six women, mean age: 60.2 ± 2.0) were studied. Of these subjects, 45 were treated with insulin, 72 with an oral hypoglycemic agent, and 20 with diet therapy alone, respectively. The mean duration of diabetes in these subjects was 14.3 ± 0.8. Diabetic nephropathy was divided into three classes according to the 24-h urinary albumin excretion (UAE): 57 normoalbuminuria (<30 mg/d) subjects, 53 microalbuminuria (30–300 mg/d) subjects, and 27 macroalbuminuria (≥300 mg/d) subjects, respectively. Sonograms were obtained by using a mechanical sector scanner with a 3.75 MHZ probe (Toshiba SSA-270A). A duplex Doppler examination was performed on the bilateral kidney. Doppler signal waveform was taken in the region of the interlobar artery in the kidney, and the RI was calculated from the following formula: Vmax − Vmin/Vmax. Serum levels of type IV collagen and laminin or sialic acid were assayed by a RIA, EIA or an enzymatic method, respectively, and plasma fibronectin by a TIA method.

Results

The clinical background and renal function in these patients are shown in Table 1. The subjects in groups of microalbuminuria (micro) and macroalbuminuria (macro) had over 9.0% of glycohemoglobin (HbA1c) and an increased level of UAE. Serum or urinary renal functions in the macro group were significantly higher than those of the normoalbuminuria group (normo, Table 1). In Table 2, the RIs and serum or plasma levels of ECM in the three groups of NIDDM and control subjects were shown. The mean RI was 0.60 ± 0.01 in the control group, however, it was 0.64 ± 0.01 in the normo group, and then increased parallel with the severity of diabetic nephropathy. The RI came to 0.73 ± 0.01 maximally in the macro group. In the changes of ECMs, serum levels of type IV collagen (7S) increased parallel with the increase of UAE. It was 5.7 ± 0.2 ng/ml

Table 1. The clinical background and renal functions in NIDDM subjects with nephropathy.

Albuminuria	Normo	Micro	Macro
N	57	53	27
M/F	27/30	22/31	15/31
Age (years)	62.3 ± 1.5	62.5 ± 2.0	65.0 ± 2.2
HbA1c (%)	7.7 ± 0.2	9.0 ± 0.3[a]	9.1 ± 0.3[a]
S-Cr (mg/dl)	0.7 ± 0.92	0.7 ± 0.02	1.1 ± 0.2[a]
BUN (mg/dl)	16.3 ± 0.7	16.8 ± 0.6	25.8 ± 3.1[a]
UAE (mg/dl)	12.0 ± 0.7	116 ± 11[a]	1175 ± 210[a]
NAG (mg/dl)	4.8 ± 0.2	5.4 ± 0.2	10.2 ± 1.6[a]

[a]$p < 0.01$ vs. normo group.

Table 2. The RIs, serum type IV collagen, laminin and sialic acid, and plasma fibronectin levels in three groups of NIDDM subjects with nephropathy and control subjects.

Albuminuria	Diabetic subjects			
	Normo	Micro	Macro	Control
Resistive index	0.64 ± 0.01	0.66 ± 0.01	0.73 ± 0.01[a]	0.60 ± 0.01
IV Collagen (7s) (ng/ml)	4.7 ± 0.1	5.1 ± 0.1	5.7 ± 0.1[a]	4.4 ± 0.1
Laminin (ng/dl)	194.6 ± 4.9	223.3 ± 8.9	303.8 ± 21.1[a]	192.0 ± 3.0
Fibronectin (μg/ml)	407.3 ± 12.8	430.4 ± 13.2	462.3 ± 24.7[a]	370.4 ± 13.0
Sialic acid (mg/dl)	63.6 ± 1.1	62.7 ± 1.2	69.7 ± 1.8[b]	60.2 ± 1.0

[a]$p<0.01$ Macro group vs. normo, micro and Control groups; [b]$p<0.01$ macro group vs. Control group.

in the macro group, and this level was significantly higher than those of other groups. A mean level of serum laminin was 194.6 ± 4.9 ng/ml in the normo group, and enhanced to 303.8 ± 21.2 ng/ml in the macro group, and this was significantly higher than those of the other groups. The serum sialic acid of the three groups did not increase parallel with the increase of UAE. The level of the macro group was significantly higher than that of the control. The plasma fibronectin increased parallel with the increases of UAE. In the macro group, the fibronectin was 462.3 ± 24.7 ng/ml, and this was significantly higher than those of other groups.

We studied the interrelationships among levels of RI, serum creatinine, UAE, type IV collagen (7S), laminin, fibronectin or sialic acid (Table 3). Serum creatinine and UAE had strong positive correlations with the RI, type IV collagen or laminin levels. Above all, there was a stronger positive relationship between type IV collagen and the laminin level in the correlations of ECMs. There were, however, no relations among glycoslated hemoglobin, glycoalbumin, RI, serum or renal functions, or ECM levels.

Table 3. The correlation coefficients in the relationships among RI, serum creatinine, urinary albumin excretion, serum type IV collagen, laminin, sialic acid and plasma fibronectin.

	S-Cr	UAE	IV-Coll	Fibron.	S-Acid	Laminin	RI
S-CR		0.463[a]	0.309[a]	0.046	−0.030	0.525[a]	0.468[a]
UAE	0.463[a]		0.601[a]	0.291[a]	0.245[b]	0.589[a]	0.528[a]
IV-Coll	0.309[a]	0.601[a]		−0.100	0.249[b]	0.708[a]	0.386[a]
Fibron.	0.046	0.291[a]	−0.100		0.241[b]	0.219[c]	−0.05
S-Acid	−0.030	0.245[b]	0.249[b]	0.241[b]		0.387[a]	0.263[a]
Laminin	0.525[a]	0.589[a]	0.708[a]	0.219[c]	0.387[a]		0.385[a]
RI	0.468[a]	0.528[a]	0.386[a]	−0.05	0.263[a]	0.385[a]	

[a]$p<0.01$; [b]$p<0.02$; [c]$p<0.05$. S-Cr: serum creatinine, UAE: urinary albumin excretion, IV-Coll: type IV collagen, Fibron.: fibronectin, S-Acid: sialic acid, RI: resistive index.

Discussion

Renal involvement in diabetes mellitus is an important biological problem. The mechanism of this injury, the underlying cause, and the nature of progressive renal insufficiency are unclear. In general, it has been proposed that diabetic nephropathy is predominantly a glomerular disease as a progressive increase in urinary albumin excretion. A pathologic lesion of diffuse glomerular sclerosis or nodular intercapillary glomerulosclerosis is typically seen in patients with advanced diabetic nephropathy [7]. The lesion mainly consists of an excess production of extracellular substances in the mesangium histologically [8]. Recently, the clinical and histological studies have revealed the increased distribution of the components of the extracellular matrices in diabetic nephropathy [9]. It has been reported that the increases of serum laminin and type IV collagen were closely related with the development of diabetic nephropathy [10], and increased steady-static levels of laminin B_1 in RNA in kidneys of long-term streptozotocin-treated rats [11].

We have reported that NIDDM subjects had elevated RI as compared to that in nondiabetic subjects [5]. The RI also rose parallel with the increases of urinary protein and albumin excretion in diabetic subjects, and increased more in hypertensive NIDDM patients with overt nephropathy [6].

In the present study, we investigated the relationships between the renal RI and changes of ECMs in NIDDM subjects with nephropathy. The results are as follows:

1) serum creatinine level and urinary albumin excretion are significantly correlated with levels of type IV collagen, laminin, sialic acid or interlobar RI of the kidney in NIDDM subjects with overt nephropathy;
2) serum type IV collagen had a strong correlation with a level of laminin (r = 0.708);
3) the RI significantly correlated with levels of type IV collagen, lamin or sialic acid; and
4) the RI, serum levels of type IV collagen and laminin, and plasma fibronectin increased parallel with the severity of diabetic nephropathy.

Thus, it is suggested that the proliferation or deterioration of ECMs in the capillary wall and/or glomerular basement membrane may contribute to the progression of intrarenal arterial resistance, and may lead to the advanced stage of diabetic renal disease.

References

1. Mauer SM, Stiffes MW, Brown DM. The kidney in diabetes. Am J Med 1981;70:603–612.
2. Østerby R, Gundersen HJG. Glomerular size and structure in diabetes mellitus. Diabetologia 1975;11:225–229.
3. Brownlee M, Cerami A, Vlassara H. Advanced glycosylation end products in tissue and the biochemical basis of diabetic complications. N Engl J Med 1988;318:1315–1321.

4. Kefalides NS. Biochemical properties of human glomerular basement membrane in normal and diabetic kidney. J Clin Invest 1974;53:403–407.
5. Hosojima H, Miyauchi E, Morimoto S, Yamamoto I. Intrarenal duplex doppler sonography in type 2 diabetic patients with nephropathy. Diabetologia Croatica 1995;24:13–18.
6. Hosojima H, Miyauchi E, Morimoto S, Yamamoto I. Evaluation of renal blood flow with renal duplex Doppler sonography in diabetic patients with nephropathy. J Jpn Diab Soc 1996;39: 765–774.
7. Mogensen CE. Diabetes mellitus and the kidney. Kidney Int 1982;21:673–675.
8. Suzuki Y. Constituents of the extracellular matrices in diabetic glomerulosclerosis. Jpn J Nephr 1989;31:47–54.
9. Pietschman P, Schernthaner G, Schnack CH, Gaube S. Serum concentrations of laminin P_1 in diabetics with advanced nephropathy. J Clin Pathol 1988;41:929–1003.
10. Högeman B, Voss B, Altenwerth FJ, Schneider M, Rauterburg J, Gerlach U. Concentrations of 7S collagen and laminin P_1, in sera of patients with diabetes mellitus. Klin Wochenschr 1986;64:382–387.
11. Poulsom R, Kurkinen M, Prockop DJ, Boot-Handford RP. Increased steady-state levels of laminin B_1 mRNA in kidneys of long-term, streptozotocin diabetic rats. J Biol Chem 1988;263: 10072–10076.

Recent Advances on the Pathogenesis and Management of Diabetes Mellitus.
S.H. Shinn, M. Shichiri and K.-W. Kim, editors.

The effect of PGE1 on symptom and vascular cell damage in diabetic patients with limb numbness

Y. Kawabata, H. Ikegami, E. Yamato, Y. Kawaguchi, T. Fujisawa, Y. Hamada, M. Hotta, H. Ueda, M. Shintani, K. Nojima, N. Babaya, J. Fu, G.-Q. Shen and T. Ogihara
Osaka University Medical School, Osaka, Japan

Abstract. Although both vascular and metabolic factors were implicated in the pathogenesis of diabetic neuropathy, the relative contribution of these factors to diabetic neuropathy is still controversial. To assess the contribution of the vascular factor to neuropathy, we investigated the effect of prostaglandin E1 (PGE1) on symptoms, ankle pressure index (API) and vascular endothelial cell damage in NIDDM patients with limb numbness. After the intravenous administration of PGE1 (80 μg/day) for 2 weeks, numbness and API improved in 88% of the subjects. In addition, plasma thrombomodulin levels, a marker for endothelial cell damage, tended to decrease. These data suggest that improvement of hemodynamics by PGE1 contributed to the amelioration of limb numbness in diabetic patients and that this effect is associated with the improvement of endothelial cell damage.

Keywords: diabetic neuropathy, endothelial cell damage, prostaglandin E1, thrombomodulin.

Introduction

Although both vascular and metabolic factors are implicated in the pathogenesis of diabetic neuropathy, the relative contribution of these factors to diabetic neuropathy is still controversial. Prostaglandin E1 (PGE1) has a vasodilatory effect and inhibitory effect for platelet aggregation, and improves red blood cell deformability. Therefore, the improvement of hemodynamics by PGE1 is expected to reduce symptoms and vascular endothelial cell damage in diabetic neuropathy.

In the present study, we investigated the effect of PGE1 on symptom and vascular endothelial cell damage in diabetic patients with neuropathy.

Subjects and Methods

Subjects

We studied eight patients (four males and four females) with non-insulin-depend-

Address for correspondence: Hiroshi Ikegami MD, Department of Geriatric Medicine, Osaka University Medical School, 2-2 Yamadaoka, Suita, Osaka 565, Japan. Tel.: +81-6-879-3852. Fax: +81-6-879-3859.

ent diabetes mellitus (NIDDM) complaining of limb numbness. The mean age was 62.6 years. The mean fasting plasma glucose level was 159 mg/dl and the mean hemoglobin A1c was 8.2%. Four patients were treated with sulfonylurea and four with insulin. Patients whose serum creatinine concentration was higher than 1.2 mg/dl and patients who had a bleeding tendency were excluded.

Methods

Patients were intravenously administered with 40 μg PGE1 (Prostandin®) twice daily for 2 weeks. Subjective symptom (limb numbness) was evaluated before and after PGE1 administration. Plasma thrombomodulin (TM) levels, as a marker of endothelial cell damage and ankle pressure index (API), were measured simultaneously. TM levels were measured with an enzyme-linked immunosorbent assay kit (MGC-01-001) established by Mitsubishi Gas Chemical Co. Ltd. (Tokyo, Japan).

Statistical analysis

Statistical analyses were performed using the Mann-Whitney U test. Results are expressed as mean ± SEM and $p < 0.05$ was considered as significant.

Results

Figure 1 shows a clinical course of a typical case treated with PGE1. The patient was a 62-year-old female. She suffered from NIDDM for 14 years and had been treated with gliclazide. She was admitted due to severe lower limb numbness. She received PGE1 from the 15th day after admission. Limb numbness improved after PGE1 administration. API improved from 0.95 to 1.20, and the plasma TM level decreased from 39.3 to 32.4 U/ml. As a whole, limb numbness improved in 88% of the patients. API improved in seven out of eight patients

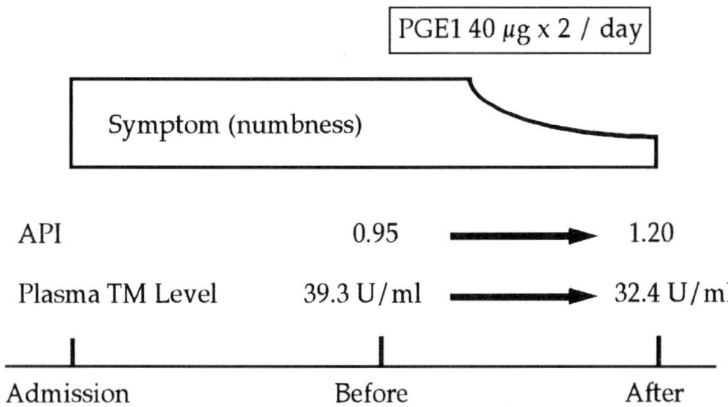

Fig. 1. Clinical course of a typical case treated with PGE1.

(88%) after PGE1 administration. Figure 2 shows changes in API by PGE1 administration. API significantly increased from 0.92 ± 0.06 to 1.01 ± 0.06. Plasma TM levels significantly decreased 7.8 ± 3.6% from the basal value after PGE1 administration (Fig. 3).

To assess the relationship between the improvement of clinical symptoms and improvement of vascular dysfunction, correlation among symptoms, API and plasma thrombomodulin levels were studied (Fig. 4). All seven patients with improvement of limb numbness after PGE1 administration showed an increase in API, and all but one showed a decrease in plasma thrombomodulin levels, indicating that the improvement of the clinical symptom was associated with amelioration of vascular dysfunction.

Conclusions

Although etiology and molecular mechanisms of diabetic neuropathy are still unclear, vascular and metabolic factors have been implicated in the pathogenesis of diabetic neuropathy. Hyperglycemia-induced polyol pathway hyperactivity accompanied by nerve sorbitol accumulation and myoinositol depletion may play a role in the pathogenesis of diabetic neuropathy [1—3]. On the other hand, impaired nerve blood flow, epineural arteriovenous shunting and a reduction in sural nerve oxygen tension have been reported as evidence suggesting the contribution of a vascular factor to diabetic neuropathy [4,5].

Prostaglandin derivatives such as PGE1 and prostacyclin analogue (iloprost) have been reported to improve the subjective symptom of peripheral sensory disturbances in diabetic patients [6,7]. A prostacyclin analogue (beraprost) has

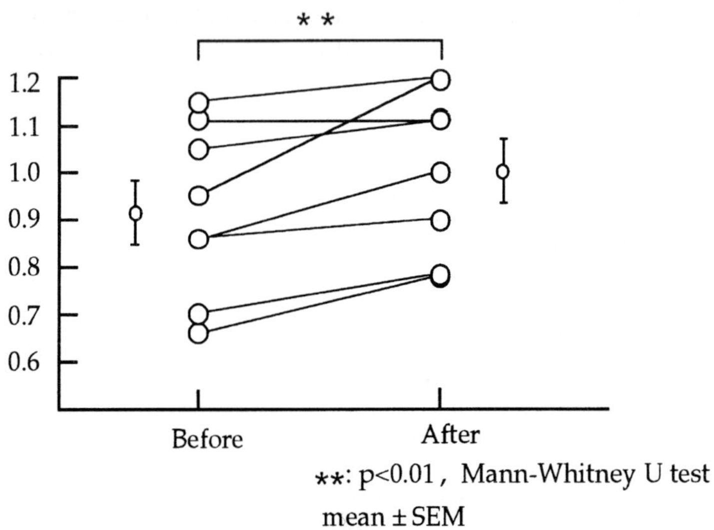

Fig. 2. Changes in API by PGE1 administration.

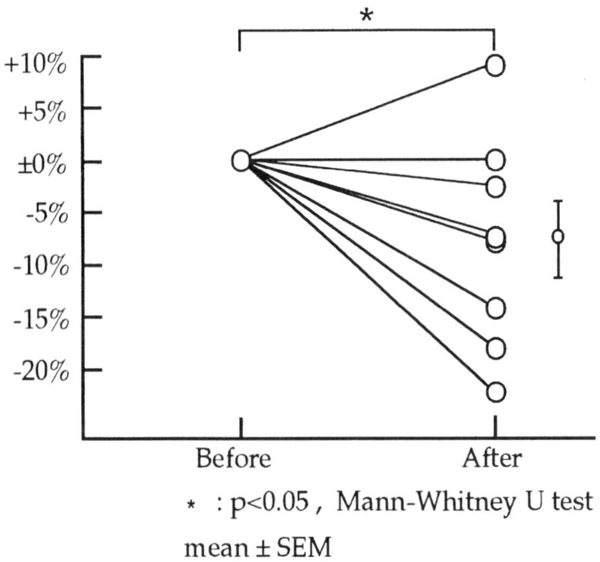

Fig. 3. Changes in plasma TM levels by PGE1 administration.

been reported to reduce plasma TM levels in NIDDM patients with microalbuminuria [8]. TM is an endothelial cell surface glycoprotein and plays an important role in the regulation of blood coagulation. Endothelial cells release TM in the vascular bed during cell destruction due to physiological metabolism or pathological disorder. TM is therefore considered as an indicator of systemic vascular cell damage [9,10]. In this study, we found that PGE1 administration reduced plasma TM levels accompanied by the improvement of limb numbness in diabetic patients. The decrease of plasma TM levels caused by PGE1 is consid-

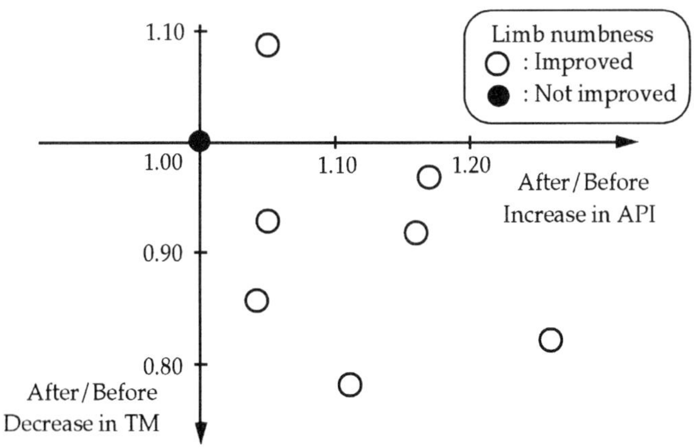

Fig. 4. Relationship among clinical symptom, API and TM.

ered to reflect the amelioration of vascular cell damage, which contributed to the improvement in limb numbness. Our data support the hypothesis that the vascular factor plays an important role in the pathogenesis of diabetic neuropathy.

In conclusion, the improvement in limb numbness by PGE1 was associated with the improvement in API and plasma TM levels, suggesting that the vascular factor, at least in part, contribute to diabetic neuropathy.

References

1. Ward JD et al. Effect of blood sugar control on the accumulation of sorbitol and fructose in nervous tissue. Diabetes 1972;21:1173–1178.
2. Dyck PJ et al. Nerve glucose, fructose, sorbitol, myo-inositol and fibre degeneration and regeneration in diabetic neuropathy. N Engl J Med 1988;319:542–548.
3. Greene D et al. Sorbitol, phosphoinositides, and sodium-potassium-ATPase in the pathogenesis of diabetic complications. N Engl J Med 1987;316:599–606.
4. Tesfaye S et al. Impaired blood flow and arterio-venous shunting in human diabetic neuropathy: A novel technique of nerve photography and fluorescein angiopathy. Diabetologia 1993;36: 1266–1274.
5. Newrick PG et al. Sural nerve oxygen tension in diabetes. BMJ 1986;293:1053–1054.
6. Goto Y et al. Evaluation of the therapeutic effect of prostaglandin E1 on diabetic peripheral neuropathy. A multicenter clinical study. J Jpn Diabet Soc 1984;27:3–11.
7. Shindo H et al. Clinical efficacy of a stable prostacyclin analog, iloprost, in diabetic neuropathy. Prostaglandins 1991;41:85–96.
8. Nishimura M et al. The effect of PGI_2 analogue on vascular endothelial function and platelet aggregation in patients with NIDDM. J Diab Comp 1995;9:330–333.
9. Amano K et al. Fluctuation in plasma levels of thrombomodulin in patients with DIC. Thromb Haemost 1992;68:404–406.
10. Iwashima T et al. Elevation of plasma thrombomodulin level in diabetic patients with early diabetic nephropathy. Diabetes 1990;39:983–988.

Recent Advances on the Pathogenesis and Management of Diabetes Mellitus.
S.H. Shinn, M. Shichiri and K.-W. Kim, editors.

Intra-arterial infusion of prostaglandin analogue in the management of diabetic foot gangrene

Sung-Nam Choi, Hyun-Chul Bae, Byoung-Ho Kong, Kwang-Suk Kim, Yeon-Sahng Oh and Soon-Hyun Shinn
Department of Endocrinology and Metabolism, School of Medicine, Chung-Ang University, Seoul, Korea

Abstract. *Background.* The laborious and costly treatment of diabetic foot often leads to destructive below-knee amputation, or more. In addition, 40% of amputees suffer a second necessary amputation within 5 years. Uniquely, Carson proposed that prostaglandin infusion may create benefits in the management of diabetic gangrene. Up to 80% of prostaglandin infused through peripheral vein is destroyed in the pulmonary circulation. Therefore, I infused prostaglandin E1 analogue by mechanical pump into the femoral artery, then I observed its influence on the level of amputation.

Methods. Five patients with diabetic foot, classified as the fourth stage in Fontain and greater than the fourth in Wagner's classification, were treated with the prostaglandin E1 analogues and triple antibiotics (cefotaxime 3 g, amikin 0.5 g and clindamycin 0.6 g a day). These were together infused into the femoral artery by teromo infusion pump. The average duration of intra-arterial PGE1 was 21 days. At this stage, orthopedic surgeons were consulted and the level of amputation determined.

Results. Only one patient suffered the below-knee amputation. The other four patients received the ray amputation (one or two toes). This clinical trial was intended to circumvent the pulmonary degradation of prostaglandin E1 and elevate the tissue concentration in situ. This treatment may prevent high-level amputation. A confinement of 3 weeks did not cause any systemic side effects. In the future, a study with a large population is needed.

Keywords: diabetic foot, prostaglandin, intra-arterial infusion.

Introduction

Diabetic foot gangrene results in a high degree of morbidity and mortality. The laborious and costly treatment often leads to destructive below-knee amputation or more. Patients undergoing below-knee amputation and more extensive procedures have on average around a 50% rate of 3-year survival. In addition, 40% of amputees suffer a second necessary amputation within 5 years. Diabetic foot is a very common problem, and more than half of nontraumatic amputees are diabetics. The longer the duration of diabetes, the higher the risk of peripheral vascular disease. Various pathologic foot changes cause the amputations. For example, ulceration, neuropathy, infection, gangrene and ischemia are all, in combination, involved in the development of diabetic foot. The traditional orthopedic gangrene management of diabetic foot has mainly depended on destructive

Address for correspondence: S.N. Choi, Chung-Ang University Medical Center, 82-1, Pil-Dong 2 Ga, Chung-Gu, Seoul, Korea. Tel.: +82-02-260-2184.

amputation, together with glucose control and antibiotics. Uniquely, Carson proposed that prostaglandin infusion may benefit the management of diabetic gangrene [3]. Prostaglandin causes vasodilation and inhibits platelet aggregation, lysosomal protease, and phospholipase activity in the necrotizing tissues. In this way, prostaglandin prevents further destruction. In addition, prostaglandin facilitates the uptake and utilization of oxygen in the peripheral tissue and fastens healing of wounds. Lastly, the prostaglandin itself has an anti-inflammatory effect. However, up to 80% of prostaglandin infused through peripheral vein is destroyed in the pulmonary circulation. Therefore, prostaglandin E1 analogue was infused by mechanical pump into the femoral artery, then its influence on the level of amputation was observed.

Material, Methods and Patients

The five patients with the diabetic foot gangrene were included. They were classified by Fontain (Table 1) or Wagner (Table 2) criteria. All the patients in this study were at stage 4 in Fontain and over grade 4 in Wagner. The total of five patients consisted of two males and three females. The mean age was 51 years and mean duration of diabetes was 12.2 years. The mean duration of diabetic foot was 12.6 days. The mean serum hemoglobin A1C and albumin were 10.5% and 1.8 g/dl, respectively. The initial leukocyte count was more than 20,000/ mm^3. The prostaglandin E1 analogues (alprostadil-α-cyclodextrin) and triple antibiotics went together into the femoral artery by infusion pump. The total daily dose of prostaglandin analogue was 20 μg. Carrier solution was normal saline. Triple antibiotics are cefotaxime 3 g, amikin 500 mg and clindamycin 600 mg a day. The average duration of intra-arterial PGE1 infusion was 21 days. At this stage, we consulted the orthopedic surgeon and determined the level of amputation.

Results

Clinical and biochemical characteristics are given in Table 3. All the patients in this study were initially recommended a below-knee amputation by an orthopedic surgeon. However, intra-arterial infusion of prostaglandin E1 analogue into the femoral artery reduced the unnecessary amputation. Finally, only one patient (the case 2 patient in Table 3) suffered the below-knee amputation, at quite a

Table 1. Fontain classification for peripheral occlusive disease.

Stage	Definition
I	Asymptomatic
II	Intermittent claudication
III	Rest pain
IV	Ischemic ulcer and necrosis

Table 2. Wagner's classification.

Grade 0	No open lesion
Grade 1	Superficial ulcer
Grade 2	Deep ulcer
Grade 3	Abscess osteitis
Grade 4	Gangrene forefoot
Grade 5	Gangrene entire foot

high level. He had controlled his diabetes with insulin injection (total daily dose, 48 IU) and his HbA1C level was 11.7%, higher compared to the other patients. Serum albumin concentration was 1.8 g/dl. He had triple diabetic complications. His clinical and biochemical characteristics were not significantly different from the other four patients. The other four patients received the ray amputation (one or two toes).

Discussion

The management of diabetic foot is laborious and costly. In general, patients with diabetic foot were treated with antibiotics and other conservative treatment modalities. If such conservative treatment failed, the patient had to undergo surgical management, including amputation. In a previous study performed by Yamamoto, the beneficial role of prostaglandin E1 analogue was proven [1]. In this study, we can also deduce the conclusion that intra-arterial infusion of prostaglandin-may reduce the unnecessary amputation in diabetic foot. The benefits of prosta-

Table 3. Clinical and biochemical characteristics of patients.

	Case 1	Case 2	Case 3	Case 4	Case 5
Age (sex)	M/42	M/49	F/54	F/59	F/51
Initial foot lesion	Whole	Sole	Metatarsal	Metatarsal	Dorsum
Duration					
Diabetes (years)	5	10	16	10	10
Gangrene (days)	10	3	10	30	10
Diabetic complication[a]	n	R, N, n	N, R	N, R	N, R
WBC (mm^3)	26300	19600	19200	31600	18400
Hb (g/dl)	9.3	11	9	9.2	13
Platelet (mm^3)	263 k	404 k	302 k	366 k	364 k
Albumin (g/dl)	1.3	1.8	2.4	1.3	2.2
Cholesterol(mg/dl)	56	114	133	301	122
GOT (IU/l)	46	18	12	13	12
GPT (IU/l)	40	19	9	12	12
BUN	39	20	34	35	11

[a]n: neuropathy; R: retinopathy; N: nephropathy.

glandin on diabetic foot management, infused through peripheral venous route had been established. However, infused prostaglandin venously has undergone 70 – 80% degradation in the pulmonary circulation. Therefore the pharmacologic effects of prostaglandin, (described previously, vasodilation, antiplatelet, anti-inflammatory, etc.) are reduced and unpredictable. Nevertheless, intra-arterial infusion of prostaglandin could increase the tissue prostaglandin concentration and circumvent the pulmonary degradation. Thus, the beneficial effect of prostaglandin on diabetic foot could be augmented. Our study potentiated the important role of vasodilating prostaglandin, especially E1 analogue. A study with intra-arterial prostaglandin infusion has been performed previously. Selected patients had black foot disease and peripheral occlusive vascular disease. The daily dose of prostaglandin analogues was from 20 to 40 μg. The beneficial effect of prostaglandin E1 analogueon on black foot disease was also observed. However, the study with intra-arterially infused vasodilating prostaglandin in the management of diabetic foot gangrene was not performed. In this study, we observed the potentially beneficial effect of vasodilating prostaglandin in the management of diabetic foot. However, the tissue concentration of prostaglandin, tissue oxygen tension before and after treatment and degree of vasodilation were not measured.

Confinement for 3 weeks did not cause any systemic side effects. In the future, a study with a large population is needed

References

1. Yamamoto F. Efficacy of intravenous infusion of prostaglandin E1 as therapy for ischemic extremities. Gendi Iryo 1981;13:2117.
2. Diehm C. Clinical effects of intravenously administered prostaglandin E1 in patients with rest pain due to peripheral obliterative arterial disease (POAD) – a preliminary report on a placebo-controlled doubled blind study. Vasa 1987;17(Suppl):52.
3. Carson LA. Intravenous prostaglandin E1 in severe peripheral vascular disease. Lancet 1976; 2:810.
4. Larsson J. Clinical characteristics in relation to final amputation level in diabetic patients with foot ulcer: a prospective study of healing below or above the ankle in 187 patients. Foot Ankle Int 1995;16:70.
5. Levin ME. Evaluating and treating diabetic peripheral vascular disease, part I. Clinical Diabet 1987;May/June:62.
6. Waugh NR. Amputations in diabetic patients – a review of rates, relative risks and resource use. Commun Med 1988;10:279.
7. Hoar CS. Evaluation of below the knee amputation in the treatment of diabetic gangrene. N Engl J Med 1962;266:440.
8. Selby JV. Risk factors for low extremity amputation in persons with diabetes. Diabet care 1995;18:509.
9. Gregory MC. Assessment and management of foot disease in patients with diabetes. N Engl J Med 1994;29:854.
10. Tawata M. Effects of a single drip infusion of lipo-prostaglandin E1 on vibratory threshold in patients with diabetic neuropathy. Prostaglandins 1995;49:27.

Recent Advances on the Pathogenesis and Management of Diabetes Mellitus.
S.H. Shinn, M. Shichiri and K.-W. Kim, editors.

Optimal dose evaluation of mexiletine in patients with diabetic painful neuropathy

Kempei Matsuoka[1], Yukimasa Hirata[2], Yasunori Kanazawa[5], Minoru Ohtake[3] and Narimitsu Kaihara[4]

[1]*Saiseikai Diabetes Center, Tokyo;* [2]*Tokyo Women's Medical College, Tokyo;* [3]*Nippon Medical School, Tokyo;* [4]*Okura National Hospital, Tokyo; and* [5]*Omiya Medical Center, Jichi Medical School, Saitama, Japan*

Abstract. *Background.* In diabetic neuropathy, spontaneous pains and severe dyschesia accompanying discomfort persist. Mexiletine hydrochloride (MX), whose structural formula is similar to lidocaine, is an antiarrhythmic drug commonly used.

Methods. A multicenter-controlled study for optimal dose evaluation of MX for shooting pain and allodynia was conducted at 40 institutes. After obtaining a written agreement, 169 patients were randomized into three groups: the placebo (59), 300 mg/day (56) and 450 mg/day (54). They were given the drug for 4 weeks after a 2-week run-in-period. The effect was evaluated using a seven-grade scale recorded by patients.

Results. At the end of the 2nd week, the ratio concerning pains of the lower legs "improved" (not including moderately improved) to 9.5, 24.3 and 35.5%, respectively ($p < 0.01$). At the end of the study it was 11.1, 23.8 and 36.1%, respectively.

Conclusion. From the above results, 300 mg/day of MX, which is the usual dosage frequently used to control arrhythmia was found to be appropriate to control painful diabetic neuropathy. No serious adverse effects were documented.

Keywords: allodynia, antiarrhythmic drug, Na-channel blocker, shooting pain.

Introduction

In dolorous neuropathy, symptoms such as spontaneous pain and severe dyschesia accompanying tremendous discomfort persists. Since they may exacerbate the quality of life of patients, treatment of these symptoms is of great importance. Acute painful neuropathy may follow after either a period of unstable glycemic control or sudden normalization of hyperglycemia, which is very annoying for patients and occasionally undermines the relationship between the patients and physicians [1]. In light of these facts, the use of symptomatic drugs, with a certain extent of immediate action, is indispensable to alleviate the complaints of patients. Mexiletine HCl (MX) is an antiarrhythmic agent commonly used in cardiology and has been found to be useful on painful neuropathy by Dejgard et al. [2]. It has a structural formula similar to lidocaine, whose main action is in-

Address for correspondence: Kempei Matsuoka MD, Saiseikai Diabetes Center, 1-4-17 Mita, Minato-ku, Tokyo 108, Japan.

hibition of Na-channel in the cell membrane and to exert analgesic effects by suppression of action potential [3,4].

Material and Methods

A trial for optimal dose evaluation for painful neuropathy such as shooting pain and allodynia was conducted at 40 institutes, and 169 patients (103 males, 66 females, 28–81 years old, duration of diabetes: 1 month to 34 years) with spontaneous pain or severe dyschesia due to diabetic neuropathy of at least 1 month duration were randomized into three groups: placebo (n = 59), MX 300 mg/day (n = 57) and MX 450 mg/day (n = 54) after obtaining a written agreement. The patients were treated for 4 weeks after a 2-week run-in-period. The efficacy was evaluated using a seven-grade score (Table 1) recorded by patients and assessed as "improved" if the score improved by 2 or more grades at the end of a 2- and 4-week study period. Overall evaluation was done by attending physicians at the end of the 4-week study period referring the record of the patients under the following criteria: "Markedly improved" if scores were 6, 5, 4, 3 to 0; "improved" if scores were 6, 5, 4, 3 to 1 or 2 and 6 to 3; "slightly improved" if scores improved by 1 or 2 except for the above; "no changes" if scores did not change at all; and "worsened" if scores were exacerbated.

Results

According to the patients' records concerning the pain of the lower extremities as shown in Table 2, the ratio of improvement, not including one score improvement after the 2-week treatment, was 9.5% in the placebo group, 24.5% in the MX 300 mg/day group, and 35.5% in the MX 450 mg/day group. After the 4-week treatment, the ratio of improvement was 11.1, 23.8 and 36.1%, respectively. However, the efficacy on paresthesia and numbness was not obtained. The result of the overall evaluation assessed by attending physicians at the end of the 4-week trial is shown in Table 3. There were no markedly improved cases in the placebo group. The ratio of "markedly improved" and "improved" was 6.8% in the placebo group, 46.4% in the MX 300 mg/day group, and 42.6% in the MX 450 mg/

Table 1. Criteria for scores of painful neuropathy.

Scores	Degree	Symptomatic expressions
6	+++	Extremely intense; the pain disturbs sleep at night
5	+++	Somewhere between 6 and 5
4	++	Intense; the pain is annoying even while working
3	++	Somewhere between 4 and 3
2	+	Weak; the pain does not interfere with daily activity
1	+	Somewhere between 2 and 0
0	–	None

Table 2. Trend of allodynia and shooting pains of the lower extremities after a 2- and 4-week study period recorded by patients.

	Disappeared	−2 scores	−1 scores	Unchanged	Worsened	p[a]
After 2 weeks						
Placebo	4 (9.5)	0 (9.5)	13 (40.5)	22	3	
MX 300 mg/day	7 (18.9)	2 (24.3)	12 (56.8)	15	0	= 0.0075
MX 450 mg/day	7 (22.6)	4 (35.5)	6 (54.8)	14	0	
After 4 weeks						
Placebo	4 (8.9)	1 (11.1)	5 (23.8)	25	2	
MX 300 mg/day	5 (11.9)	5 (23.8)	9 (45.2)	22	0	= 0.0077
MX 450 mg/day	9 (25.0)	4 (36.1)	8 (958.3)	5	0	

( ): Cummurative %. [a]Cochran-Armitage test: improved with −2 scores or better vs. placebo group.

day group ($p < 0.01$ vs. placebo). There was no significant difference between the MX 300 mg/day and MX 450 mg/day groups. Adverse events on this trial are shown in Table 4. The incidence of the adverse events was 18.6% in the placebo group and about 28% in patients treated with MX. However, no serious side effects were documented in the MX group except for upper gastrointestinal symptoms which were already known about in the patients treated for arrhythmia.

Discussion

Clinical usefulness of MX against painful neuropathy has been reported by the results of several studies in the past [4,5]. Improvement was noted in many subjects after increasing the dose to 300 or 450 mg/day, suggesting that the optimal dose for painful neuropathy is almost the same as that used for arrhythmias [6]. In this trial, due to the overall evaluation by physicians, MX 300 mg/day was found to be appropriate for the management of painful neuropathy when the assessment was limited to allodynia and shooting pain which are typical to somatic, diabetic neuropathy. Symptomatic effects on paresthesia were obscured,

Table 3. The ratio of improvement by an overall evaluation.

	n	Markedly improved	Improved	Slightly improved	Unchanged	Worsened	p
Placebo	59	0 (−)	9 (6.8)	18 (40.7)	25	4	
MX 300 mg/day	56	3 (15.3)	23 (46.4)	11 (66.1)	15	1	= 0.0019
MX 450 mg/day	54	8 (14.8%)	15 (42.6%)	6 (53.4)	19	0	

p: Cochran-Armitage test vs. placebo. (%): Cummurative in "markedly improved" + "improved group".

Table 4. Adverse events on a trial of Mexiletine.

Symptoms	Placebo	300 mg/day	450 mg/day
Dizziness	1	2	2
Nausea	2	4	3
Stomach distress	2	9	5
Anorexia	2	0	1
Generalized fatigue	2	0	0
Others	7	14	12
Cases developed	11 (18.6%)	16 (28.6%)	15 (27.8%)

possibly because paresthesia, which patients complain about occasionally, mean abnormal sensations including numbness and tingling, and is a very vague and nonspecific expression to be an independent parameter. Neurological tests such as deep tendon reflexes, vibratory perception threshold and motor and sensory nerve conduction velocity were carried out, but there were no significant differences between the MX and placebo groups. Within 2–4 weeks of the trial, the Na-blocking effect was not influenced to functional improvement of the nerve fibers. Recently, Kamei et al. [7] reported that MX involves a Δ-1 opioid receptor with antinociceptive effect by an animal experiment. The safety of MX has already been established by its extensive use in cardiology. In addition, the results of our current study also suggest that MX can be safely applied to diabetic patients with painful neuropathy.

Conclusions

Mexiletine HCl whose chemical formula is similar to lidocaine, inhibits the Na-channel in the cell membrane and exerts an analgesic effect by suppressing action potentials. By a multicenter double-blind trial for optimal dose evaluation, at the end of the 2-week administration, the ratio of symptomatic improvement was 9.5% in placebo, 24.3% in 300 mg/day, and 35.5% in 450 mg/day. By overall evaluation, there was no significant difference between the MX 300 mg/day and MX 450 mg/day groups. From the result, 300 mg/day, which is the most common dosage for controlling arrhythmia, appears appropriate for diabetic painful neuropathy. No serious adverse events except for stomach symptoms were documented.

References

1. Matsuoka K. Management of diabetic painful neuropathy. J Jpn Med Assoc 1990;104:143–146.
2. Dejgard A et al. Mexiletine for treatment of chronic painful diabetic neuropathy. Lancet 1988; (January 2–9):9–11.
3. Hohnloser S et al. Effects of mexiletine on steady state characteristics and recovery kinetics of Vmax and conduction velocity in guinea pig myocardium. J Cardiovasc Pharmacol 1982;4: 232–239.

4. Chabal C et al. The use of oral mexiletine for the treatment of pain after peripheral nerve injury. Anesthesiology 1992;76:113–117.
5. Suzuki Y et al. Double blind crossover trial of mexiletine in diabetic painful neuropathy. Sinyaku to Rinsho 41:113–117.
6. Hirata Y et al. Clinical usefulness of MX-PDN in painful diabetic neuropathy. Igaku to Yakugaku 1996;35:749–763.
7. Kamei J et al. Antinociceptive effect of mexiletine in diabetic mice. Res Commun Chem Pharmacol 1992;77:245–248.

Recent Advances on the Pathogenesis and Management of Diabetes Mellitus.
S.H. Shinn, M. Shichiri and K.-W. Kim, editors.

Preventive effect of cilostazol on the reduced sciatic nerve blood flow in the streptozotocin-induced diabetic rat

Y.D. Song, Hari Lee, S.W. Park, H.C. Lee, B.S. Cha, S.K. Lim, K.R. Kim and K.B. Huh
Division of Endocrinology, Department of Internal Medicine, Yonsei University College of Medicine, Seoul, Korea

Abstract. In this study the effect of chronic cilostazol treatment on the sciatic nerve blood flow of streptozotocin-induced diabetic rats was investigated. Nerve blood flow was assessed using laser flowmetry. The results showed that the diabetic group had a significant reduction in nerve blood flow when compared with controls. The chronic cilostazol treatment of diabetic rats significantly improves the deficit in nerve blood flow observed in diabetic rats after 8 weeks of diabetes mellitus and could completely restore the deficit as compared to the control group. It is suggested that cilostazol is a potent vasodilator of rat peripheral nerves, and the treatment of diabetic rats with cilostazol may improve or prevent the changes of nerve blood flow.

Keywords: cilostazol, diabetic neuropathy, nerve blood flow.

Introduction

One view of diabetic neuropathy suggests that reduced nerve blood flow (caused by rheological changes coupled with vasa nervorum microangiopathy) leads to endoneural hypoxia which is sufficient to impair nerve function [1]. The nerve dysfunction may be prevented or corrected by vasodilator treatment or improvement of Na+,K+-ATPase activity. Therefore, we evaluated the effect of cilostazol (which blocks platelet aggregation and is a vasodilator on the sciatic nerve blood flow) in order to determine whether it would be helpful in improving experimental diabetic neuropathy.

Material and Methods

Male rats of inbred Sprague-Dawley, with a mean body weight of approximately 300 g, were used in the experiments. Diabetes was induced by a single injection of streptozotocin at a dose of 45 mg/kg in the tail vein. Diabetic rats were allowed free access to water and rat chow (normal or cilostazol supplementation was provided as a gift by Otsuka Pharmaceutical Co. Ltd., Tokoshima, Japan). We separated the rats into three groups. Each group received their respective

---

Address for correspondence: Young Duk Song MD, Department of Internal Medicine, Severance Hospital Yonsei University College of Medicine, #134 Shinchon-dong Seodaemun-ku, Seoul 120-752, Korea. Tel.: +82-2-361-5422. Fax: +82-2-393-6884. E-mail: endosong@yumc.yonsei.ac.kr

Table 1. Effect of diabetes and oral supplementation of cilostazol for 8 weeks on sciatic NBF.

	Group I	Group II	Group III
N	10	8	8
Nerve blood flow (ml/min/100 g)	40.1 ± 3.4	32 ± 2.4	39 ± 4.2

Group I, control receiving normal diet; group II, STZ receiving normal diet; group III, STZ receiving cilostazol supplementation. Values are mean ± SD.

diets for a total of 8 weeks: group I (n = 8) controls received a normal diet; group II (n = 8) STZ received a normal diet; and group III (n = 8) STZ received (0.1%) a cilostazol diet. Eight weeks afterwards, the rats were anaesthetized and the sciatic nerve was exposed, and blood flow was assessed using Advance laser blood flowmeter ALF21 (Advance Co. Ltd., Tokyo, Japan). Flow values were expressed in ml/min/100 g of tissue.

Results

No differences between the three groups in the values of mean blood pressure, heart rate, pH, PO_2, PCO_2, were found at the time of killing. The sciatic nerve blood flow of the three groups revealed significant differences. The vehicle-treated diabetic group (group II) had a significant reduction in nerve blood flow when compared with controls ($p < 0.005$). The treatment of streptozotocin-induced diabetic rats with cilostazol significantly ameliorated the deficit in nerve blood flow that was observed in vehicle-treated diabetic rats after 8 weeks of diabetes mellitus ($p < 0.001$), and could completely restore the deficit as compared to the control group (Table 1).

Discussion

We observed that the sciatic nerve blood flow decreased in diabetic rats 8 weeks after induction of diabetes, which is compatible with the other reports [2–5]. The nerve blood flow in the cilostazol-treated group increased independently of blood glucose, blood pressure, temperature, pH, PO_2 and PCO_2 and was similar to the control group. Our results suggested that cilostazol may be a potent vasodilator of rat peripheral nerves, and the treatment of diabetic rat with cilostazol may prevent the changes of nerve blood flow. The model described in this paper may be helpful in the search for a better insight into the blood flow regulation of the peripheral nerve and perhaps in the pathogenesis of diabetic neuropathy. Further research (especially controlled clinical studies in human diabetic neuropathy) is necessary to unravel the pathogenesis of diabetic neuropathy and the exact mechanism of action of cilostazol.

References

1. Low PA, Tuck RR, Takeuchi M. Nerve microenvironment in diabetic neuropathy. In: Dyck PJ, Thomas PK, Asbury AK, Winergrad AI, Porte D Jr (eds) Diabetic Neuropathy. Philadelphia, PA: Saunders, 1987;266–278.
2. Yasuda H, Sonobe M, Yamashita M, Terada M, Hatanaka I, Huitian Z, Shigeta Y. Effect of prostaglandin E1 analogue TFC 612 on diabetic neuropathy in streptozotocin-induced diabetic rats. Diabetes 1989;38:832.
3. Cameron NE, Cotter MA, Low PA. Nerve blood flow in early experimental diabetes in rats: relation to conduction deficits. Am J Physiol 1991;261:E1–E8.
4. Kihara M, Schmelzer JD, Poduslo JF, Curran GL, Nickander KK, Low PA. Aminoguanidine effects on nerve blood flow, vascular permeability, electrophysiology, and oxygen free radicals. Proc Natl Acad Sci USA 1991; 88:6107.
5. Hotta N, Kakuta H, Fukasawa H, Koh N, Sakakibara F, Komori H, Sakamoto N. Effect of niceritrol on streptozocin-induced diabetic neuropathy in rats. Diabetes 1992;41:587.

Recent Advances on the Pathogenesis and Management of Diabetes Mellitus.
S.H. Shinn, M. Shichiri and K.-W. Kim, editors.

Erythrocyte aldose reductase level and the progression of diabetic retinopathy

Yoshiatsu Takahashi[1], Tomokazu Tachikawa[2], Shinichiro Takayama[2], Takashi Ito[2], Yasue Omori[2] and Yasuhiko Iwamoto[2]
[1]Diabetes Center, Tokyo Women's Medical College, Tokyo; and [2]Mitsubishi Gas Chemical Company, Tokyo, Japan

Abstract. To investigate the role of the aldose reductase protein level on the progression of diabetic retinopathy, the erythrocyte aldose reductase protein level was determined in 76 NIDDM patients by a two-site ELISA using recombinant human aldose reductase. Among 25 patients with proliferative retinopathy, which was developed within 5 years of the diagnosis of diabetes, the level of erythrocyte aldose reductase was significantly higher than that of 51 patients with no or mild retinopathy more than 8 years after the diagnosis and with prolonged hyperglycemia. The age at examination was younger and the maximum body mass index in the past was higher in patients with proliferative retinopathy than that in patients with no or mild retinopathy. These results indicate that the level of erythrocyte aldose reductase protein in NIDDM patients is associated with the progression of retinopathy irrespective of glycaemia control and diabetes duration.

Keywords: diabetes duration, glycaemia control, NIDDM.

Introduction

Prolonged hyperglycemia has been thought to be the primary cause of diabetic complications, and good glycaemia control can delay the onset of diabetic complications in NIDDM as well as IDDM [1]. However, it is well known that some diabetic patients develop severe complications early in the duration of diabetes, while some patients have no or mild complications even after many years of diabetes with hyperglycemia.

Aldose reductase is a key enzyme of polyol pathway and the activation of polyol pathway is well known to be one of the causes of diabetic complications [2,3]. The aim of this study was to investigate the role of the aldose reductase protein level on the progression of diabetic retinopathy irrespective of glycaemia control and diabetes duration.

Materials and Methods

Seventy-six patients fulfilling the following criteria were included in the study:
1. NIDDM patients with preproliferative or proliferative retinopathy ("severe

Address for correspondence: Y. Takahashi MD, Diabetes Center, Tokyo Women's Medical College, Kawada-cho, Shinjuku-ku, Tokyo 162, Japan.

retinopathy" group), which was developed within 5 years of the diagnosis of diabetes.

2. NIDDM patients who have no or simple mild retinopathy more than 8 years after the diagnosis of diabetes and with prolonged hyperglycemia (mean HbA1c $>8.7\%$, "no or mild retinopathy" group).

The patient's record forms included age at examination, known duration of diabetes, mode of treatment, body mass index (BMI) at examination and maximum BMI in the past, history of habitual smoking or drinking and with or without hypertension. Color fundus photographs were taken at 50° with a Canon fundus camera (Canon, Tokyo, Japan). If diabetic retinopathy was detected, both fundi were examined by one or two ophthalmologists specializing in diabetic retinopathy and performed the grading. The HbA1c level was determined every month in all patients using high-performance liquid chromatography (Hi-AutoA1c HA8121, Kyoto Daiichi, Kyoto, Japan; normal range: 4.3—5.8%). We calculated the mean of all measurements and the median number of HbA1c measurements per patient to be 56 (range 5—120).

For the determination of the erythrocyte AR level, hemolysate was prepared from erythrocyte fractions isolated from heparinized blood samples, and AR in the lysate was directly measured by the two-site enzyme immunoassay [4]. The hemoglobin concentrations in each lysate were determined by the hemoglobincynamide method [5]. All results are expressed as mean ± SD unless otherwise cited. Clinical characteristics between the two groups were compared using the Student's t test, Fisher's exact test and Wilcoxon's U-test (all two-tailed). Logistic regression analysis was used for the prediction of severe diabetic retinopathy and $p<0.05$ was considered statistically significant.

Results

The clinical demography of the diabetic patients is shown in Table 1. Between the two groups, there is no difference in sex, mean level of HbA1c in the past, BMI at examination, the level of diabetic neuropathy and smoking or drinking habits. However, the patients with severe retinopathy were younger at the time of examination, had a higher maximum BMI in the past, a higher level in erythrocyte AR content and higher frequency of hypertension than those with no or mild retinopathy.

Logistic regression analysis revealed that the age, hypertension and erythrocyte AR level were significant and independent factors for the prediction of diabetic severe retinopathy (Table 2).

Discussion

This study shows a significant difference in the erythrocyte AR protein level between the two groups, i.e., higher in the patients with severe retinopathy than those with no or mild retinopathy. Since the patients with severe retinopathy had

Table 1. Comparison of clinical features and erythrocyte aldose reductase (AR) level between the NIDDM patients with no or mild retinopathy and those with severe retinopathy.

	Diabetic retinopathy		Significance (p)
	No/mild (51)	Severe	
Age (years)	59 ± 8.6	49 ± 9.4	0.0006
Sex (m/f)	35/16	17/8	ns
Maximum BMI in the past	25.8 ± 4	29.7 ± 5.1	0.0001
BMI at examination	22.4 ± 3	23.7 ± 3.5	ns
Treatment of diabetes[a]	1:25:25	9:6:10	<0.002
Hypertension (−/+)	39/12	10/15	0.0001
Diabetic neuropathy[b]	6:45	6:19	ns
Erythrocyte AR level (ng/mgHb)	8.7 ± 1.8	12.2 ± 5.1	<0.0001
Duration of diabetes (years)	15 ± 6.6	2.5 ± 1.6	0.0001
Mean HbA1c in the past (%)	9.7 ± 1.2	8.6 ± 2.5	ns

[a]Diet:OHA:insulin; [b]no/mild:definite; ns: not significant; BMI: body mass index. Values are given as mean ± SD.

a shorter duration of diabetes than those with no or mild retinopathy and no difference in long-term glycaemia control, the erythrocyte AR level is associated with the progression of retinopathy independently to the duration of diabetes and glycaemia control.

It has been reported that the AR level in erythrocyte is not affected by age [4] and glycaemia control (from our data, not shown in this study). Therefore, the erythrocyte AR level could be determined genetically, and it has been recently supported in some papers, reporting the significant association between the polymorphism of allele in the AR gene and the progression of diabetic complications [6,7].

Our results also indicate that the maximum BMI in the past in the patients with severe retinopathy is higher than those with no or mild retinopathy. Therefore, it may imply that total glycaemia control in those patients could actually be much worse than those with no or mild retinopathy. The duration of diabetes as well as glycaemia control are well known to be the discrete factors affecting the devel-

Table 2. Predictive factors for the progression of severe diabetic retinopathy independent of duration of diabetes and glycemic control by logistic regression analysis.

Factor	β	SE	Odds ratio	95% C.I.	p-value
Age	−0.219	0.069	0.804	1.28 ~ 3.76	0.0041
AR	0.787	0.274	2.20	1.28 ~ 3.76	0.0017
Hypertension	3.51	1.088	33.45	4.0 ~ 282	0.0013
ΔBMI	0.196	0.108	1.217	0.985 ~ 1.50	0.0683

$P = 1/1 + \exp^{-}$ (0.616 − 0.219 age + 0.787 AR + 3.51 HT + 0.196 ΔBMI) $\chi^2 = 58$ ($p < 0.0001$). Model sensitivity: 92%, specificity: 75%, predictive accuracy: 87%. ΔBMI indicates maximum body mass index in the past minus present body mass index.

opment of diabetic complications. However, the factor of maximum BMI and also ΔBMI, which indicates maximum BMI in the past minus present BMI, was omitted by the logistic regression analysis for the significant predictor of severe diabetic retinopathy.

Therefore, our results may imply that among patients with equivalent duration of diabetes and glycaemia control, those with high AR levels are more susceptible to severe diabetic retinopathy. In other words, NIDDM patients who have a low level of erythrocyte AR may be resistant to develop severe retinopathy.

In conclusion, it is assumed that measuring the AR level in erythrocyte may be useful for predicting severe diabetic retinopathy in NIDDM patients.

References

1. The Diabetes Control and Complications Trial Research Group. The effect of intensive treatment of diabetes on the development and progression of long-term complications in insulin-dependent diabetes mellitus. N Engl J Med 1993;329:977–986.
2. Yamaoka T, Nishimura C. Acute onset of diabetic pathological changes in transgenic mice with human aldose reductase cDNA. Diabetologia 1995;38:255–261.
3. Robinson WG, Kador PF. Retinal capillaries: Basement membrane thickening by galactosemia prevented with aldose reductase inhibitor. Science 1993;221:1117–1179.
4. Nishimura C, Hamada Y. Enzyme immunoassay for erythrocyte aldose reductase. Clin Chem 1994;49:889–894.
5. Van Kampen EJ, Zijlstra WG. Standardization of hemoglobinometry. II. The hemoglobincyanide method. Clin Chem Acta 1961;6:538–544.
6. Ko BCB, Lam KSL. An (A-C)n dinucleotide repeat polymorphic marker at the 5′ end of the aldose reductase gene is associated with early-onset diabetic retinopathy in NIDDM patients. Diabetes 1995;44:727–732.
7. Heesom AE, Hibberd ML. Polymorphism in the 5′-end of the aldose reductase gene is strongly associated with the development of diabetic nephropathy in Type 1 diabetes. Diabetes 1997;46: 287–291.

Index of authors

Keyword index